AGING:
The Health Care Challenge

*An Interdisciplinary Approach
to Assessment and Rehabilitative
Management of the Elderly*

AGING: The Health Care Challenge

An Interdisciplinary Approach to Assessment and Rehabilitative Management of the Elderly

CAROLE BERNSTEIN LEWIS, R.P.T., M.S.G., M.P.A., Ph.D.

CO-DIRECTOR OF PHYSICAL THERAPY SERVICES OF
WASHINGTON, D.C.

ADJUNCT ASSISTANT PROFESSOR OF PHYSICAL THERAPY
UNIVERSITY OF PITTSBURGH COLLEGE OF MEDICINE
PITTSBURGH, PENNSYLVANIA

INSTRUCTOR OF HEALTH EDUCATION
UNIVERSITY OF MARYLAND
DEPARTMENT OF HEALTH EDUCATION
COLLEGE PARK, MARYLAND

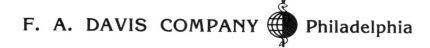

F. A. DAVIS COMPANY ⚕ Philadelphia

Library of Congress Cataloging in Publication Data
Main entry under title:

Aging, the health care challenge.

  Includes bibliographies and index.
  1. Aged—Diseases. 2. Aged—Rehabilitation. 3. Aged—Care and hygiene. 4. Gerontology. I. Lewis, Carole Bernstein. [DNLM: 1. Aging. 2. Geriatrics. WT 104 A2684]
RC952.5.A48 1985   362.1'9897   84-12688
ISBN 0-8636-5614-9

DEDICATION

This book is dedicated to our parents with love and respect and our sincerest wishes for their healthy aging.

Ben and Peggy Bernstein
Ann and Sandy Campanelli
Richard and Nancy Coffin
Stanley and Elizabeth Crump
Melvin and Alta Dunn
Johnny and Ester Friedland
Jenievieve and Steven John Gudas
Andrew and Julia Habasevich
Mildred and Pierce Hills
Ruth and William Hoste
Wallace and Regina Kapuscinski
Jim and Rita Laflin
Albert and Ann Leonard
Jack and Mary O'Hara
Nathan and Lena Pillberg
Mary and Fred Schaefer
Jim and Dal Schunk
Henry Charles and Rosemary Hunter Singleton

ACKNOWLEDGMENTS

I would like to thank all my wonderfully tolerant and delightful older patients for all their feedback, encouragement, and love as well as my fine professors and rehabilitation peers for encouraging me by their sharing and questioning of ideas.

C.B.L.

CONTRIBUTORS

LINDA CAMPANELLI-KATZ, M.A.
Associate Director, Adult Health and Developmental Program, University of Maryland, College Park, Maryland

CAROLYN E. CRUMP, M.A.
Associate Research Scientist, Advanced Research Resources Organization, Rockville, Maryland

STEPHEN A. GUDAS, R.P.T., M.S.
Assistant Professor, Medical College of Virginia, Virginia Commonwealth University, Department of Physical Therapy, School of Allied Health Professions, Richmond, Virginia; Consultant to the Cancer Rehabilitation and Continuing Care Program, Medical College of Virginia, Richmond, Virginia

ROBERT A. HABASEVICH, M.S., R.P.T.
Director, Massachusetts Bay Rehabilitation Associates, Duxbury, Massachusetts

KATHLEEN HOSTY, M.A., C.C.C./S.P.
Speech-Language Pathologist, Metropolitan Speech Pathology Group, Inc., Washington, D.C.

Z. ANNETTE IGLARSH, R.P.T., Ph.D.
Assistant Professor, University of Maryland, School of Medicine, Department of Psychiatry, Baltimore, Maryland; Associate, Burch, Rhoads, and Loomis P.A., Baltimore, Maryland

KAREN S. JORDAN, O.T.R.
Director, Occupational Therapy Services, Hyattsville, Maryland

MOLLY LAFLIN, M.S.
Instructor, Bowling Green State University, School of Health Physical Education and Recreation, Bowling Green, Ohio; Consultant, Committee on Aging, American School Health Association

ANTONIA LEONARD, O.T.R.
Chief Occupational Therapist, St. Joseph's Hospital, Stamford, Connecticut; Consultant, Hospice of Stamford, Stamford, Connecticut

CAROLE BERNSTEIN LEWIS, R.P.T., M.S.G., M.P.A., Ph.D.
Co-Director of Physical Therapy Services of Washington, D.C.; Adjunct Assistant Professor of Physical Therapy, University of Pittsburgh College of Medicine, Pittsburgh, Pennsylvania; Instructor of Health Education, University of Maryland, Department of Health Education, College Park, Maryland

GAIL HILLS MAGUIRE, Ph.D., O.T.R.
Chairperson, Occupational Therapy Department, College of Allied Health Sciences, Howard University, Washington, D.C.

NANCY M. O'HARA, M.A.
Visiting Assistant Professor, University of South Carolina, Columbia, South Carolina

SHELLEY PILBERG, M.S., C.C.C./S.P.
Speech-Language Pathologist, Metropolitan Speech Pathology Group, Inc., Washington, D.C.

KATHRYN SCHAEFER, M.P.A., R.P.T.
Co-Director of Physical Therapy Services of Washington, D.C.

CAROL R. SCHUNK, R.P.T., M.S.
Assistant Professor, Pacific University, Department of Physical Therapy, Portland, Oregon

JEROME F. SINGLETON, M.T.R.S., Ph.D.
Assistant Professor, School of Recreation, Physical and Health Education, Dalhousie University, Halifax, Nova Scotia, Canada

DIANE WHITE, P.D.
Registered Pharmacist Consultant to the University of Maryland School of Pharmacy, Baltimore, Maryland; Consultant to "Elder-Ed" (Drug Use and Abuse for Senior Citizens), Baltimore, Maryland

CYNTHIA COFFIN ZADAI, M.S., R.P.T.
Director, Chest Physical Therapy, Beth Israel Hospital, Boston, Massachusetts

CONTENTS

INTRODUCTION

CAROLE BERNSTEIN LEWIS,
R.P.T., M.S.G., M.P.A., Ph.D.

One of the most frequent questions rehabilitation professionals ask me is, "What's so different about treating the older person? A hip is a hip." My response is similar to the purpose of this book. It is true that a hip is a hip; however, if you can expand your focus and look at the whole picture—that is, the person, the support system, living environment, and history—you have a much better idea of what is involved.

When I lecture I like to give the following example. A friend of mine returned from the mountains with a beautiful photograph of a mountain goat, and far to the right in the background was the earnest excited face of a baby goat. I told my friend that I loved the picture and wanted a copy. He said, "Sure, but I'll crop out the extra features and center the goat." I was aghast. The little goat's expression was the essence of the picture. This experience taught me the importance of guiding others to see the whole picture. This focus on the wholeness of events is crucial to the rehabilitation of the elderly, and it is the approach taken in this text. The various sections do not deal solely with the physiologic systems but also explore the diverse aspects of the older person.

There is a definite need for a text on rehabilitation of the elderly. Rehabilitation professionals are becoming more and more aware of the comprehensive clinical-oriented health care programs for the elderly. Their concerns lead to a need for more information on the subject. This book was written in response to that need and because of the increased need for improved health care that is arising in the elderly population.

The statistics on aging are startling. In the late 1800s, 3 percent of the population was age 65 or older. Today it is approximately 11 percent. In the year 2020,

1

it could be as high as 30 percent of the population. In addition, health care needs of the elderly make the older person a major consumer of the various forms of health care. For example, elderly persons have twice as many hospital stays, and the stays last twice as long. In addition, people over age 65 visit the doctor 43 percent more often than those under age 65. Also, the variety of health care settings currently available and needed are much greater for the elderly than for other segments of the population; for example, elderly people use hospitals, long-term care settings, rehabilitation facilities, outpatient clinics, respite centers, home care, hospices, and day care centers.

Rehabilitation professionals are concerned about the above settings, learning how to update their skills, and providing the best services in different settings. They are acutely aware of the statistics on the elderly and the need for improved health care.

This book addresses innovative health care techniques for managing the increasing health care needs of the elderly. Suggestions for optimizing care in the multiple settings are addressed in several chapters.

Another thread running throughout the book is the importance of achieving and maintaining independence for the elderly. This concept, along with the concern for improving and optimizing the older person's quality of life, runs through most of the chapters. This focus on functional approaches emphasizes quality of life and independence through understanding and integrating all the aspects of the elderly patient.

Additional positive aspects of this text are the clear simple writing styles of all the authors. Updated research and information have been included, but the research language has been deleted. The emphasis here is threefold: (1) to provide the most information possible in the simplest way; (2) to encourage the reader to use the information in the daily clinical setting and to think of it and to share it with the patients; and (3) to serve as a role model to the readers in the importance of communicating with each other, not creating distance between each other by the use of jargon and anecdotes. This text could be used by someone who has no experience with elderly patients. Not only does this book provide clinical skill modifications, it also provides excellent baseline level information on the elderly.

Some additional comments as to the purpose, focus, and factors of the book that I feel must be shared relate to what makes the older person different.

Another classic response that I commonly use when describing the uniqueness of the elderly is the multiplicity of problems that can be seen in this population. For example, as most geriatric practitioners know, the common finding on the chart of a newly admitted elderly patient is a list of diagnoses ranging from diabetes to depression. Often, the diagnosis is only the tip of the iceberg and may not even address the real problem, which could be the "difficulty with walking because of improper foot care." So to be a "top notch" rehabilitation professional in the field of aging takes a strong investigative skill along with the ability to recognize and to treat potential problems.

I once heard a quote that I feel is extremely relevant to the treatment of elderly patients: "The eyes cannot see what the mind does not know." Therefore, this book provides background information for health professionals to use on a daily basis when assessing the total picture of the elderly patient, especially those health professionals not trained in aging who think that "a hip is a hip."

Another unique aspect of the elderly is the tremendous amount of variation that exists in this population. Even though this text describes an average for changes that occur with age, the reader is encouraged to see the extremes that can exist in younger people and how people vary more as they age and will, therefore, have much more variation in clinical symptoms and responses.

This concept of variation is also useful in encouraging the reader to use carefully thought out labels. A label can be helpful in some contexts and harmful in others. It is obvious that this book "walks" a fine line in this area but does provide useful information that will not be used as a means of labeling for the purposes of denying care to older persons.

As part of the introduction, I would like to discuss the purposes and theoretic frameworks of the major sections of the text. Initially, the text provides general information on values, theories, and psychologic aspects of aging to encourage the reader to explore the nontangible parameters of approaching the elderly patient. Then the various aspects of function and independent living are explored in terms of activities of daily living and communication and leisure skills. These three areas are crucial aspects of designing a rehabilitation program that focuses on improving the quality of life.

The middle section of the text might be thought of as the tangible section. The approach is one of a review, exploring the areas of the five senses, muscles, bones, the nervous system, the cardiopulmonary system, and the field of oncology. In each of the above sections, specific changes with age are explored, ways of integrating information are discussed, and ways of modifying treatment programs are explained as well as avenues of future investigations suggested.

The final section discusses additional aspects of the elderly person and really puts the aging patient into a more wholistic picture. Some controversial yet crucial areas of rehabilitation are explained in detail. The new concept of stress is defined and discussed. Implications for creative programming are given.

Drugs as variables to patient outcome are described along with the complications and the importance of understanding how drugs can affect the patient's independent functioning.

Sex is explored in the sense that sexuality is more than just sexual intercourse; it is a touch, a wink, or a smile—something we all experience throughout our lives. In this particular chapter, the focus is on understanding sexuality and learning how to enhance it, to maintain it, and even to increase it in later years.

It is hoped that the research chapter will provide impetus to further study of the health care needs of the elderly. Special considerations are given that emphasize how aging research can be different from other research designs.

Another controversial chapter in this section concerns dying. No time in life is dying more apparent than in the stage of old age. As Elisabeth Kübler-Ross says, "Death is a final stage of growth," and what we need to do is to learn how to plan for it and to accept it and to help others and our patients with this particular stage of life.

Finally, the last two chapters give a broader perspective of the realm of aging in the community and in the government. The financial supports and the legislative considerations are addressed in these chapters. It was my hope when designing and planning this text to pull together the best clinicians, educators, and writers to design a text that would be the most comprehensive in the area of rehabilitation and the aging. It is meant to provide the clinician with information on how to investigate multiple areas, how to integrate these ideas, and how to provide this information to clinicians, students, and educators.

It is obvious that rehabilitation professionals are realizing the importance of a multiple approach to patient care. This book uses this ideology in the presentation of its material.

One final hope that I have for this book is that it will end the scenario of my sitting down to breakfast with a rehabilitation professional and hearing, "So what's so different about treating the elderly person? A hip is a hip." I hope that many will read this book and will be able to share ideas on ways of improving health care for the elderly and devising new and more challenging areas of exploration for health professionals working with the elderly.

SECTION 1

THEORIES AND PSYCHOSOCIAL ASPECTS OF AGING

CHAPTER 1

THEORIES OF AGING

LINDA CAMPANELLI-KATZ, M.A.

BEHAVIORAL OBJECTIVES

Upon completion of this chapter, the reader will be able to
1. List four principal theories of aging.
2. Describe two differences and similarities in the four theories of aging.
3. Identify a factor in each principal theory of aging that influences physiologic change that may have impact on rehabilitation.
4. Describe two ways to differentiate between genetic theories and nongenetic theories.
5. Discuss the concept that there is no universal theory of aging.
6. Summarize the concept that aging is developmental and not a sudden occurrence.

"In the beginning . . ."

The search for the elixir of that nemesis called "old age" has led many scientists to the laboratory drawing board. Because the study of gerontology is relatively young, the excitement of exploring its new territory has seduced many scientific minds.

Although several theories have been proposed, only the principal theories of aging will be reviewed. There are several underlying assumptions regarding theoretic gerontology, and the following fundamental considerations are an important basis upon which to build further knowledge.

FUNDAMENTAL CONSIDERATIONS

Aging is developmental. This concept is very simple but easily forgotten. Basically, we are reminded that we do not suddenly age. Our aging time capsules do not go off at 65! We develop into more mature adults and grow older developmentally, not chronologically. This is why later life is unique among all developmental stages. One who is 70 years old chronologically may have the physiologic age of a 50-year-old person. Yet a 50-year-old person may have enough chronic diseases to parallel the physiologic decline of a 90-year-old person.

Old age is a gift of 20th-century modern technology and scientific advancement. This concept is credited to the gerontologist James Birren, who makes the point that experiencing the extended life expectancy that we now have is really a gift of modern medicine and modern technology.

Since the discovery of insulin, the vaccine, a decline in infant mortality, and the development of modern surgical techniques and advanced treatment modes for formerly fatal diseases, we are blessed with longer lives. Also, we are staying *older* longer, not younger longer, in the 20th century. The whole phenomenon is new.

The effects of normal aging versus pathologic aging must be differentiated if possible. Often we assume that a functional decline is due to aging. But pathology (disease) may often cause functional decline, which is not a normal aging process. For example, if one has adult-onset diabetes, then the probability of cardiovascular disease increases, owing to the effect of the diabetes. However, it is not "normal" to get diabetes; it is a function of a lifestyle and heredity in North America. An example of normal aging is the acquisition of cataracts. Anyone who lives long enough will develop cataracts. Thus, senile cataracts are normal age changes caused by the progressive opacity of the lens of the eye.

There is no universally accepted theory of aging. Although aging is a universal phenomenon, no one really knows what causes it or why we age at different rates. There is much speculation, but it is difficult to point to a single theory without using any others as backups; hence the diversity of opinions and the lack of support for one major theory.

Aging theories can be divided into two major categories: genetic and nongenetic. Genetic theories focus on the mechanisms for aging located in the nucleus of the cell. Nongenetic theories focus upon areas otherwise located, such as in organs, tissues, or systems. In order to understand the theories, a basic understanding of the three somatic cell types is necessary.

BACKGROUND INFORMATION

Not all somatic cells age at the same rate, nor do they have similar aging characteristics. Somatic cells are divided into three major categories: continuously proliferating cells, reverting postmitotic cells, and fixed postmitotic cells.[1]

Continuously proliferating cells never cease to replicate themselves, and injury done to these cells is healed through regeneration. Such cells can be found as superficial skin cells, red blood cells, cells of the lining of the intestine, and bone marrow cells. Reverting postmitotic cells have a slower rate of division than the continuously proliferating cells; but when there is injury, the rate of division is speeded up and regeneration is possible. An example of these are kidney and liver cells. The final type of somatic cells, the fixed postmitotic cells, never replicate once the cells reach maturity.[1,2] Muscle cells and nerve cells are primary examples of fixed postmitotic cells. In our adult life, therefore, nerve and muscle cells repair themselves only if the nucleus is intact. Because the postmitotic cell will not replicate itself, no new vital cells are produced. Therefore, the need for residual fixed somatic cells to remain vital and in "good shape" is crucial to the well-being and life expectancy of the individual.

A HISTORIC PERSPECTIVE

The study of cellular aging has been retarded to an extent by a historic event in biologic science. Beginning in 1912, Carrel and Ebeling conducted a series of experiments using normal chick embryo fibroblasts cultured in vitro. The in vitro experiments are conducted in an artificial environment, such as in a test tube, as opposed to in vivo experiments, which are conducted within the body.

Based on Carrel's series of experiments, it was thought that fibroblasts could replicate indefinitely and so virtually remain immortal. It was not until much later that replication by others of Carrel's studies did not render the same results. Scientists later discovered that the method of preparation of the chick embryo extract was continuously contaminated with fresh embryonic cells. The result was erratic miotic activity coinciding with the periodic addition of chick embryo extract.[2] In other words, these cells lived forever because young embryo cells were mixed with the older prepared culture. Recently one of Carrel's laboratory assistants, now in her nineties, admitted to this.

In 1961, a landmark study by two then unknown cell biologists, Hayflick and Moorehead,[3] turned the study of senescence of cultured cells completely around. They had concluded from their in vitro studies of fetal fibroblast cells (lung, skin, muscle, heart) that human fibroblasts have a limited lifespan in culture.[3] Their experiment, illustrated in Figure 1-1, is clearly described by Fries and Crapo.[1]

> Placed in a flask with liquid tissue culture medium, the cells were grown until they formed a layer across the bottom of the flask. After formation of this primary culture, the enzyme trypsin was added to break the attachments between the cells, which were then divided in half and cultured again to confluence in two new flasks. This subcultivation produces a population doubling, since just enough cells to cover the bottom of one flask become just enough to cover the bottom of two flasks. And the process can be repeated until the cells no longer proliferate.

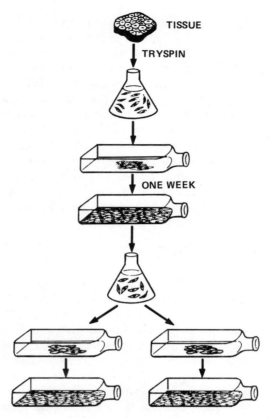

Figure 1-1. This is a schematic drawing of the Hayflick and Moorehead serial cultures of human fibroblasts. (From Fries and Crapo,[1] with permission.)

The Hayflick and Moorehead experiment was christened the cellular biology of the aging movement and remains a classic among the biologic studies in aging. In essence, they were among the first scientists to change the philosophy of modern biology.

HAYFLICK LIMIT THEORY

The limited number of cell population doublings ranges from 40 to 60, the average doubling being 50. The developmental senescence process of cultured cells is graphically described in Figure 1-2. Hayflick and others have repeatedly shown that Phase III is nearly always between 40 and 60 population doublings for embryo cells. Does that tell us that the "Hayflick limit" is intrinsic for embryo cells

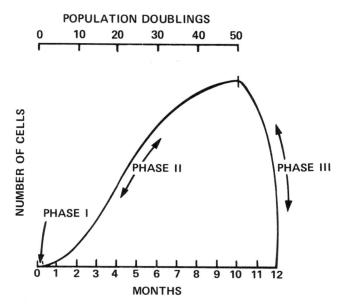

Figure 1-2. This graph shows growth characteristics of human embryo fibroblast cultures in vitro. Notice the rapid cell proliferation in Phase II and the final cessation of division in Phase III. Note that this entire schema represents one individual's entire lifetime. (From Fries and Crapo,[1] with permission.)

or that we are mortal because studies in vitro are applicable to humans in vivo? Probably not.

Hayflick noted alterations and degeneration within the cells before they reached their growth limit.[4] These alterations were evident in cell organelles, membranes, and genetic material. What Hayflick may have shown us in these studies is that functional changes within cells are responsible for aging and that the cumulative effect of improper functioning of cells and eventual loss of cells in organs and tissues is responsible for the aging phenomenon.

Hayflick's limit has served as a model to others who have shown that population doubling potential is a function of donor age;[5] that is, an inverse correlation exists between donor age and the population doubling potential.[6] Evidence of the Hayflick limit has also been seen in cultures taken from individuals with progeria (Hutchinson-Guilford syndrome) and Werner's syndrome. Inasmuch as progeria is a premature aging syndrome, the decreased lifespan of the donors' cells shows a lower Hayflick limit, as expected.[1] Finally, although not as reliable as originally thought, the length of the longest lifespan for different species and the number of population doublings are correlated. For example, the Galapagos tortoise has a maximum lifespan of 175 years with a maximum doubling number of 125, whereas man has a maximum lifespan of 110 years, with a maximum doubling number of 60.[7]

ERROR THEORY

The Error Theory, also known as the Error Catastrophe Theory, was first presented by Orgel in 1963. The theory specifies that "any accident or error in either the machinery or the process of making proteins would cascade into multiple effects."[8] A decrease in the fidelity or accuracy of protein synthesis was specifically hypothesized to be caused by errors in proper initiation of the pairing of messenger RNA condon with an anticondon of transfer RNA. However, "it may not be possible to distinguish between contributions to cellular aging caused by errors in protein synthesis from those due to an accumulation of somatic mutations."[9] Is inaccurate protein synthesis distinguishable from inaccurate DNA synthesis? Is the accuracy of both processes dependent on the fidelity of the other? Are intracellular and extracellular mechanisms of aging coupled, since inaccurate protein synthesis affects extracellular events? The interdependence and cumulative effects of errors remain deeply intertwined and somewhat indistinguishable.

Recent experiments contradict Orgel and no longer lend support to the Error Theory. Experiments have shown that not all aged cells accumulate misspecified molecules and that aging is not necessarily accelerated when misspecified molecules are purposely introduced.[9] However, from a historical standpoint, it was important to test these hypotheses in order to move toward a more plausible theory.

REDUNDANT DNA THEORY

Medvedev[10] has devised a theory that may be coupled to the Error Theory. He believes that biologic age changes are a result of errors accumulating in functioning genes; but as these errors accumulate reserve, genetic sequences with identical information take over until the system's redundancy is exhausted. This theory is known as the Redundant Message Theory. Medvedev[10] believes that different species' lifespans may be a function of the degree of *repeated* genetic sequences. If error occurred in a nonrepeated gene sequence, the chance of preserving intact a final gene product during evolution or a long lifespan would be lessened.

Redundancy seems to protect mammals from losing vital genetic information during the lifespan.[10] The major criticism of this theory is that it fails to explain other possible aging factors, such as radiation-induced aging and quantitative aspects of normal aging.

TRANSCRIPTION THEORY

Other scientists have developed theories focused specifically on stages of genetic processing. One of these processes, transcription, is the first stage in the transfer of information from DNA to protein synthesis. It entails the formation of messenger RNA so that it contains, in the linear sequence of its nucleotides, the genetic information located in the DNA gene from which mRNA is transcribed.

This theory, according to Hayflick,[9] maintains that

(1) with increasing age, deleterious changes occur in the metabolism of differentiated post-mitotic cells
(2) the alterations are the results of primary events occurring within the nuclear chromatin
(3) there exists in the nuclear chromatin complex a control mechanism responsible for the appearance and the sequence of the primary aging events
(4) this control mechanism involves the regulation of transcription although other regulated events may occur.

There appears to have been insufficient experimentation regarding this hypothesis, but, as Hayflick[9] suggests, this should not imply that the hypothesis is wrong.

When contemplating these theories thus far, one must ask, "How come some cells, such as germ cells and some cancer cells (HeLa and other strains) never age or die?" Hayflick[9] suggests that "in order to maintain immortality, genetic information is exchanged between these cells in the same way that the genetic cards are reshuffled when egg and sperm fuse." The reshuffling of a fused sperm and egg cell leads to a fixed lifespan. As with all species, there appears to be a specific time for decrement and eventual death. Hayflick[9] and others refer to this as "mean time to failure." Perhaps species-related genetic apparatus runs out of correctly programmed material and some species-related repair systems are better than others because they have a longer lifespan. If so, does that mean we are programmed to age as nature intended it? Is there a Programmed Theory of Aging, per se?

NONGENETIC THEORIES

Crosslinkage Theory

In 1942, Johan Bjorksten[11,12] first related the concept of crosslinkage to developmental aging. Prior to the 1940s, crosslinking was used as a method to stabilize macromolecules for individual purposes, such as vulcanizing rubber. Basically, Bjorksten looked at large reactive protein molecules within the body—such as collagen, elastin, and DNA molecules—and regarded their crosslinkage as responsible for secondary and tertiary causes of aging.

According to Bjorksten,[11]

Crosslinking reactions result in the union of at least two large molecules. A bridge or link between these is usually formed by a crosslinking agent: a small, motile molecule or free radical with a reactive hook or some other mechanism at both ends, capable of reacting with at least two large molecules. It is also possible for two large molecules to become crosslinked by the action of their own side chains or reactive groups present on one or both of them, or pathologically formed by ionizing radiation.

Figure 1-3 shows the conceptual crosslinkage of DNA.

The implications of crosslinking are enormous. Bjorksten[12] implies that it is the primary cause of sclerosis, failure of the immune system, and loss of elasticity. Aging of the skin is perhaps the most obvious example of crosslinking. Since crosslinking is a tanning process, exposure to solar radiation promotes it. Tanning is the same process used by native North Americans to toughen hides for clothing and shelter. The long-term effect of chronic sun exposure without the use of a sunscreen accelerates aging and promotes significant loss of elasticity of the dermal superficial and deeper layers.

It was once thought that the inflexibility of the body with age was primarily due to the crosslinking of tendon, bone, and muscle tissue. It has since been noted that more active individuals remain more flexible despite constant exposure to crosslinking agents. A combination of exercise and proper dietary considerations seems to help inhibit the crosslinking process.

The popularity of the theory stems from the fact that potential crosslinking agents are ubiquitous. Unsaturated fats, polyvalent metal ions (Al, Mg, Zn), and exposure to radiation are a few. The prophylactic use of vitamin E as an antioxidant has been recommended,[13] as well as dietary and drug restrictions of compounds containing crosslinking agents. Such agents are contained in antacids, baking powder, and coagulants, all of which contain aluminum. There is presently considerable controversy over vitamin E supplementation with respect to

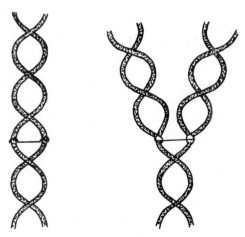

Figure 1-3.   This is a representation of crosslinkage splitting a protein molecule. (From Bjorksten,[11] with permission.)

dosage and possible adverse side effects. Selenium and lecithin have also proven to be effective crosslinking inhibitors (antioxidants); however, the extent of their effectiveness in vivo is not certain.[11]

Free Radical Theory

Basically, free radicals are highly charged ions whose outer orbits contain an unpaired electron. Free radicals have been shown to damage cell membranes, lysosomes, mitochondria, and nuclear membranes through a chemical reaction called lipid peroxidation. Both membrane damage and crosslinking of biomolecules result from free radical chain reactions.[14] The net result of free radical reactions, as summarized by Leibovitz and Siegel,[15] is a decline in cellular integrity caused by reduced enzyme activities, error-prone nucleic acid metabolism, damaged membrane functions, and accumulation of aging pigments (lipofuscin) in lysosomes.

The accumulation of age pigments does not refer to the dark brown spots on one's hands. Age pigments (lipofuscin) are seen at microscopic levels in self-selected tissues of the body, such as nerve and muscle tissue. The rate of accumulation of age pigments is a good index of chronologic age and perhaps one of the few aging phenomenons universally demonstrated in mammals. Age pigments as an entity are examples of degenerative change. When accumulated in tissue, they choke off oxygen and nutrient supplies to surrounding areas, causing further degeneration and eventual death of tissue.

The free radical theory of aging is attributed to Harmon,[16] whose studies have a history of almost 30 years. There is much support for free radical reactions and their implications in the aging process as well as their probable pathologic effects as a hypothesized cancer-causing and atherosclerosis-causing agent.

Extensive research has been done regarding the use of antioxidants with free radicals. Vitamin E, vitamin C, selenium, and gluthathione peroxidase and superoxide dismultase have been used as free radical and lipid peroxidase inhibitors.[15] The implication is that there appear to be effective free radical inhibitors that may prevent further cellular degeneration, such as reduced accumulation of age pigments.

Autoimmune Theory

Several theories have been hypothesized to explain the phenomenon of autoimmunity. According to these theories, the regulatory machinery of the immune system allows cells reactive against self-antigens to flourish by suppressing immune cells reactive against non-self-antigens. In other words, the immune system no longer recognizes some of its own members and becomes self-destructive by literally reacting against itself.

Autoimmune diseases include those affecting the young (for example, lupus erythematosus and scleroderma) and those affecting the old (for example, adult-onset diabetes and senile amyloidosis).[16] Hayflick[9] points out that

> Although this hypothesis has much to recommend it, it may not be universally applicable since age changes occur in nonvertebrates that lack an immune system. Also, known alterations in the immune system with age may be caused by more fundamental changes in the genetic apparatus of its constituent cells.

What we see, then, is a possible genetic explanation as the basis for a nongenetic theory.

Hormonal Theories

D. donner Denckla, an endocrinologist recently turned gerontologist, believes that the seat of aging is located in the brain.[17] His theory is based on past studies of hypothyroidism, a disease that mimics mature aging. Hypothyroidism can be fatal if untreated with thyroxin, inasmuch as all the manifestations of aging are evidenced, such as a depressed immune system, wrinkling of the skin, gray hair, and a slowed metabolic rate.

The pituitary gland controls the thyroid gland, and thus the secretion of thyroxin. Thyroxin is the master rate-controlling hormone within the body. However, it is not the release of thyroxin upon which Denckla is focusing. The focus of this theory is the proposed ability of the pituitary to release a blocking hormone labeled DECO (decreasing oxygen consumption), which blocks the cell membrane from taking up thyroxin. Denckla has not isolated the antiaging serum, but what Denckla has given us is an alternative philosophic point of view in theoretic gerontology: the in vivo versus the in vitro controversy. Denckla believes that the aging process in vitro is an artifact and unrelated in any meaningful way to true aging.

> Denckla says, "I don't care what happens to cells in tissue culture. What IS important is what people die of." He believes that for good evolutionary reasons—to ensure the turnover of generations so that mutations can take place that enable a species to adapt to a changing environment—nature cannot trust to chance (wear and tear). There must, therefore, exist "an absolutely failsafe killing mechanism without which the species would not survive."[17]

There have been other theories proposed with regard to functional decline of various organs and systems. As Hayflick[9] notes, (1) they may simply be the result of more fundamental causes, or (2) the organ system in question may not be universally present in all aging animals.

Data attempting to relate endocrine function to aging do not lend satisfactory evidence to substantiate a significant contribution of endocrine gland function to the process of aging.[18] For example, in response to stress and trophic hormones, the adrenal cortex and thyroid gland remain intact. For women, menopause is a hormone-mediated event that chronicles but does not regulate aging.[18] The ovary is the sole endocrine gland whose functional capacity predictably declines with normal aging. On the other hand, androgen production by the testis is not as predictable because there are individual differences.

WHAT WE HAVE ACCOMPLISHED

In summary, we have two major camps of scientific investigators: the genetic theorists and the nongenetic theorists. Differences of opinion exist regarding the use of in vitro methods (continued experiments under glass) and in vivo methods (within the body observations).

Although Hayflick's limit is the greatest contribution to the history of cellular biology within the past 25 years, Harmon and Toppel's work regarding free-radical theory and Bjorksten's work regarding crosslinking theory also have contributed plausible mechanisms for the implications of their theories. For example, the accumulation of lipofuscin and destruction to cell membranes and organelles may result from free radicals. And crosslinking may play a role in the development of arteriosclerosis and the eventual sclerotic processes seen in scleroderma and progeria patients.

Gerontology has evolved into a more sophisticated science in the sense that we are now able to distinguish between logical, plausible explanations and Ponce de Leon type searches for the fountain of eternal youth. But the question remains, Does a panacea exist?

Frolkis, a Soviet gerontologist, was quoted as saying that "the number of hypotheses is generally inversely proportional to the clarity of the problem."[17] The brief overview of theories presented should confirm the complicated nature of theoretic gerontology. Therapists and health providers should not take the concept of the complexity of this stage of life lightly. Theoretic implications will affect how we minister to our patients. Although there is no universal aging theory, there does exist a universal aging phenomenon of which we are a part. One day we, too, will be older.

REFERENCES

1. FRIES, I AND CRAPO, L: *Vitality and Aging*. WH Freeman, San Francisco, 1981.

2. HAYFLICK, L: *Senescence and cultured cells*. In SHOCK, N (ED): *Perspectives in Experimental Gerontology*. Charles C Thomas, Springfield, IL, 1966.

3. HAYFLICK, L AND MOOREHEAD, PS: *The serial cultivation of human diploid all strains*. Exp Cell Res 25:585, 1961.

4. HAYFLICK, L: *The cellular basis for biological aging*. In FINCH, C AND HAYFLICK, L (EDS): *The Handbook of the Biology of Aging*. Van Nostrand Reinhold, New York, 1977.

5. MARTIN, GM, SPRAGUE, CA, EPSTEIN, CJ: *Replicative lifespan of cultivated human cells.* Lab Invest 23:26, 1970.

6. SCHNEIDER, EL AND MITSUI, Y: *The Relationship Between In Vitro Cellular Aging and In Vivo Human Age.* Proceedings of the National Academy of Sciences 73:3584, 1976.

7. STANLEY, JF, PYE, D, MACGREGOR, A: *Comparison of doubling numbers attained by cultural animal cells with life span of species.* Nature 255:158, 1975.

8. SONNEBORN, T: *The origin, evolution, nature and causes of aging.* In BEHNKE, J, FINCH, C, MOMENT, G (EDS): *The Biology of Aging.* Plenum Press, New York, 1979, p 341.

9. HAYFLICK, L: *Theories of aging.* In CAPE, R, COE, R, RODSTEIN, M (EDS): *Fundamentals of Geriatric Medicine.* Raven Press, New York, 1983.

10. MEDVEDEV, Z: *Possible role of repeated nucleotide sequences in DNA in the evolution of life spans of differential cells.* Nature 237:453, 1972.

11. BJORKSTEN, J: *The crosslinkage theory of aging: Clinical implications.* Compr Ther II:65, 1976.

12. BJORKSTEN, J: *Crosslinkage and the aging process.* In ROCKSTEIN, M (ED): *Theoretical Aspects of Aging.* Academic Press, New York, 1974, p 43.

13. BJORKSTEN, J: *The place of vitamin E in the quest of longevity.* Rejuvenation 3:37, 1975.

14. TAPPEL, AL: *Lipid peroxidation damage to cell components.* Fed Proc 32:1870, 1973.

15. LEIBOVITZ, BE AND SIEGEL, B: *Aspects of free radical reactions of biological systems: Aging.* J Gerontol, 35(1):45, 1980.

16. HARMON, D: *Prolongation of life: Roles of free radical reactions in aging.* J Am Geriatr Soc 17:721, 1969.

17. WALFORD, RL: *The immunologic theory of aging: Current status.* Fed Proc 33:2020, 1974.

18. ROSENFELD, A: *Are we programmed to die?* Saturday Review 10(2):10, 1976.

19. DAVIS, PJ: *Endocrinology and aging.* In BEHNKE, A, FINCH, C, MOMENT, G (EDS): *The Biology of Aging.* Plenum Press, New York, 1979, p 273.

CHAPTER 2

PSYCHOSOCIAL ASPECTS OF AGING

CAROLE BERNSTEIN LEWIS, R.P.T., M.S.G., M.P.A., Ph.D.

BEHAVIORAL OBJECTIVES

Upon completion of this chapter, the reader will be able to
1. List five psychosocial changes that occur with age.
2. List three symptoms of depression and three appropriate interventions.
3. Define hypochondriasis and list two appropriate treatment modifications.
4. List 10 suggestions to motivate older persons to exercise.
5. Discuss the types, causes, evaluating tools, and treatments for organic brain syndrome.
6. Identify psychosocial changes with age and integrate psychosocial modifications into treatment programs for the geriatric patient.

If you are a man and you are prejudiced against women, you will never know how a woman feels. If you are white and you are prejudiced against blacks, you will never know how a black person feels. But if you are young and you are prejudiced against the old, you are indeed prejudiced against yourself, because you, too, will have the honor of being old some day.

—Unknown

Rehabilitation with any age group involves more than just physical assessment and treatment. The psychosocial component of rehabilitation is crucial in de-

19

signing effective programs, achieving goals, and enhancing motivation of our elderly patients. Becoming familiar with and using the psychosocial components of rehabilitation not only provides insight into persons receiving the care but encourages creative ideas for persons providing the care.

The information provided in this chapter is designed to highlight psychosocial areas specific to the older population, such as attitudes toward older persons and the effects of social myths, losses, stress, common problems, and pathology.

UNDERSTANDING ATTITUDES TOWARD THE ELDERLY

One method for understanding attitudes is to review various theories and views on old age and to examine which ones reflect our attitudes, the attitudes of our patients, and the attitudes of our fellow workers.

The following questions can also help clarify the global question of attitudes.

1. Which theories do I accept for myself? Which theories do I accept for my patients?
2. Is my goal setting influenced by my beliefs?
3. Is my communication influenced by my beliefs?
4. What means am I implementing to achieve maximum communication and understanding according to these theories?
5. Can I change my attitude?
6. What events have influenced my attitudes?

Eric Erikson developed one of the first psychology of personality theories in the area of aging. Erikson viewed the entire process of human development as a series of stages one goes through in order to develop fully one's ego. Erikson describes eight stages of ego development from infancy to old age.[1] Each of his stages represents a choice of crises in the expanding ego. The tasks in adult life begin with intimacy versus isolation. In this task, the person must develop close relations with another person or people. If the person does not, that person will be isolated and not learn or experience love. The following task is generativity versus stagnation. In this area, the person seeks to find a vocation or avocation where he or she can help others or in some way contribute to society. Good examples may be raising children or working as a physical therapist. In both of these examples, there is a helping and a giving of self and the individual learns and experiences caring. The final task outlined by Erikson is ego-integrity versus despair. This task, the task of old age, is to review life and to gain a sense of uniqueness, accomplishment, and life integration. One should gain a feeling that if one could live life all over again, one would do it in a similar fashion. The person develops active concern with life even in the face of death and learns and experiences his or her own wisdom. The integration of the ego at this stage of life implies an ability to develop in many areas—art, religion, politics, science—and to accept leadership in one or several of these areas. The opposite of ego-integrity is despair, in which the person feels unhappy and bitter about life as he or she has led it. Death to them is something to be feared.

As therapists, we can try to give our patients outlets to express their life experiences. Older persons have unique, exciting stories to share. According to Erikson, the sharing of these experiences and acceptance of leadership roles help strengthen the sense of ego integrity. The patient may be experiencing depression and despair.

The next theory, developed by Cummings and Henry,[2] is the disengagement theory, which was widely accepted into the 1950s. The premise of this theory is that when a person reaches old age, he or she begins to withdraw from society and that society in turn withdraws from the individual. Many examples of this can be seen in our society. Older people are less "important" in the nuclear family, in business, and in the social arena in general. According to the disengagement theory, this is a very natural occurrence. Without it, there would be havoc at the death of these people, who would hold such important positions in society. For the older person, this becomes a time of freedom; there is now no emphasis on achievement or responsibility. The disengagement theory may help explain patients who are indifferent to their care. This theory may also help us choose our mode of interaction. This theory states that a pleasant yet not binding type of relationship is needed in working with older people who are disengaging.[2]

In recent years, Cummings and Henry have disagreed with their own theory and now feel that persons do not naturally disengage.[2] This withdrawal is more a manifestation of depression and should *not* be thought of as normal but as a problem needing psychologic intervention which will be discussed later in this chapter. Rehabilitation professionals must be aware that people in areas of medical and social care may use the theory of disengagement as a justification for minimal or substandard treatment of older persons.

Another aging theory takes a totally opposite view from the disengagement theory. This is the activity theory developed by Robert Butler, who was the director of the National Institute on Aging. His theory states that older people must stay active and involved to continue to maintain their own integrity.[3] The nature of the activities may change by becoming, for example, less physically stressful. However, they must be as important as other previous activities were in the person's life. This idea has tremendous implications when one views the loss of activities and choices experienced by many nursing home residents. If a person loses the closeness of family interactions, a close tie with a staff member may keep this person active. Another example is the loss of family customs, such as a glass of wine with dinner. This little ritual can be easily implemented into a nursing home. To many residents, such gestures mean a lot. An example of this theory on a physical level would be the substitution of a less strenuous activity for a more strenuous one, for example, walking for one hour a day instead of playing tennis.

The fourth theory, the subculture theory, simply states that older people actually become a group unto themselves with jokes, norms, and feelings that only older people will understand.[4] In other words, older persons are the ones who understand what it is like to be old. This theory relates the importance of encouraging communication and sharing between older persons and can be used when older patients do not seem to be communicating with a young therapist because they feel that the therapist can't really understand what it's like to be old. A positive approach to this problem is to use older staff and volunteers to explore and to communicate with believers in this theory.

The final theory presented here is Bernice Neugarten's. She presents various tasks that the older person must accomplish to age successfully. The following are some of these tasks.

1. Accepting the increasing imminence and reality of death.
2. Coping with genuine, sometimes painful, severely disabling, physical ill health.
3. Coordinating the necessary dependence on medical, domestic, and family support and making an accurate estimation of the available independent choices that can still be made in order to achieve maximum satisfaction.
4. Giving and obtaining emotional gratification from friends and relatives.[5]

Which of the above theories do you accept? Which of the theories do you accept for your clients? If you accepted the disengagement theory, are you setting appropriate goals? If you accepted the subculture theory, how effective are your communication skills?

THE EFFECTS OF ATTITUDES AND LOSSES

There are other important factors that can affect the psychosocial perspectives of aging. These include the social forces of attitudes and losses.

American society holds a negative view of aging. Indoctrination into this negative view begins at an early age. Young children see older people as witches or hags in various fairy tales. As we get older, older people may be described as "crocks" or senile, and the concept of the "mother-in-law" and the "old maid" are continually held up for ridicule. Negative feelings toward older people are enhanced by the lack of visibility given to older persons in the media. Older people are infrequently seen on television shows or commercials. Our society likes to keep the undesirables out of sight and thus prohibits its members from learning about the group to contradict any myths.

The reason American society was stressed in the previous paragraph is that in many other societies increased age increases prestige. The older person is thought of as an "elder," or someone who is looked up to for advice and guidance. In an advanced society such as ours, technology is changing so quickly that material and past knowledge loses its relevance, therefore the advice of older persons becomes less important. The field of physical therapy is a perfect example. Many of the old techniques—such as the Payvex machine, bakers, and infrared lamps—are no longer used, and persons having extensive skill in these areas can contribute very little to what a new graduate finds meaningful. It makes you wonder if the concept of proprioceptive neuromuscular facilitation and ultrasound will be as irrelevant to the future generations.

You can begin to imagine how these influences affect the older person's opinion of his or her self and the health care practitioner working with the elderly.

There are many losses that begin to affect people as they age and that cause deprivation. The concept of retirement brings with it many changes. Work represents more than providing an income; it bestows status on a person, regulates the pattern of activity, fixes a pattern of association, and offers a meaningful set of life experiences.[6] For example, a working occupational therapist (OT) has the status of being an occupational therapist, a professional. He or she has a daily pattern of activity, that is, working from nine to five. This person also knows that he or she will see certain coworkers and patients in the daily work environment. Finally, the occupational therapist has meaningful life experience by helping rehabilitate the patients. Many retired persons, on the other hand, may not know what they will do from day to day, who they'll see, or how society views them. The loss of these interactions can be just as devastating as a visual or hearing loss. It is difficult for anyone to function without defined norms.[7] Work provides a fixed way of responding, and for many people it is very difficult to learn new response patterns. Do our facilities provide this for our patients?

Besides the experience of retirement, the older person may be deprived of the closeness and interaction of a loved one owing to illness or death.

A method for understanding and assessing the psychosocial losses and problems in aging is imperative to help provide effective treatment intervention.

One method is based on Hans Selye's theory of stress. Selye defines stress as "a nonspecific response of the body to any demand made upon it."[8] He feels that, in the aged, not only are more stresses made upon the body but the waste products from dealing with previous reactions clog the system.[8] The topic of stress and methods for evaluating and treating it are discussed in detail in the chapter on stress.

COPING WITH STRESS

Seyle feels the most successful aged persons are those who continue to receive satisfaction and recognition throughout life.[8] Being involved in activities is extremely important. Taking stress off one system can often be accomplished by putting stress on another. A well-documented example is the positive effect on depressed patients of running.[9] We can also easily see the ill effects of those who lament over their problems and illnesses and appear to increase the symptoms with each thought. The importance of this can be seen in rehabilitation departments where a person attempts even the smallest task and receives satisfaction.

Even though the chapter on stress and aging (Chapter 12) specifically describes the stress phenomenon and how it relates to the older person, the remainder of this chapter can be more easily understood by keeping in mind that stress may be a contributing factor to some of the psychosocial problems of the aged.

Common Problems

DEPRESSION

Depression leads to some of the less effective methods of coping with stress. Depression is so very common in the elderly that some studies quote that 50 percent of the elderly population are depressed.[9] Signs of depression include unhappiness, pessimism, lower self-esteem, lower estimation of potential, loss of interest, fatigue, and withdrawal.[10]

Another manifestation of depression can be seen in a study involving horseshoes. In the study, it was found that elderly depressed persons not only predicted they would do poorly on a horseshoe throw but still thought they had done poorly after they had thrown the horseshoes.[11] On the other hand, the control, or normal, group of elderly people scored very close to the depressed group on throws of the horseshoes but had a much more realistic view of their task.[11]

This study indicates a treatment modification for the rehabilitation professional working with the older person. This modification is to provide increased feedback to depressed older persons so that they can begin to have more realistic and less pessimistic views of their accomplishments.

Some other suggestions in working with depressed older persons are explained below.

Encourage them to ventilate their problems, and let them know that depression at times is normal. This can be done by allowing and encouraging group interactions, especially in the area of feelings. Reward can be a very powerful stimulus and can help bring people out of depressions. This can be accomplished by special activities, staff recognition, and award ceremonies. Family involvement and participation have also been shown to be helpful with older people. Helping others can have a very positive effect. Many times the sense of accomplishment and the altruistic feeling from this activity can counteract the depression. The positive effects of music can also promote positive feeling with any depressed person.[9]

Remotivation therapy is another treatment approach for depression as designed for use in extended care facilities and nursing homes. The steps involved in this therapy are

1. Establishing a climate of acceptance. The goal of this step is to have a warm friendly atmosphere within the group.
2. Developing a bridge to reality. This is accomplished by reading nonfiction stories and discussing current events.

3. Engaging in sharing the world. Topics are developed from ideas discussed in step 2 above. Props are often used in this step.
4. Encouraging an appreciation of the work of the world. Patients are stimulated to think about work in relation to themselves.
5. Fostering a climate of appreciation. This final step encourages the patients to express their enjoyment of getting together or to express anything that they enjoyed in the session.[3]

These steps are used in accomplishing simple tasks for the older person and provide good results.

Hypochondriasis

Another coping mechanism commonly seen in the stressed elderly is hypochondriasis. This is an overconcern with the body or some portion of it whether an illness exists or not.[12] Many times the cause stems from negative feelings, guilt, depression, narcissistic pleasure, or the desire to control. Our society shuns psychologic weakness, and physical illness is seen as a more acceptable excuse for nonperformance. When people no longer are able to contribute to society, they may develop physical complaints. This way, they can say, "I'm sick, and I need to be taken care of."

The treatment for hypochondriasis is a very difficult one. First we must realize the underlying reasons. In many cases, people want to be "taken care of." Our goal is not to cure their medical problem but to make them as independent as possible and to assist them in seeking help to focus on the underlying problem.

In many cases the care itself may be the only treatment needed. If one feels not as worthwhile as one used to be, life review is a very successful method of treatment. Life review is a reviewing of the person's entire life to the present time. This process enables older people to share all their accomplishments and to view their lives more positively.[4]

Some other pointers to keep in mind with hypochondriacal patients are that they will try to test you by asking you how long they will be coming for treatment. If you give them a time limit, they will know that the treatment will end, and they may develop new pains or complaints to prolong treatments. Try to treat incrementally; tell them that there may not be 100 percent recovery but that you are working to help them be as independent as possible, even with the disability. Finally, let them know you care and that you really want to help.

Lack of Motivation

Another area that is closely related to depression is motivation. Depression often causes a lack of motivation. Frequently therapists working with the elderly are plagued with unmotivated patients. The following is a list from Dr. Raymond Harris's book, *Guide to Fitness After 50*.[13] Although this list was developed for leaders of fitness classes, it is useful for any professional attempting to motivate an older person to exercise.

1. Recognition that the approach requires mental, emotional, and physical engagement.
2. Individualization of the program to the group and to the person.
3. Satisfaction of some of the participant's basic psychic needs.
4. Provision of choice elements and alternatives.
5. Social support and reinforcement.
6. Continuous reproductive measurement certifications from the beginning by assessment devices.
7. Incorporation of creative opportunities such as novelty, change of pace, improvisations.
8. Engagement of recreational elements; play and game qualities.
9. Personal projections of the leader as a concerned, interested, competent, and helpful person.
10. Attention to the aesthetics of the environment and to the propitious atmosphere.
11. Counseling to some degree as an adjunct.

Several of the suggestions in the list cited above have specific application to the rehabilitation settings and so deserve specific explanation. Providing a choice to elderly rehabilitation patients during a daily routine can be very motivating and easy to incorporate. Simply ask the patient to

1. Choose a time of day for treatment (for example, early morning or late morning). The use of an appointment is helpful.
2. Decide an order for the program (for example, work first with weights or ambulate first).
3. Elect to work in a group or singly.
4. Choose a therapist or aide to work with. Often these choices are made for the patient, and with minimal inconvenience the options can be left to the patient.

The use of reproducible measurement certifications is almost always used in the clinical setting but infrequently shared. Good examples of reproducible measurements are goniometric measurements, heart rate, blood pressure, and steps walked. Sharing initial measures and improvements in these measures can be very motivating.

Providing the appropriate environment can encourage any person to work harder. For the older person the appropriate environment can be extremely varied. For an older person suffering from hearing loss, a room with minimal distraction is preferred. This quiet setting allows the elderly patient with a hearing problem to listen and to focus clearly on the main stimulus, the rehabilitation program. For the older person who receives little stimulation, a busy, bright, exciting setting may provide more impetus to work at a program. For optimal rehabilitation of the older person, both settings should be available.

MANIFESTATIONS OF PATHOLOGY

Organic Brain Syndrome

Another behavioral manifestation seen in older persons that is frequently discussed in aging literature is organic brain syndrome (OBS). This term is preferred over senility because of the image of irreversibility, ineffective treatment, and futility that is frequently associated with the senility. Organic brain syndrome is a neuropsychiatric disorder, based in the central nervous system and diagnosed through behavior.[11] The OBS brain shows plaques, lipofuscins, neurofibrillary tangles, and ischemic changes at autopsy.[14] There is tremendous controversy over the labeling and categorizing of OBS. The classifications vary from researcher to researcher. The categorization presented in this chapter is a blending of several theories. There are basically two types of organic brain syndrome: acute and chronic.

ACUTE BRAIN SYNDROME

Examining acute brain syndrome (ABS) first, we see that it is reversible and usually sudden in onset. Some of the various causes of ABS are alcohol, drugs, sensory and sleep deprivation, stress, malnutrition, metabolic and electrolyte imbalances, and cerebrovascular accidents (CVA).[15]

The treatment for ABS is to identify the cause and to take steps to alleviate its effects. For example, an older person may be confused from an unexpected drug reaction. The treatment would be to stop or to change the drug dose that is causing the confusion. If the cause is identified and appropriately altered, symptoms may cease in two to four weeks. What we must keep in mind, however, is that ABS is on a continuum with chronic brain syndrome (CBS). The longer the person has the ABS, the more structural damage will be done to the central nervous system; therefore, early detection and intervention of ABS is essential.

CHRONIC BRAIN SYNDROME

Chronic brain syndrome (CBS) is not reversible.[16] CBS can be divided into two types. The first type, *arteriosclerotic*, affects twice as many men as women. It is due to ischemic changes in the brain and is more closely associated with cerebrovascular accidents than with arteriosclerosis. Autopsy of brains displaying CBS show small cerebral infarcts. Persons with hypertension and diabetes are more prone to this type of OBS. The type of mental decline associated with arteriosclerotic OBS is in a steplike pattern in which the person drops in cognition, stabilizes at that level, drops again, and then stabilizes again. These drops and stabilizations repeat themselves until the person dies. Eighty percent of the people diagnosed with this type of CBS die within two years after the diagnosis.[15]

The next type, *Alzheimer's*, affects three times as many women as men, and it is characterized by plaques and neurofibrillary tangles.[16] The cause is unknown, but some researchers theorize that its causes are genetic, a slow virus, or metabolic.[17] The person's cognition level tends to decline at a gradual rate rather than in the steplike decline seen in the arteriosclerotic type of OBS.

RECOGNITION OF ORGANIC BRAIN SYNDROME

In dealing with both acute and chronic brain syndromes, a mnemonic device may be helpful in recognizing the behavior changes. The mnemonic device is the word JAMCO.

> J—Judgment. The person may show inappropriate behavior as a result of poor choices. For example, the older person may talk loudly during a lecture or appear in public areas inappropriately clothed.
> A—Affect. The person may cry or laugh easily, inappropriately, or uncontrollably. For example, patients may cry uncontrollably after a therapist tells them that they could do better with their exercises. Or the affect may be much flatter, that is, patients may become unresponsive.
> M—Memory. The person may lose short-term, then long-term, memory. For example, the patient may remember back to the age of six but does not know where he or she is now.
> C—Cognition. Cognitive levels may fluctuate. The person may be lucid one moment and confused the next. For example, patients may know where they are at the beginning of a treatment session and at the end may think they are in another country.
> O—Orientation. There may be a loss of orientation to time, place, then person. For example, the person may lose the knowledge of the time of day early in the disease process. Then as the disease progresses, the patient may lose the knowledge of where he or she is. In the final stages of the disease, the person may even forget who he or she is.

In ABS, behavior changes noted above are more sudden and fluctuating than in CBS.[18] In CBS, especially Alzheimer's, the person's affect is much flatter and the use of monosyllabic words is more common.

TREATMENT

The treatment for these brain syndromes begins with accurate assessment. Several tests are available for testing cognitive impairment of the older person. One excellent, quick test is the Mini Mental State Exam developed at Johns Hopkins University.[19] This test takes only 20 minutes to administer. It provides the clinician with information on the patient's cognitive function, as well as information on the patient's ability to understand and to execute commands and some activities of daily living. From this test, a practitioner can evaluate the patient's ability to follow one-, two-, and three-step commands, to read and to execute written words, to identify small and large objects, to calculate using subtraction, to remember certain objects and then to recall these objects. This test should be given in a quiet setting. Patients should be allowed ample time to respond to questions (1 to 2 minutes each). The maximum score attainable is 30. A score of less than 24 points indicates possible cognitive impairment.[19]

Rehabilitation professionals may not have enough time to administer the entire test; therefore, if time is a limitation, practitioners wishing to use this test to evaluate cognitive changes in their elderly patients may want to use only the last section (language). This section provides information that will assist the practitioner in providing improved care. For example, a patient may be able to do a task such as rising to ambulate, however, that patient may need to have the task broken up into two-step commands. The Mini Mental State Exam assesses this deficit initially and can help both the staff and the patient avoid frustration and possible inaccurate assessment of the situation (Fig. 2-1).

Despite what instrument is used, if any, during the initial evaluation, a careful, accurate history should be taken from the patient and the family, checking to make sure that the patient does not have ABS. If the patient does have ABS, the cause should be treated. If the person has a CBS, then the following treatment suggestions may be helpful.

1. Simplify the environment to decrease confusion for the CBS patient.
2. Support the CBS patient in any and all tasks that he or she successfully accomplishes or even attempts.
3. Provide support and education to the family of elderly persons with OBS.[20] Alzheimer's support groups may be found in many communities to provide this assistance.
4. Use touch as much as possible. Touch is very important because it puts two people in the same place at the same time. The use of touch helps orient any person to place and person.

CONCLUSION

Rehabilitation professionals evaluate and treat many older persons for a variety of disabilities. It is difficult to separate the psychosocial component from the physiologic aspect of disability, and, therefore, a thorough investigator would be careless to ignore the psychosocial aspects of any disability, but especially in the aging. To provide a total picture for care of the elderly, this chapter highlighted

DATE _____

	Maximum Score	Score
ORIENTATION		
What is the (year) (season) (date) (month)?	5	( )
Where are we (state) (country) (town) (hospital) (floor)?	5	( )

REGISTRATION

Name three objects. Allow yourself 1 second to say each, then ask the patient to repeat all three after you have said them.   3   ( )

Give 1 point for each correct answer. Then repeat them until the patient learns all three. Count trials and record.

Trials _____

ATTENTION AND CALCULATION

Serial 7s. 1 point for each correct answer. (Subtract 7 from 100 five times). Alternatively spell *world* backward.   5   ( )

RECALL

Ask the patient to recall the three objects repeated above. Give 1 point for each correct answer.   3   ( )

LANGUAGE

Identify a pencil and a watch (2 points).   9   ( )

Repeat the following: "No ifs and/or buts" (1 point).

Follow a three-stage command, for example, "Take a paper in your right hand, fold it in half, and put it on the floor" (3 points).

Read and obey the following: "Close your eyes" (1 point).

Write a sentence (1 point).

Copy a design (1 point).

TOTAL SCORE _____

Assess level of consciousness along a continuum.

Alert	Drowsy	Stupor	Coma

Figure 2–1.   Mini Mental State Exam (From Rabins and Folstein,[19] with permission.)

the effects of attitudes, social myths, and losses, as well as stress, common problems, and pathology frequently seen in the elderly population.

In conclusion, rehabilitation of the elderly client is one of the most challenging tasks for health care professionals because of the unique and complex nature of the older individual. Working with these people requires a sharp investigative skill to uncover multiple physical as well as psychologic complications.

REFERENCES

1. NEUHAUS, R AND NEUHAUS, R: *Successful Aging*. John Wiley & Sons, New York, 1982.

2. POON, L: *Aging in the 1980s: Psychological Issues*. American Psychological Association, Washington, DC, 1980.

3. EBERSOLE, P AND HESS, P: *Toward Healthy Aging*. CV Mosby, St Louis, 1981.

4. BUTLER, R AND LEWIS, N: *Aging and Mental Health: Positive Psychosocial and Biomedical Approaches*. CV Mosby, St Louis, 1982.

5. NEUGARTEN, B: *Middle Age and Aging*. University of Chicago Press, Chicago, 1975.

6. LOETHER, H: *Problems of Aging*. Dickerson Publishing, Encino, CA, 1967.

7. HOWARD, J: *Adapting to retirement*. J Am Geriatr Soc 30(8): 489, August, 1982.

8. SELYE, H: *Stress and aging*. J Am Geriatr 28(9): 668, September, 1970.

9. BLAZER, D: *Depression in Late Life*. CV Mosby, St Louis, 1982.

10. BECK, A: *Depression Causes and Treatment*. University of Pennsylvania, Philadelphia, 1982.

11. ZARIT, S: *Aging and Mental Disorders*. Free Press, New York, 1981.

12. FREEDMAN, N: *Depression in a family practice elderly population*. J Am Geriatr Soc 30(6):371, June, 1982.

13. HARRIS, R: *Guide to Fitness After 50*. Plenum Press, New York, 1977.

14. WOOLANTIN, MO AND FREDICH, P: *Care of the patient with a true dementia*. In WOOLANTIN, MO AND FREDICH, P: *Confusion*. CV Mosby, St Louis, 1973.

15. FEIGHNER, GP, ET AL: *Diagnostic criteria for use in psychiatric research*. Arch Gen Psychiatry 26:57, 1972.

16. BURNSIDE, IM: *Alzheimer's disease: An overview*. Journal of Gerontological Nursing 5(4):14, 1979.

17. HAYTER, J: *Patients who have Alzheimer's disease*. Am J Nurs 74:1460, 1974.

18. FOWLER, RS: *Adapting care for the brain damaged patient*. Am J Nurs 72:2056, November, 1972.

19. RABINS, P AND FOLSTEIN, M: *Psychiatric evaluation of the elderly patient*. Primary Care 16(3):609.

20. MACE, N AND ROBINS, P: *The 36 Hour Day*. Johns Hopkins University Press, Baltimore, 1981.

BIBLIOGRAPHY

ALLEN, R: *Investigations in Stress Control*. Burgess Publishing, Minneapolis, 1981.

BARTOL, M: *Dialogue with dementia: Nonverbal communication in patients with Alzheimer's disease*. Journal of Gerontological Nursing 5:21, July/August, 1979.

BIRKETT, M: *Nursing care study, secondary dementia*. Nursing Mirror 136:34, January, 1973.

BOTWENICK, J: *Aging and Behavior*. Springer, New York, 1973.

BRODIE, NH, McGHIE, RL, O'HARA, H, VALLE-JONES, GC, SCHIFF, AA: *Anxiety depression in elderly patients*. Practitioner 215:660, November, 1975.

CROMWELL, HA: *Management of anxiety/depression in geriatric patients*. Med Times 101(1):47, January, 1973.

EISDORFER, C AND COHEN, D: *The cognitively impaired elderly: Differential diagnosis*. In STORANDT, M, SIEGLER, I, AND ELIAS, M (EDS): *The Clinical Psychology of Aging*. Plenum Press, New York, 1978.

EISDORFER, C AND FRIEDEL, R: *Cognitive and Emotional Disturbance in the Elderly*. Year Book Medical Publishers, Chicago, 1977.

EVERLY, G: *The Nature and Treatment of the Stress Response*. Plenum Press, New York, 1981.

GARFUNKEL, F AND LANDAU, G: *Short-term memory course for the well older adult*. Perspect Aging 8:19, January/February, 1979.

HAYMES, S: *Epidemiology of Aging*. US Department of Health and Human Services, Washington, DC, 1980.

ISAACS, B: *The evaluation of drugs in Alzheimer's disease*. Age Ageing 8:115, 1979.

KNIGHT, B: *Psychotherapy and behavior change with the non-institutionalized aged*. Int J Aging Hum Dev 9:221, 1978–1979.

LEAF, A: *Long lived population*. J Am Geriatr Soc 30(8):485, August, 1982.

PFEIFFER, E: *A short portable mental status questionnaire for the assessment of organic brain deficit in elderly patients*. J Am Geriatr Soc 23:433, 1975.

SCHAIE, J AND SCHAIE, W: *Psychological evaluation of the cognitively impaired elderly*. In EISDORFER, C AND FRIEDEL, R (EDS): *Cognitive and Emotional Disturbance in the Elderly*. Year Book Medical Publishers, Chicago, 1977.

SCHULTZ, J: *The Economics of Aging*. Wadsworth Publishing, Belmonte, CA, 1976.

SCHWENCK, M: *Reality orientation for the institutionalized aged: Does it help?* Gerontologist 19:373, 1979.

SHANAS, E AND BENSTOCK, R: *Handbook of Aging and Social Science*. Van Nostrand Reinhold, New York, 1976.

WEG, R: *The Aged Who, Where, How Well*. Ethel Percy Andrus Gerontology Center, 1979.

WOODRUFF, D AND BIRREN, J: *Aging*. D. Van Nostrand, New York, 1975.

SECTION 2

PHYSICAL ASPECTS OF AGING

CHAPTER **3**

ACTIVITIES OF
DAILY LIVING

GAIL HILLS MAGUIRE, Ph.D., O.T.R.

BEHAVIORAL OBJECTIVES

Upon completion of this chapter, the reader will be able to
1. Identify the range of activities included under activities of daily living (ADL).
2. List methods to measure independence in ADL.
3. Identify the categories of ADL included in the Maguire Trilevel ADL Assessment (MTAA).
4. Score a sample MTAA.
5. Describe three common functional problems of the elderly, including (1) reduced strength and endurance, (2) decreased joint mobility, and (3) increased danger of accidents.
6. Discuss a practical suggestion for each of the common functional problems.

Health status may be defined in physical, mental, or social terms[1,2] but usually has one of two meanings in relation to the elderly: (1) the absence of death, disease, disability, dysfunction, or discomfort,[3,4] or (2) the degree of functional capacity or disability. This chapter will concern the latter meaning, which permits measurement in relation to departures from normal life roles or activities rather than medical or biologic criteria.[5,6] Explaining health in terms of functional capacity in daily activities is germane, because the core problem in geriatrics is the continuous loss of adaptive capacity[4] coupled with an increase in chronic conditions.

A large number of people aged 65 to 75 years and particularly those over age 75 have substantial limitations in physical and emotional performance. Furthermore, many disabled persons over age 65 years need mobility or personal care assistance for independent living. This group includes a large portion of the elderly population, and the problem can only increase as the number of elderly persons in general and those over age 75 in particular continue to increase.[7]

Kuriansky and Gurland[8] report that measurement of self-care functions originated in medicine to guide treatment programs and to document the progress and adaptive ability of physically disabled patients. Such evaluations have been useful in diagnosis, prognosis, prevention, and treatment of elderly patients.

Williams[9] and Chappell[3] note that independence in daily activities is often used to assess functional ability. In a study of institutionalized geriatric patients, Kuriansky and Gurland[8] found that the more independent persons are in activities of daily living (ADL), the better their chances are for survival and early discharge.

The goal of rehabilitation is to assist patients to be as independent as possible in their functioning. This chapter will deal with the role of ADL in the rehabilitation of the elderly.

The discussion will include (1) definition of activities of daily living, (2) Maguire's Trilevel ADL Assessment, (3) common functional problems for the elderly—reduced strength, joint mobility, and safety, and (4) practical suggestions for ADL.

DEFINITION OF ACTIVITIES OF DAILY LIVING

One individual flies across the country to see her daughter and grandchildren, while another leaves her home only when she is escorted and chauffeured by family or friends. Still another person is happily engaged in activities alone or with others, while someone else responds that she does "nothing much," feels "poorly," and rarely hears from her family or friends. These are all people over the age of 65, and yet their activities of daily living are very different. Since the concept of ADL was first introduced almost 40 years ago, there has been a great variance of opinion about the definition.[4] One approach sees all activities—including recreation and work—in the scope of ADL; another focuses only on self-care activities, and other approaches define ADL as a combination of the two extremes.

Leering[4] defines functional capacity in terms of needs for food, safety, body temperature, and hygiene. He has proposed that a hierarchical design beginning with the autonomic nervous system (ANS), followed by activities of daily living, mobility, and household activities, follows the evolutional stages of life. This design also assumes that motion is necessary in all parts of the body for functional capacity.

Katz and Akpom[10] suggest that patients recovering from illness or disability pass through three successive stages of recovery, beginning with feeding and continence, then transferring and toileting (social and cultural aspects), followed by dressing and bathing. This pattern has some elements in common with Leering's[4] design. Pedretti[11] defines ADL to include mobility, self-care, management of environmental hardware and devices, communication, and home management activities. Grover[12] is developing a standardized index of physical functioning, including validity and reliability studies.

This controversy over the content and methods to measure ADL is reflected in the forms or indexes used in evaluation, which range from a dozen items to 85 or more. Often individual items are grouped into categories for ease of evaluation and recording, but even the categories are not uniform. The measures to determine level of performance in these categories also vary. In the past, researchers have measured functional capacity through rank-ordered descriptions such as independent, independent with aids, requires some supervision/assistance, or dependent. This approach leads to complicated decisions as to the degree and effect of equipment and/or assistance.[13] For instance, how do you rate an elderly person who uses a bathrail for safety but, if necessary, could manage without it? This inconsistent use of criteria by the same or different evaluators is a potential source of unreliability.[13]

MEASURING INDEPENDENCE

In all the various ADL instruments, usually one of the following three methods has been utilized to measure independence in activities of daily living: (1) self-reports by the patient, (2) direct examination of a group of sample activities,[8] or (3) ratings of the patient's performance by a trained observer, such as a therapist or a nurse.

Researchers concerned with classification of large groups of people into similar categories have utilized the first method, and the second method has often been used as a screening device. Self-reports can be heavily influenced by the patient's psychologic state. These methods give an impression of the total level of independence but do not give the detailed profile that is often necessary to plan a specific treatment program. Therefore, most therapists utilize the trained observer method for therapeutic intervention. However, observer ratings are often difficult to standardize and to interpret without lengthy comments. The Revised Kenny Self-Care Evaluation[14] is an attempt to give a numerical measure to observer ratings. It measures only self-care in the home or protected environment and does not include home management duties such as washing dishes, cooking, and so forth.

MAGUIRE'S TRILEVEL ADL ASSESSMENT

Leering[4] has mentioned that the field of geriatrics would benefit from a uniform system to determine functional capacity. Without a structured system, the same items may be listed under many different headings so that it is impossible to compare treatments and assessments worldwide.

The following model, Maguire's Trilevel ADL Assessment (MTAA), is a systems approach that divides the tasks of daily living into six categories: (1) communication, (2) eating, (3) mobility, (4) hygiene, (5) dressing, and (6) organization. Each category is divided into three environmental levels: (1) personal, (2) home or sheltered environment, and (3) the community (Fig. 3-1). The MTAA is an initial attempt to conceptualize a developmental analysis of components in each of the categories of activities and is not a research instrument. Items such as organization which are often observed but not formally recorded have been included. It can be used as a self-report or observed checklist. No validity or reliability studies are available, and there has been no attempt to differentiate which skills are most critical.

Most therapists devise simple or complex ADL evaluation procedures and/or forms based on the needs dictated by their environment and patient population. Individual sections of this model can be selected based on the needs of a specific patient population.

The following sample of the MTAA shows how it can be used for an elderly client who is living in the community. Mrs. Smith was mainly independent but needed help to identify the necessary assistance and adaptation of her environment that would ensure her independence as long as possible. Limited intervention with an elderly patient can make the difference between maintaining an optimal level of functioning or the steady increase in psychologic and physical dependency.

Scoring the MTAA

The scoring method for the MTAA is a modification of the system used for the Revised Kenny Self-Care Evaluation.[14] Scoring is based on two steps. The first step is a traditional descriptive rating; the second step is a quantitative scoring of functioning on each of the three levels (self-care, home, and community). If the patient is obviously on a very independent level, the therapist can ask if he or she is totally independent in a task such as eating. If the answer is yes, mark *independent* and move to the next section. Another approach is to follow that question with a question regarding a more difficult item in the category, such as whether the patient can cut with a knife.

In the first step the rater assigns one of the following ratings to each task:

> I = totally independent
> S = needs any degree of supervision

NAME *JANE SMITH*   AGE *75*   DATE *2'7'85*

DIAGNOSIS *RHEUMATOID ARTHRITIS;*   DATE OF ONSET *1965*

HYPERTENSION R CATARACT SURGERY c̄ CONTACT

DATE OF ADMISSION *2/7/85 OUT PATIENT*

EYEGLASSES *✓* SPECIAL LENS (TYPE) *R CATARACT* HEARING AIDS ___ R ___ L *✓*

SCORING

1. Rate each task under colum R as
   I = totally independent
   S = any supervision
   A = any assistance
   D = totally dependent
   NA = not applicable

2. Score each level under subtotal as
   4 = all Is in level
   3 = 1 or 2 As or Ss; Others all Is or equipment essential to function or safety
   2 = all other configurations
   1 = 1 or 2 As or Ss or 1 I; others all Ds
   0 = all tasks rated D

3. Transfer scores to MTAA Score Sheet
   Write summary of each category.

Envi-ronment	Cate-gories	Tasks	Evaluation Date:		Progress Rounds:		Progress Rounds:	
		COMMUNICATION	R		R		R	
Person-al	Communi-cation	Follows verbal directions	I					
		Communicates verbally/sign language	I					
		Follows written directions	I					
		Writes name	I					
		Operates signal light	I					
		Operates TV/radio	I					
		Equipment List	✓	L HEARING AID R CATARACT GLASSES				
		SCORE	3	INDEPENDENT c̄ EQUIPMENT				
Home	Communi-cation	Types/writes written communication/correspondence	I					
		Uses telephone	I	REJECTED AMPLIFIER				
		Opens and seals envelopes	I					
		Opens/locks doors	I					
		Operates light switch	I					
		Operates door bell	I					
		Equipment List	✓	SEE PERSONAL				
		SCORE	3	INDEPENDENT c̄ EQUIPMENT				

**(c) 1983 Maguire, G. H. Used with permission.

Figure 3-1. Shown here is the Maguire Trilevel ADL Assessment (MTAA).

(Figure continues on pp. 40–47.)

Environment	Categories	Tasks	Evalution Date: 2/7/85		Progress Rounds:		Progress Rounds:	
Community	Communication	Maintains personal contacts	I	MAINLY PHONE				
		Maintains business contacts	I					
		Equipment List	✓	SEE PERSONAL				
		SCORE	3	INDEPENDENT ? EQUIPMENT				

EATING

Personal	Eating	Finger foods	I					
		Use of utensils	I					
		Pour from container	I					
		Drink (cup/glass/straw)	I					
		Cuts with knife	I					
		Takes medication	I					
		Equipment List	N/A					
		SCORE	4					

Home	Eating-Cooking	Operates faucets	I	NEEDS NEW WASHERS				
		Lights match/gas burner	I					
		Operates appliance controls	I					
		Handles hot foods/liquids	I					
		Used sharp utensils	I					
		Reaches and transports items refrigerator/cupboards	I	NO HIGH SHELVES				
		Opens containers/pkg. foods	I					
		Opens manual/electric can opener	I					
		Opens screw jars	I					
		Breaks an egg	I					
		Peels/cuts vegetables	I	CUTS SM. PIECES AT TIME				
		Washes/drys dishes	I					

Figure 3-1. *Continued.*

Envi-ronment	Cate-gories	Tasks	Evaluation Date: 2/7/85		Progress Rounds:		Progress Rounds:	
Home	Eating Cooking	Uses measuring devices	I					
		Uses hand (electric) beater	I					
		*Rolls pastry	/					
		Weekly menu/shopping list	I					
		Diet (type) LOW SALT	S	DIDN'T UNDERSTAND; REFERRED TO DIETICIAN				
		Equipment List	N/A	REJECTED REACHER				
		SCORE	3	NEED SUPERVISION 8 DIET				
Comm-unity	Eating	Food shops	A	NEEDS TRANSPORTATION				
		Equipment List	N/A					
		SCORE	3	DAUGHTER DRIVES HER				

MOBILITY

Envi-ronment	Cate-gories	Tasks	Eval		Progress		Progress	
Person-al	Moving in bed	Shift position	I					
		Turn to left side	I					
		Turn to right side	I					
		Turn to prone	I					
		Turn to supine	I					
		Equipment List	N/A					
Person-al	Rising and Sitting	Come to sitting position	I					
		Maintain sitting balance	I					
		Legs over side of bed	I					
		Move to edge of bed	I					
		Legs back onto bed	I					
		Equipment List	N/A					
Person-al	Sitting Trans-fer	Shift bed to chair	N/A					
		Shift chair to bed	N/A					
		Equipment List	N/A					

*optional activity

Figure 3-1. *Continued.*

Environ-ment	Cate-gories	Tasks	Evaluation Date: 2/7/85		Progress Rounds:		Progress Rounds:	
Person-al	Stand-ing Trans-fer	Slide forward	I					
		Position feet	I					
		Stand	I	GREAT EFFORT LOW SOFT CHAIR				
		Pivot	I					
		Sit	I					
		Equipment List	✓	FIRM HIGH CHAIR				
Person-al	Toilet Trans-fer	Position (paper sanitary supplies, etc.)	I					
		Manage equipment	I					
		Transfer to commode	I	RAISED SEAT BETTER				
		Undress	I					
		Dress	I					
		Transfer back	I					
		Equipment List	✓	GRAB BAR—TOILET SEAT—MUCH SAFER				
Person-al	Bath-ing Trans-fer	Tub/shower approach	I					
		Use of grab bars	I					
		Tub/shower entry	I					
		Tub/shower exit	I					
		Equipment List	✓	HAS STALL SHOWER SEAT + GRAB BAR—EASIER				
		SCORE	3	INDEPENDENT Ē EQUIPMENT				

Home	Loco-mot-ion	Travels 30'	I					
		Travels 100'	I					
		Turns	I					
		Carries object	I					
		Opens/travels through door	I					
		Picks up object from floor	I	DIFFICULT				
		Gets down/up from floor	I	DIFFICULT				
		Stairs ____ with rails ____ without ____ goes down/up ramp	I	RAILS HELPFUL				

Figure 3-1. *Continued.*

PHYSICAL ASPECTS OF AGING

Environ-ment	Cate-gories	Tasks	Evaluation Date: 2/7/85		Progress Rounds:		Progress Rounds:	
		Equipment___w/c ✓ other (specify) *CANE/SUPPORT*	✓					
		SCORE	3	*INDEPENDENT Ē CANE*				
Home	Wheel Chair Mobi-lity	Positions chair	N/A					
		Brakes on/off						
		Arm rests on/off						
		Footrests on/off						
		Positions transfer board						
		Equipment List	↓					
		SCORE	N/A					
Commu-nity	Loco-motion	Crosses street with traffic light	S	*TOO SLOW TO BE SAFE*				
		Operates elevator	I					
		Transfers in/out car	I					
		Transfers equipment/w/c in/out car	N/A					
		Uses public transportation	A	*DIFFICULTY Ē BUS STEP, FEAR*				
		Operates w/c on rough surfaces	N/A					
		Equipment List	✓	*CANE*				
		SCORE	3	*UNSAFE IN TRAFFIC/BUS*				

HYGIENE

Environ-ment	Cate-gories	Tasks						
Person-al	Face Hair and Arms	Handkerchief, tissue	I					
		Wash face	I					
		Wash hands and arms	I					
		Brush teeth and dentures	I					
		Shaving/make-up	I					
		Manicure	I					
		Equipment List	N/A					
Person-al	Trunk and Peri-neum	Wash back	I	*LONGHANDLED BATHBRUSH EASIER*				
		Wash buttocks	I					
		Wash chest	I					

Figure 3-1. *Continued.*

ACTIVITIES OF DAILY LIVING   **43**

Environ-ment	Cate-gories	Tasks	Evaluation Date: 2/7/85	Progress Rounds:		Progress Rounds:	
Person-al	Trunk and Peri-neum	Wash abdomen	I				
		Wash groin	I				
		Equipment List	✓ LONG BRUSH EASIER, NOT NECESSARY				
Person-al	Lower Extrem-ities	Wash upper legs	I				
		Wash lower legs	I				
		Wash feet	I LONG-HANDLED BRUSH				
		Pedicure	D TOO PAINFUL TO STAY BENT				
		Equipment List	✓ LONGHANDLED BRUSH HELPFUL				
Person-al	Bowel Pro-gram	Suppository	N/A				
		Digital stimulation					
		Equipment care					
		Cleaning self					
		Equipment List					
Person-al	Blad-der Pro-gram	Stimulation					
		Equipment care					
		Cleaning self					
		Catheter care					
		Equipment List					
		SCORE	3 NEEDS PEDICURE LONG-HANDLED BATH BRUSH HELPFUL				
Home		Make bed	I				
		Change bed	I LOOSE ELASTIC FITTED SHEETS				
		Dust floor	I FLEX MOP HELPFUL				
		Wet mop floor	I DOESN'T DO OFTEN				
		Vacuum	N/A NO CARPET — WOOD FLOORS				
		Clean bath	I LONG-HANDLED SPONGE				
		Dust	I				
		Equipment List	✓ SEE ABOVE				
		SCORE	3 INDEPENDENT c EQUIPMENT				

Figure 3-1. *Continued.*

Environ-ment	Cate-gories	Tasks	Evaluation Date: 2/7/85	Progress Rounds:	Progress Rounds:
DRESSING					
Person-al	Upper Trunk and Arms	✓ Hearing aid ✓ eyeglasses	I		
		Front opening on/off	I		
		Pullover on/off	I		
		Bra on/off	I		
		Corset/brace on/off	N/A		
		Equipment/prosthesis/on/off	N/A		
		Sweater/shawl on/off	I		
		Equipment List	N/A		
Person-al	Lower Trunk and Legs	Slacks/shirt on/off	I		
		Underclothing on/off	I		
		Belt on/off	I		
		Braces/prosthesis on/off	N/A		
		Girdle on/off	N/A		
Person-al	Feet	Stockings on/off	I		
		Shoes/slippers on/off	I — SLIP-ON SHOES LONG-HANDLED SHOE		
		Braces/prosthesis on/off	N/A — HORN HELPFUL, NOT NECESSARY		
		Wraps/supports hose on/off	N/A		
		Equipment	✓ SEE ABOVE		
	SCORE		3 — INDEPENDENT C̄ EQUIPMENT		

Home	Laun-dry	Hand washing	I		
		Hang clothes rack/line	I		
		*Iron	N/A		
		Fold clothes	I		
		Washing machine	I		
		Dryer	I		
		*Polish/clean shoes	/		
	Sew-ing	*Thread needle and make knot	I		
		*Sew on button	I		
		*Mend	/		

*Optional activity

Figure 3-1. *Continued.*

ACTIVITIES OF DAILY LIVING   **45**

Environ-ment	Cate-gories	Tasks	Evaluation Date: 2/7/85	Progress Rounds:	Progress Rounds:
Home	Sewing	*Sewing machine			
		*Cut with shears	I DIFFICULT		
		SCORE	4 INDEPENDENT		

Commu-nity		Clothes shopping/orders by phone	I USES CATALOG, NEEDS TRANSPORTATION		
		Equipment			
		SCORE	3 NEEDS TRANSPORTATION		

ORGANIZATION

Person-al	Plan-ning	Daily activity schedule	I		
		Identifies needed assistance	S DENIED NEEDING ASSISTANCE INITIALLY		
		Budget/money management	I		
		Appointments - bank, medical, etc.	I NEEDS TRANSPORTATION		
		Equipment			
			3 NEEDS TRANSPORTATION		

Home	Manage-ment	Household bills, etc.	S DAUGHTER BAL-ANCES CHECK BOOK		
		Plans activities with families/others	S STOPPED INITIATING		
		Fosters interpersonal rela-tionships	S MAINTAINED PHONE CONTACT, STOPPED PERSONAL CONTACT		
		Heavy household tasks/repairs	D FAMILY ASSISTS		
		Child care (if applicable)	N/A		
		Personal leisure activities	S NEEDS TO LEAVE HOUSE		
		Religious activities	A NEEDS TRANSPORTATION		
		Equipment			
		SCORE	2		

Commu-nity	Manage-ment	Job/professional affairs			
		Community leisure activities			

*Optional activity

Comments: MAINLY INDEPENDENT WITH TRANSPORTATION, EQUIPMENT AND MINIMAL ASSISTANCE. PT. REPORTS DEPRESSED BY RECENT ↑ IN R.A. RESULTED IN ↑ DEPENDENCE ON DAUGHTER + RELUCTANCE TO GO OUT. AGREED TO ACCEPT SR. CITIZEN TRANSPORTATION AND GO TO LOCAL CENTER ON TRIAL BASIS.

Figure 3-1. *Continued.*

MTTAA SCORE SHEET

CATEGORIES	LEVELS	LEVEL SCORES
Communication	Personal	3
	Home	3
	Community	3
		3
Food	Personal	4
Needs	Home	3
	Community	3
		3+
Mobility	Personal	3
	Home	3
	Community	3
		3
Hygiene	Personal	3
	Home	3
	Community	3
		3
Dressing	Personal	3
	Home	3
	Community	4
		3+
Organization	Personal	3
	Home	2
	Community	2
		2

Figure 3-1. *Continued.*

A = needs any degree of assistance
D = totally dependent
NA = not applicable

This step of the scoring requires the rater to make only two choices regarding the patient's performance: Is the patient totally independent, or does the patient require some assistance and/or supervision? Does the patient require equipment for functioning or safety? The rater does not have to make a judgment on the degree of necessary assistance and/or supervision. If the patient is independent when using the equipment, the therapist marks *I* and then lists the equipment under Comments. If the patient needs supervision or assistance in addition to the equipment, an *S* or *A* is marked and the equipment is listed. If the patient is obviously on a very dependent level, the therapist can give a descriptive rating to only those applicable tasks—such as communication, eating, and bed mobility on the personal level—and stop at this point. The rating of other tasks can be continued later. (Note: A later rating should be entered, with the date, under the progress note column.)

The next step requires the therapist to give a quantitative rating to each level (personal, home, community) of each of the six categories (communication through organization). The ratings are recorded on the form as follows:

4 = all tasks in the level rated *I*
3 = one or two *A*'s or *S*'s; others all *I*'s or equipment *essential* to function or safety
2 = all other configurations
1 = one or two *A*'s or *S*'s or one *I*; others all *D*'s
0 = all tasks rated *D*

After completing the rating of each level, the therapist should transfer the scores to the MTAA score sheet. This gives a summary of the patient's functioning level in each category. An average score for each category may be done. For purposes of reporting, a descriptive summary of each level on completion of the MTAA might be as follows:

4 = totally independent
3 = mainly but not quite independent; requires equipment or extra time
2 = all other combinations; the specific degree of assistance and/or supervision/equipment should be described
1 = mainly dependent with one or two exceptions
0 = totally dependent

If you look at the completed score sheet for Mrs. Smith (see Figure 3-1), you will note that she needs some equipment or assistance in all areas and that the tasks in the area of organization require the most assistance. A summary statement might read as follows:

> The patient functions alone in her own home with the following equipment: hearing aid, R cataract lens, glasses, long-handle bath brush, shoehorn, slip-on shoes, bathroom grab bars, tub seat, raised toilet seat, 19″ high firm chair, railings on stairs, fleximop, and swivel sponge. Mrs. Smith needs assistance with transportation to food store, appointments, supervision or assistance paying bills, maintaining family contacts, heavy household tasks/repairs, and interaction with people other than her daughter. She has agreed to attend the local senior citizen center twice a week and to use their transportation for some appointments and such trips as to the library. A ride has been arranged for church activities. This should reduce her feelings of resentment and dependency on her daughter, who is busy with a job and a family. All recommendations, including energy conservation, were discussed when the patient and daughter were together. Role conflicts between the two were discussed.
>
> Mrs. Smith should be reevaluated in three months to determine whether she is less depressed, whether she is following her low salt diet, to check the progress of ulnar drift on her hands, and to see whether she is maintaining contacts outside the home.

Problems in Rating the MTAA

In any evaluation taken at a particular point in time, there is always the question, Am I measuring the patient's actual ability? The therapist must always rate only the observed performance and then note on the score sheet any conditions, such as fatigue or mental state, that seemed to affect performance. This should be followed by a reevaluation at another session.

Some tasks or whole levels of any activity are not applicable to a patient. Mark NA (not applicable) on the score sheet; it cannot be scored and is ignored in judgments. For example, under mobility, a person may do a standing transfer and not a sitting transfer. Mark items under sitting transfer NA and score only the standing transfer section.

Whenever equipment or an inordinate amount of time is essential—not just helpful—for safe performance of any tasks within a level, the score for that level is a 3 and the equipment is described under comments. This is consistent with the concept of supervision or assistance; the patient is not totally independent in a nonadapted environment.

If there is only one item that can be scored in a level, the ratings are as follows: one $I = 4$; one $D = 0$, one A or $S = 2$. This situation falls within the rules because a single I is treated as "all I's"; a single D is "all D's"; and an A or S falls within "all other configurations." Scoring for only two items in a level is similar:

Two *I*'s are 4, two *D*'s are 0, one *I* and one *A* or *S* are 3, one *I* and one *D* are 1, and one *D* and one *A* or *S* are also 1.

COMMON FUNCTIONAL PROBLEMS FOR THE ELDERLY

A comprehensive but not exhaustive list of ADL tasks has been presented to highlight the magnitude of potential daily activities for any individual. However, the unique problem in rehabilitation of the elderly is treatment of acute or chronic conditions in the context of a gradual but continuous loss of adaptive capacity. The older the age the more this combination of pathology superimposed on a general decline in function can lead to disability.

The purpose of the following summary of suggestions and techniques is to give you some general ideas about how to solve three of the most common functional problems of the elderly: (1) reduced strength and endurance, (2) joint problems, and (3) increased safety problems.

Many times the therapist must design or adapt techniques or equipment to solve individual patient problems. In fact, many of the devices presently sold by rehabilitation equipment companies were originally designed by occupational therapists or patients. Retraining in ADL is a mutual process, and clients should be freely involved in adapting situations or equipment to their particular needs.[11] The reader is referred to the references and bibliography at the end of this chapter for information in relation to specific handicaps.

Reduced Strength and Endurance

There is a gradual decline in strength and endurance with increasing age, particularly after age 75; yet most people wish to remain as independent as possible. The following is a summary of energy conservation and work simplification techniques. When the occupational therapist is designing such a program for an elderly patient, the therapist must balance the program so that the goal of maintaining full range of motion (ROM) and maximum independence is not compromised by work simplification techniques to reduce fatigue. Work simplification and energy conservation techniques are often recommended for rheumatoid arthritic and cardiac patients but can be utilized successfully by anyone, particularly the elderly. Individuals will make choices about adopting such techniques based on their personal and physical resources and values.

ENERGY CONSERVATION AND WORK SIMPLIFICATION TECHNIQUES

1. Review the normal schedule of activities and eliminate the unnecessary ones.

2. Determine if work efficiency can be enhanced by combining, rear-ranging, or simplifying procedures.
3. Identify equipment or people necessary to the task.
4. Plan activities so that there is a balance of heavy and light tasks throughout the day, week, and month.
5. Alternate work sessions with sufficient rest periods to avoid over-fatigue.
6. Avoid rushing, which increases tension and fatigue. A moderate steady pace is more productive.
7. Utilize proper body mechanics at all times.
8. Organize storage and work areas according to function. Assemble all necessary supplies and equipment before beginning a task.
9. Maintain a good posture. Sit rather than stand, and avoid bending and stooping whenever possible.
10. Use lightweight equipment and energy-saving appliances.[11,15]

Decreased Joint Mobility

In addition to a decrease in strength, many elderly individuals have deterioration of their joints, which causes decreased mobility and discomfort. The following principles of joint protection can be utilized to reduce joint stress and discomfort and to preserve joint structures. These recommendations are even more crucial for conditions such as rheumatoid arthritis.

JOINT PROTECTION

1. Maintain full active range of motion in all joints. During daily activities, each joint should be actively moved through the full range of motion. For example, light objects can be stored at various heights to encourage full range of motion when reaching such objects. Activities such as dusting or sweeping the floor can be done in smooth, long sweeping motions. This must be planned as part of the total program to prevent undue fatigue.
2. Avoid unnecessary pressure on joints. Utilize the largest joint whenever possible. For example, rather than using the fingers, the whole palm of the hand can be used to push off from the chair before standing. Large objects can be carried by the arms rather than by the hands. Equipment such as a jar opener, an electric can opener, and enlarged utensil handles can reduce stress on fingers caused by a tight grasp (Fig. 3-2).
3. To reduce strain on joints, use proper body mechanics whenever lifting or pushing an object.
4. Avoid static motions that require sustained muscle contractions over a long period of time. Such positions are very fatiguing. For example,

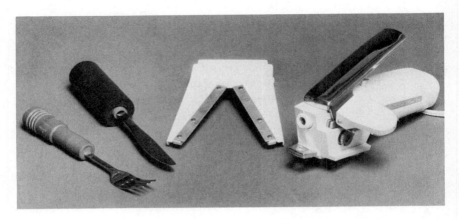

Figure 3-2. Shown here is adaptive equipment: (left to right) large-handle fork, large-handle knife, jar opener, and one-handle can opener.

holders can be utilized for holding a book or the telephone (see Figure 3-2).[11,15,16,17]

Increased Danger of Accidents

The combination of joint limitations, a slowed reaction time, and decreased vision, hearing, strength, and endurance can lead to a greater risk of household accidents for the elderly. Slippery or uneven surfaces, stairs or steps, the kitchen, and the bathroom are potentially hazardous areas for the elderly. The elderly usually avoid icy or uneven surfaces whenever possible but often take risks by standing on chairs to do things, such as to hang curtains. Such individuals should be encouraged to identify someone who could assist them with such chores. One method is to trade a service, such as babysitting or baking, for jobs that are too risky. Stairs should be well lighted at all times and equipped with nonskid surfaces and a handrailing. A physical therapist should evaluate ambulation problems and recommend proper equipment. Canes, walkers, and crutches should not be purchased and used by the patient without proper fitting and training. Elderly persons should never descend stairs in stocking feet or floppy slippers with soft soles, which increase the chances of slipping. Accidents in the kitchen often involve the use of appliances. It may help forgetful persons to set a timer to remind them when stove burners or ovens need to be turned off.

The bathroom is the most common area for accidents. The occupational therapist can do an evaluation to determine whether the patient can transfer independently or requires supervision or assistance. The tub or shower should be measured to determine the best type and location of equipment, such as grab bars or bathtub seats (Fig. 3-3).

PHYSICAL ASPECTS OF AGING

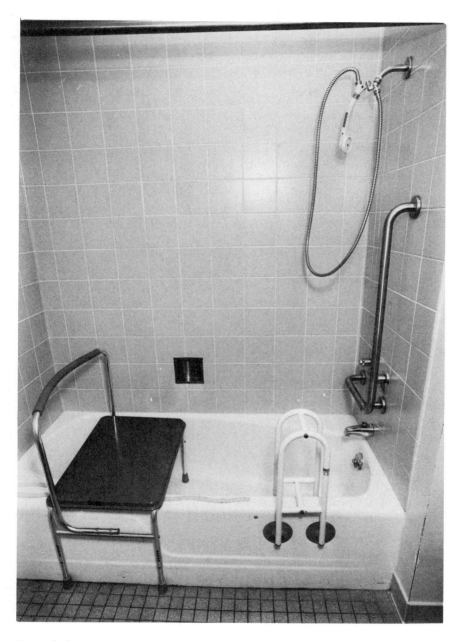

Figure 3-3. Shown here is a bathroom with adaptive equipment: (left to right) bath seat, grab bars on tub, wall grab bars, and hand-held showerhead.

Because the recovery time following an injury is usually longer for the elderly than for younger persons, a conservative approach to safety measures is advisable. In many families the fear that the older member will fall and break a hip and thus become dependent is so great that the family members discourage the elderly person from being as independent as possible. Anyone can have an accident while he or she is alone, but the risk is greater and the results can be more serious for an elderly person. Therefore, the following steps are recommended when making decisions regarding safety in performance of ADL.

1. Evaluate the patient and determine the safest method to perform an activity, including necessary equipment.
2. Give training in the method and use of equipment.
3. Determine whether the patient can consistently perform the activity in a safe manner independently, with supervision, or with assistance.
4. Arrange for someone to regularly assist with tasks the patient can not perform safely.
5. If the person is alone, assist the patient to arrange for a family member or volunteer to check regularly on his or her welfare by telephone or visit.
6. After arrangements have been made for the safety of the patient, the individual and family should be encouraged to permit the patient to be as independent as possible within the established safety guidelines.

PRACTICAL SUGGESTIONS FOR ADL PROBLEMS

With joint limitation and reduced strength and the consequent problems of safety, the following may be used:[11,15]

1. Large buttons or fastenings
2. Loose-fitting, front-opening garments
3. Velcro
4. Long-handle shoehorn, bath brush, and so forth
5. Slip-on shoes or elastic shoelaces
6. Sock or stocking aids
7. Reacher
8. Built-up utensil handles
9. Hand-held showerhead
10. Safety grab bars on tub/shower
11. Nonskid rubber mat or strips on tub/shower
12. Bathtub/shower seat
13. Raised toilet seat
14. Book/telephone holder
15. Lever-type faucets/doorknob extensions
16. Padded handles on ambulation equipment (crutches, cane, walker)

17. Suction mat to anchor dishes, bowls, and so forth
18. Electric typewriter.

The primary goal of health professionals working with the elderly should be to assist them to maintain maximum independence in activities of daily living. This is not a simple task, because the elderly are at greater risk of decreased independence owing to the subtle continuous loss of adaptive capacity coupled with an increase in chronic conditions. The expectation of reduced ability can cause both the elderly and health professionals to ignore subtle changes in functional capacity until there are major problems. It is optimal to identify problems early, to recommend modifications in the environment or performance to maximize independence and safety, and then to allow the person to function as autonomously as possible. Limited intervention only as needed can encourage psychologic and physical independence and the sense of control over one's life. Even though a "cure" might not always be possible, anything that will improve the quality or "wholeness" of the elderly person's life is worth the effort of the health professional.

REFERENCES

1. SHANAS, E AND MADDOX, GL: *Aging, health and the organization of health resources.* In BINSTOCK, RH AND SHANAS, E (EDS) *Handbook of Aging and the Social Sciences.* Van Nostrand Reinhold, Toronto, 1976.

2. STEWART, A, WARE, JE, AND BROOK, RH: *The meaning of health: Understanding functional limitations.* Med Care 15:939, 1977.

3. CHAPPELL, NL: *Measuring functional ability and chronic health conditions among the elderly: A research note on the adequacy of three instruments.* J Health Soc Behav 22:90, 1981.

4. LEERING, C: *A structural model of functional capacity in the aged.* J Am Geriatr Soc 27:314, 1979.

5. REYNOLDS, WJ, RUSHING, WA, AND MILES, DL: *The validation of a functional status index.* J Health Soc Behav 15:271, 1974.

6. SULLIVAN, DF: *Conceptual problems in developing an index of health.* US Department of Health, Education and Welfare, Washington, DC, 1966.

7. EBERSOLE, P AND HESS, P: *Toward healthy aging.* CV Mosby, St Louis, 1981.

8. KURIANSKY, J AND GURLAND, B: *The performance of activities of daily living.* Int J Aging Hum Dev 7:343, 1976.

9. WILLIAMS, MG: *Independent living and older people.* Rehabilitation 47:69, 1981.

10. KATZ, S AND AKPOM, CA: *Index of ADL.* Med Care 5 (Suppl) 14:116, 1976.

11. PEDRETTI, LW: *Occupational therapy practice skills for physical dysfunction.* CV Mosby, St Louis, 1981.

12. GROVER, PL: *Rehabilitation status index project: Executive summary.* The Fox Chase Cancer Center, Philadelphia, 1982.

13. JETTE, A: *Functional status index: Reliability of a chronic disease evaluation instrument.* Arch Phys Med Rehabil 61:395, 1961.

14. IVERSON, IA, ET AL: *The revised Kenny self-care evaluation.* Sr. Kenny Institute, Minneapolis, 1973.

15. TROMBLY, CA AND SCOTT, AD: *Occupational therapy for physical dysfunction.* Williams & Wilkins, Baltimore, 1977.

16. CODERY, JC: *Joint protection: A responsibility of the occupational therapist.* Am J Occup Ther 19:285, 1965.

17. MELVIN, JL: *Rheumatic disease: Occupational therapy and rehabilitation.* FA Davis, Philadelphia, 1977.

BIBLIOGRAPHY

AMERICAN HEART ASSOCIATION: *Up and Around.* Pamphlet.

ANIANSSON, A, RUNDGREN, A, AND SPERLING, L: *Evaluation of functional capacity in activities of daily living in 70-year-old men and women.* Scand J Rehabil Med 12:145, 1980.

BERG, WE, ATLAS, L, ZEIGER, J: *Integrated homemaking services for the aged in urban neighborhoods.* Gerontologist 14 (5 pt. 1):388, 1974.

BERRINGTON-JONES, N: *Activities for the elderly.* R Soc Health J 95:96, 1975.

CLARKE, M AND WAKEFIELD, LM: *Food choices of institutionalized vs. independent-living elderly.* J Am Diet Assoc 66:600, 1975.

Cleo Living Aids Catalogue. 3957 Mayfield Road, Cleveland, OH, 44121.

Drive-Master Corporation Catalog. 16 Andrews Drive, West Paterson, NJ 07424.

Fashion-Able Catalog. Rocky Hill, NJ 08553.

Be OK Self-Help Aids Catalog. Fred Sammons, Inc., Box 32, Brookfield, IL 60513.

Functionally Designed Clothing and Aids Catalog. Vocational Guidance and Rehabilitation Services. 2239 East 55th Street, Cleveland, OH 44103.

GRAUER, H AND BIRNBOM, FA: *Geriatric functional rating scale to determine the need for institutional care.* J Am Geriatr Soc 23:472, 1975.

How to keep the elderly at home. Mod Health Care 3(4):29, 1975.

JA Preston Corporation Catalog. 71 Fifth Avenue, New York, NY 10003.

KAUFERT, JM, ET AL: *Assessing functional status among elderly patients: A comparison of questionnaire and service provider ratings.* Med Care 17:807, 1979.

KLINGER, JL: *Mealtime manual for people with disabilities and aging.* Campbell Soup Co., Camden, NJ, 1978.

LAMB, HR: *An educational model for teaching living skills to long-term patients.* Hosp Community Psychiatry 27:875, 1976.

LECHT, S (ED): *Orthotics etcetera.* Waverly Press, 1966.

LOWMAN, E AND KLINGER, J: *Aids to independent living.* McGraw-Hill, New York, 1969.

Maddak, Inc., Catalog. Pequannock, NJ 07440.

MAGID, S AND HEARN, CR: *Characteristics of geriatric patients as related to nursing needs.* Int J Nurs Stud 18(2):97, 1981.

Malick, MH and Sherry, B: *Life work tasks.* In Hopkins, HL and Smith, HD (eds): *Willard and Spackman's Occupational Therapy,* ed 5. JB Lippincott, Philadelphia, 1978.

Manning, AM and Means, JG: *A self-feeding program for geriatric patients in a skilled nursing facility.* J Am Diet Assoc 66:275, 1975.

Nagi, S: *An epidemiology of adult disability in the United States.* Ohio State University, Columbus, OH 1975.

Neubauer, H, et al: *Assessing functional health and sociability of aged persons: The development and validation of two Guttman scales* (abstr). Aktule Gerontol 9:91, 1979.

North, AJ and Ulatowska, HK: *Competence in independently living older adults: Assessment and correlates.* J Gerontol (Suppl) 36:576, 1981.

Pierce, CH: *Recreation for th elderly: Activity participation at a senior citizen center.* Gerontologist 15:202, 1975.

Rehab Aids Catalog. Box 612, Tamiami Station, Miami, FL 33144.

Salter, CL and Salter, CA: *Effects of an individualized activity program on elderly patients.* Gerontologist 15 (5 pt. 1):404, 1975.

Schlettwein-Gsell, D, et al: *Guttman scales for impairment due to old age in average daily activity* (abstr.) Aktule Gerontol 9:87, 1979.

Sidney, KH and Shephard, RJ: *Activity patterns of elderly men and women.* J Gerontol 32:25, 1977.

Smith, CE, et al: *Differences in importance ratings of self-care geriatric patients and the nurses who care for them.* Int J Nurs Stud 17(3):145, 1980.

Staff, PH: *ADL-assessment.* Scand J Rehabil Med (Suppl) 7:153, 1980.

Stafford, JL and Bringle, RG: *The influence of task success on elderly women's interest in new activities.* Gerontologist 20:642, 1980.

Sullivan, DF: *Disability components for an index of health.* US Department of Health, Education and Welfare, Rockville, MD 1971.

CHAPTER 4

COMMUNICATION AND THE ELDERLY

SHELLEY PILBERG, M.A., C.C.C./S.P.
KATHLEEN HOSTY, M.S., C.C.C./S.P.

BEHAVIORAL OBJECTIVES

Upon completion of this chapter, the reader will be able to
1. Identify the effects of "normal" aging on the communicative process.
2. Recognize when to refer an aged individual to a speech-language pathologist or to an audiologist because of communication problems.
3. Analyze an elderly patient's communication abilities.
4. Communicate more effectively with the elderly population.
5. Recognize how communicative changes in the elderly affect their lives and the lives of their families.
6. Classify various disease processes that influence communication which are prevalent among the elderly.

Communication is one of the most critical human needs because it is the primary means by which people interact with their world and relate to each other. Although the ability to communicate efficiently diminishes in old age, the need to communicate remains unchanged.

Communication difficulties caused by aging are frustrating and often puzzling, both for the affected older person and for those with whom the person interacts. In part this is because age-related communication changes and disorders happen slowly over an extended period of time. They may go unnoticed and untreated until unusual behavioral responses call direct attention to the difficulty. Initially, communication problems can occur inconsistently and may develop into annoying or difficult behaviors in some instances long before the existence of the underlying communication-based dysfunction is diagnosed. The time of onset of communication problems varies widely. Some individuals begin to experience difficulties in late middle age (65), and others have no problems until late old age (75). The types and degrees of communication difficulties vary with each individual. Most people experience some communication difficulties as they approach old age.

This chapter discusses the problems that the elderly face in communication breakdowns caused by normal aging and age-related diseases. The components of normal communication, the effects of age on this mechanism, pathologic age-related communication disorders, and their effects on human interaction are addressed. The elements of communication that are investigated include speech, language, and hearing. Management considerations and specific strategies for improving communication with the elderly for the non-speech-language pathologist are described.

COMPONENTS OF COMMUNICATION

Communication is an interactive process, a dynamic coding of human experience into language for use both internally and externally.[1] Language is used internally when we talk to ourselves while executing a task or when thinking through a problem. Externally, language is used when we communicate with others.

Through the speech, language, and hearing process people organize perceptions, plan, recall, share feelings, control events, learn, code new information into memory, and utilize that information. With old age, these communication functions often become less efficient or impaired. This section describes the complex process of normal communication and the breakdowns that occur in this process as a result of aging.

It is important to remember throughout this discussion that communication behavior is intimately related to a person's individuality.[2] Communication style and the aging process are dependent upon a variety of factors, including health, personality, income, education, and culture.[3] Therefore, as a person grows old, his or her communication process is affected in an idiosyncratic way.

Speech, language, hearing, reading, and writing are the chief components of communication. These are the primary modes through which ideas, feelings, and information are transmitted, received, and understood.

Speech

Speech is a complex motor process involving the rapid coordination of the lungs, larynx, palate, tongue, teeth, and lips which results in a recognizable stream of phonemes (the smallest unit of speech sounds) which form words in a given language. Intact oral, respiratory, pharyngeal, and laryngeal structures, as well as unimpaired sensory-motor systems, are essential for normal speech. These processes are coordinated both centrally and peripherally. Examples of central and peripheral disorders, respectively, are verbal apraxia (a motor planning disorder which involves speech difficulty although the speech mechanism itself functions normally for nonspeech functions such as coughing, chewing) and dysarthria (general muscle weakness or lack of coordination of the external speech organs which interferes with speech). Both of these disorders are discussed in detail later in the chapter.

Speech production relies on the function and coordination of several physiologic systems: respiration (for the airstream), phonation (for voice), resonance (for quality and intelligibility), and articulation (for specific sound formation).

RESPIRATION

Speech is produced on expired air. In order to sustain phonation, the respiratory capacity of the lungs must be sufficient. In the aged, even this initial phase of the speech process can be impaired. Reduced vital capacity of the lungs contributes to a slower speech rate owing to frequent pauses for breath.[4] During periods of physical exertion older people will have a greater difficulty talking. In addition, owing to the normal deterioration of the muscles involved in respiration, older people have greater difficulty controlling expiration, which results in a tremulous, or shaky, voice.[5] The shaky voice one often hears in older people reflects an aging breathing mechanism. This is not a sign of respiratory difficulty but of reduced control of the airstream.

PHONATION

During the process of phonation, the airstream generated by the lungs vibrates the vocal cords of the larynx, which creates sound. In the aging person, normal stiffening of the vocal cords results in pitch changes. In the male, the vocal pitch tends to get higher after the age of fifty.[6] The female voice may remain the same or may drop in pitch and become slightly deeper.[7] It is believed that reduced production of sex hormones for both males and females results in these voice changes.[4] In general, the male voice becomes more feminine and the female voice becomes more masculine as the result of normal aging.

Older people often suffer from chronic hoarseness, which may be the result of the normal stiffening vocal cord joints accompanying old age.[4] Mucous secretions in the trachea and larynx, which increase with age, contribute to frequent throat clearing and hoarseness. Refer individuals with hoarseness to a specialist for differential diagnosis, because hoarseness is also a symptom of laryngeal carcinoma.

It is important to keep in mind that the vocal tone of an aged person's voice is not necessarily reflective of a person's personality but may reflect the aging process. Voices are an important part of the total pattern of self-concept and communication.[8] In voice alone, people differentiate maleness or femaleness and identify happiness or sadness, patience or irritability. Voice quality and loudness communicate much to the listener.

Another vocal change that occurs with aging is use of a louder voice. It is unclear why this occurs, but it is not necessarily indicative of a hearing loss.[7] This is an aspect of aging that is fairly easy to manage by periodically reminding a loud speaker to use a softer voice.

RESONANCE

Resonance, which refers to the quality of the voice and includes aspects of nasality and denasality, is usually not affected significantly by normal aging. This is because the nasopharynx and soft palate remain relatively unchanged in old age.

ARTICULATION

Articulation is the final step in speaking. The articulators (tongue, teeth, lips, and jaws) compress the airstream with a variety of small adjustments to form the speech sounds of language. Articulation affects the intelligibility of speech. Normally articulatory adjustments are accomplished in rapid succession with little conscious effort. Changes in articulation which occur with old age include reduction in the speaking rate caused by reduced speed of the articulators. Also a slight slurring of speech may occur, owing to imprecise articulation. This can be compounded by missing teeth or ill-fitting dentures. The mouth changes with old age, and dentures that once fit well may no longer be comfortable. After stroke, for example, a dental consultation to assure proper denture fit is appropriate. Properly aligned teeth and dentures are necessary for precise articulation and in some cases can significantly assist a person with intelligibility difficulty in compensating for the problem.

A listener who pretends to understand someone's speech gives the speaker a false sense of communicative competence. A request for a repetition is a more productive option for both parties than a false indication of understanding. Expressing interest in what a person is trying to communicate and willingness to make the necessary effort to find out what he or she is trying to say demonstrates care about that person. When a person develops articulation problems and is not intelligible, referral to a speech-language pathologist is advised.

Language

Language is a system of symbols that, when expressed and understood, transmits thoughts, desires, ideas, emotions, and information.[2] For descriptive purposes, it is useful to divide language into receptive and expressive processes. Reception refers to understanding what is heard or seen; expression refers to what is said or written.

RECEPTIVE LANGUAGE

The process of reception is dependent upon intact and unimpaired sensory channels, that is, vision for written material, and hearing for verbal material. As people approach old age, these systems can deteriorate, resulting in hearing loss and subtle language problems.[9]

In order to comprehend, or to obtain meaning from, sound, it is first necessary to distinguish spoken language from other sounds in the environment. One must recognize the speech signal and tune out irrelevant environmental noise. The auditory system is most capable in its ability to tune in and out simultaneous and competing sound stimuli. The cocktail party phenomenon is a good example of the remarkable sophistication of this system. Cocktail party conversation requires a listener to receive and to process several conversations simultaneously and to tune in and out depending on interests.

Another important element in language comprehension is memory. Immediate sensory memory holds an auditory image until it is processed in short-term memory, where meaning is attached. It is then later cataloged into storage in long-term memory for future use. Memory is employed to hold the beginning of a speech message while listening to the remainder. Older people do not appear to have significant problems with this particular area; however, all receptive processes appear to slow down and lose accuracy with age.[7]

Other components of language reception include understanding of vocabulary, grammar, syntax, and sentences. These comprehension factors are not significantly affected during normal aging, except that the process may be slightly slower than it once was. Hearing changes caused by phonemic regression frequently cause a major portion of the language comprehension problems experienced by the aged. This type of comprehension problem is fully addressed in a later section.

One method of detecting language comprehension deficiencies is by giving verbal directions without providing nonverbal cues. For example, say, "Please put the green cup next to the television, and then close the door." Then observe the listener's response. By giving a few directions and varying the length and complexity of the commands and avoiding contextual cues by glance, facial expression, or gesture, it is possible to obtain a gross measure of a person's auditory memory capability and comprehension ability.

When a person exhibits mild comprehension problems, understanding can be improved by using some simple techniques. One can use shorter sentences and speak at a slightly slower rate. By providing additional processing time, comprehension can be facilitated greatly. Studies have demonstrated that the elderly population's listening behaviors—in terms of time it takes auditory signals to reach the brain—closely correlate with those of kindergarten and early elementary school children's performance on similar listening measures.[10] Thus, when communicating with those elderly people who are having difficulty with comprehension, it would be of benefit to use less complicated language, shorter phrases, and a slower rate of presentation. Bear in mind, however, that this suggestion refers to the rate of presentation, not to the content or level of the message. Facial expressions and gestures are also good comprehension amplifiers. Therefore, while speaking, be sure that your face is visible and at the eye level of the individual to whom you are speaking.

EXPRESSIVE LANGUAGE

The other major component of language is expression, which begins with an idea and its translation into appropriate vocabulary, grammar, and syntax. With aging, the time taken for language formulation increases; therefore, there may be some delay between a request and a reply. Word finding can also be a problem for older people. They may not be able to retrieve from their memory storage the exact word needed to communicate a particular idea. They may use a word that is inexact or related. For example, "I saw a specialist, ... Dr. ... you know ... well, the doctor ... for my back." It is not useful to routinely complete the speaker's sentences. If the elderly person does not respond immediately, it may be due to an increased need in processing time. All that may be required is for the listener to wait. A useful approach is to provide adequate response time and then, perhaps, to suggest the word they might be looking for; for example, "Did you see Dr. Hite?"

Language expression involves the formulation and sequencing of sentences to suit the meaning to be communicated. Sentences are then simultaneously monitored, as they are spoken, for their adequacy in terms of word choice (vocabulary), meaning (semantics), pronunciation (articulation), grammar, and syntax. Under normal circumstances this occurs automatically and with little awareness of the process. Internal self-monitoring of speech assures that the message is appropriate and free of errors. When an error is recognized, it is automatically modified and corrected. For example, the speaker inserts a phrase such as "I meant to say" or pronounces correctly a word formerly mispronounced. These monitoring skills can become less efficient with age, resulting in a variety of subtle language difficulties, such as maintaining the topic, observing social conventions of turn taking, and interrupting in conversation.

When speaking to an individual who is having difficulty maintaining a topic or finding words, assistance may be provided by suggesting, "Did you mean ...?" Cues to establish the general topic, a visual description or category can be helpful. If used in a conversational manner, these cues are nonthreatening and can often trigger the desired response. When a person goes off a topic inappropriately, one might suggest, "Weren't we just talking about .... I had something else to say about that."

Hearing and Aging

Hearing is the primary way in which we receive spoken information. Sound waves collect in the outer ear. They are then conducted by vibration of and through the tiny bones of the middle ear to the inner ear. These vibrations cause the fluid of the inner ear to vibrate in a highly systematic manner, stimulating the cochlea, where the auditory nerve is housed. It is in the inner ear that the auditory signal is converted from mechanical to electric energy.

Some degree of hearing loss is experienced by 40 percent to 60 percent of individuals 65 years of age or older.[7] Presbycusis is both the most common communication problem in old age and the most common auditory disorder in the population.[11] Presbycusis involves reduced sensitivity to high-pitched sounds—sh, s, t, ch, v, f—although lower and some middle pitches are relatively unaffected.[11] This deterioration occurs across races, most cultures, and both sexes during aging.[11] Aging appears to be the only cause of this type of hearing loss.

Four of the important observations about the incidence of presbycusis are (1) hearing sensitivity for pure tones decreases, (2) hearing loss is similar bilaterally, (3) the loss is most prominent in high frequencies, and (4) it is typically more severe in men than in women.[11] Probably the most vexing disability and handicapping aspect of presbycusis, however, is the auditory distortion experienced by the person. This hearing loss is not simply a diminution in auditory sensitivity but confusion and jumbling of the auditory signal. The person's classic complaint is, "I can hear, but I don't understand." The family's classic lament is, "He hears when he wants to!" This "discrimination deficit" results from the pure tone configuration of the loss, wherein the high frequencies are affected more severely than mid or low frequencies. Very often, however, the problem is not peripherally based in the end organ of hearing—the cochlea—but is caused by generalized deterioration in the central auditory pathways in the brain owing to aging. In these very common cases, the person cannot understand speech regardless of how loud the signal is.

This common characteristic of hearing loss in the aged has been called phonemic regression.[12] It is the most difficult and challenging aspect of the problem and requires and deserves careful analysis and consultation by an audiologist as well as patience and understanding by communication partners. The problem is not corrected with hearing aid amplification, although hearing aid use is typically indicated for presbycusis to compensate for the peripheral sensitivity loss.

Clearly, audiologic consultation and auditory training and rehabilitation are important services for these people. This is a frustrating and confusing type of hearing loss. For example, when someone says, "How are you?" and the elderly person answers, "Seventy-one," the inappropriate responses can raise questions regarding mental status. It is important to remember that although the person can hear someone speaking, the person may not be able to understand exactly what has been said.

For those aged people with hearing loss, communication may become so frustrating that they lose interest in communication and become withdrawn and isolated. Feelings of anger and depression are common. It is important to remember that these behavioral characteristics of hearing loss can mimic those of confusion and must be clearly differentiated for appropriate intervention. The "confused" or "uncooperative" behaviors of the person with hearing loss also can lead others to limit their contact with the person and can cause further negative reactions.[12]

The challenge in management of hearing loss in the elderly involves many strategies. Early detection is an important first step in the treatment of the hearing impaired. All elderly persons should be routinely screened for hearing and communication problems, because the progression of hearing loss in the elderly occurs in small degrees over a long period of time. Behavioral signs of hearing loss include inattentiveness, inappropriate responses, difficulty following directions, speech that is unusually loud, habitually turning one ear to the speaker, frequent requests for repetition, irrelevant comments, and a tendency to withdraw from activities that require verbal communication.[11]

A quiet environment enhances communication with a hearing-impaired individual to some degree. Communication difficulty increases significantly whenever room noise equals or exceeds the strength of the speech signal or when a speaker talks rapidly. For a person with presbycusis, the epitome of unintelligibility is the soft-voiced speaker with a highly pitched voice who talks rapidly in background noise. Ironically, most collective environments for the elderly are noisy places (average sound levels of 65dB[13]—like a moderately loud radio) staffed primarily by females with soft high-pitched voices who are in a hurry with their patients.

Generally speaking, hearing aids do not always help those who have presbycusis. Owing to the complex nature of presbycusis, some individuals may receive only partial benefit from hearing aids.[14] The issue of hearing aids for people with presbycusis is not a simple one. The function of a hearing aid is simply to amplify sound—to make it louder. Hearing aids do this in a highly sophisticated manner, but that is all they do. They do not make sound clearer or unscramble distorted signals, and understanding is a major difficulty of the person with presbycusis. Other factors relevant to hearing aid use are the social stigma associated with hearing aids; low tolerance for extensive testing and trial; difficulty learning to adjust to amplification; inability to manipulate the small controls of the aid, particularly for those with arthritic hands and fingers.

Another important adjunctive method of treating hearing loss in the elderly is aural rehabilitation offered by a speech-language pathologist or an audiologist. In most cases persons having a hearing loss will benefit from aural rehabilitation. This method of remediation helps the person maximize residual hearing and learn to use other sensory channels, such as vision, to aid auditory comprehension. Aural rehabilitation is beneficial for persons with hearing aids or without. Speech reading (lipreading) skill can be developed with practice. Aural rehabilitation teaches people with hearing losses to pay closer attention to nonauditory language cues—body language, gestures, facial expression, contextual cues—which provide additional information about what is being said and can enhance significantly a person's understanding.[15] Since many hearing losses result in individual problems, aural rehabilitation can also provide instruction on the most effective means of communicating in particular environments.

There are a variety of means to enhance communication with the hearing-impaired person which can be accomplished by the non-speech-language pathologist or audiologist. Surroundings should be well lighted, as quiet as possible, and free from distractions. If glasses and hearing aid have been prescribed, the person should be wearing them. It would be appropriate to check the aid to make sure it is working and adjusted properly. When initiating speech, secure the attention of the listener by calling his or her name and/or by touching the person. Speak at eye level. For example, if the speaker is standing and the person with a hearing loss is in a wheelchair, the angle to view the speaker's face is not favorable for speech reading. In this case the speaker should also be seated before beginning to speak. A normal rate, tone, and volume are preferred, because shouting or overarticulating sounds distorts visual and auditory cues. If the message is not understood the first time, rephrase the message in different words. Persist in the communication to let the person experience success.

MEDICATION

There are drugs frequently prescribed for the aged that result in side effects which interfere with communication. It has been estimated that the elderly, although representing only 11 percent of the population, receive 25 percent of all prescription drugs.[16] Therefore, some communication problems that are seen in the elderly may be drug induced rather than pathologic. Drug-related communication problems can be mitigated through prescription changes. It is important to be aware of the potential problem of drug-induced communication deficiencies and to explore these with the physician. For example, digitalis may result in mental confusion, depression, and impaired communication; antihypertensive drugs can result in diminished communication by inducing depression; antipsychotic drugs can result in slurred speech and bizarre verbal output.[16] Depression caused by drugs can masquerade as dementia in older people. Differential diagnosis is critical to assure appropriate treatment because depression is often reversible, but dementia, at this time, appears irreversible.[17]

PATHOLOGIC AGE-RELATED COMMUNICATION DISORDERS

Aphasia

Aphasia is a language disorder caused by brain damage and characterized by complete or partial impairment of language comprehension, formulation, and use. Most commonly aphasia results from stroke, a sudden loss of brain function resulting from interference with the blood supply to a part of the brain. Seventy-five percent of people who suffer strokes are 65 years of age or older.[18] Tumors, brain infection, or head trauma can also cause aphasia.[18]

Aphasic symptoms differ considerably from person to person, depending upon the cause of the stroke, the amount and extent of damage suffered, and the area of the brain damaged.[19] People with more damage have a poorer prognosis for improved language function than those with less. In addition, aphasic persons with multiple medical problems—for example, heart disease, hypertension—will have a poorer prognosis for improvement than if they were in good health.[20]

There are a number of general behavioral characteristics associated with aphasia. Inconsistent ability is typical.[21] At one time the person may be capable of a certain performance but at another time incapable. Variations in ability to respond are inevitable and can be compared with normal variability in performance that affects us all. Variability can be very frustrating for the aphasic as well as for others. Other people can become frustrated with the person for withholding his or her best performance and nag to "try harder, you could do it yesterday." Treat this inconsistency in language performance with patience and support. Stress that results from frustrating interactions serves to reduce the residual efficiency of communication efforts. A relaxed atmosphere facilitates communication.

It is also important to remember that intelligence and sensibilities are generally well preserved. Although aphasic speech may resemble that of a child (for example, restricted vocabulary, impaired grammar, poor articulation), these people are very much the people they were premorbidly. The aphasic patient should not be addressed as a child or treated as if he or she is not present. This is demeaning, and it can result in anger and a lack of cooperation because the patient feels that his or her true capabilities are not being accurately assessed. Even if the aphasic person is not following conversation very well, he or she is often able to comprehend the tone and intent. Except for the early stages following onset of the stroke, most aphasic patients are oriented, learn new information, resume many self-care activities, and exercise good judgment. Perseveration is also sometimes associated with aphasia and consists of the continuation of a speech act after it is no longer useful. It is an involuntary continuation of behavior.

There are several different language syndromes in aphasia described by the site of lesion. The two most common classifications are Broca's aphasia and Wernicke's aphasia. There are different language manifestations in each type.

Broca's aphasia is characterized by restricted vocabulary and grammar and intact auditory comprehension. A person with Broca's aphasia generally knows what he or she wants to communicate and demonstrates a good ability to understand what is said. However, comprehension difficulty increases as length and complexity of input increases.[19] The chief difficulty is one of verbal production. Agrammatic speech patterns consist of noun + verb constructions with few grammatical markers (such as -ed and -ing). These patients also omit small words such as *is* and *on*. A typical sentence for such a patient might be, "Phone—Ruth—

office—late," meaning, "Ruth called and said she would be late at the office to-night." This type of speech is also often described as telegraphic, because it is condensed into only those words essential to convey meaning. Agrammatic sentences are spoken at a slow rate and with some pauses between words. Broca's is a non-fluent aphasia.

Patients with Broca's aphasia and anomic aphasia commonly have difficulty saying the exact word intended. Sometimes they will describe or define the word in an attempt to recall the word desired, for example, "The thing you tell time with; a round thing, you know, with hands." These patients often describe their difficulty as one in which they know what they want to say but just cannot think of the exact word or "get it out." Needless to say, when this occurs frequently, it is very frustrating. Patients with anomic aphasia have the most favorable prognosis. Patients with Broca's aphasia often make a good recovery with treatment and become adequate functional communicators with listener assistance.[19] However, if the problem is very severe, even with treatment they may never be able to use speech easily; nevertheless, such individuals usually can respond to questions and communicate, because comprehension remains relatively unimpaired. Writing is also often affected.

Techniques that facilitate communication with these patients include being patient and giving the person ample time to respond. A listener can repeat the aphasic patient's message, which allows the aphasic person to confirm or to revise the communication. For example,

Aphasic patient: I saw my granddaughter, Sandy, yesterday.
Other: You saw your daughter?
Aphasic patient: No, my granddaughter.
Other: Oh, you saw your granddaughter, Sandy, yesterday. How nice.

This lets the asphasic patient know that his or her effort at communication was successful, which can mean a great deal to a person experiencing little success in communication. This rephrasing technique provides realistic conversational feedback about the communication in a natural manner. Ask questions requiring short answers or provide multiple choices so that the aphasic person will not have to formulate a lengthy utterance. Keep paper and pencil available so that the patient can write the response or an initial letter of a word, if he or she is unable to verbalize for the moment.

The other major type of aphasia, Wernicke's aphasia, is marked by a fluent, flowing verbal output that is low in information. For example, "I, my daughter, well, she's, I'll say it's really something, well, I like to, you know, well, I guess you understand." People with Wernicke's aphasia usually have impaired comprehension and cannot recognize or correct their own verbal errors. There is a failure in the monitoring system to identify and to correct the inadequacy of the message sent. Persons with Wernicke's aphasia who suffer from severe impairment speak almost exclusively in fluent nonsense and jargon and have difficulty even at the one-word level of comprehension. More mildly impaired Wernicke's aphasia is characterized by a profusion of speech consisting of real words and wordlike speech, but with little meaning. Verbal output may also include paraphrasic errors, such as the use of *chair* for *table* or *flable* for *table*. The language may be devoid of specific content and have an abundance of general or indefinite words, so that the listener hears speech but does not understand what is said.[19] The comprehension abilities of persons with Wernicke aphasia varies from occasional difficulty understanding lengthy, complex speech to inability to respond to simple direct questions, such as, "Do apples grow on trees?" These patients sometimes become angry when they are not understood because they do not always perceive the communication problem as their own.

There are a variety of techniques to facilitate communication with this type of aphasia. Speech can be adjusted in rate, length, and complexity to a level at which the person responds with success. Use of more familiar and concrete vocabulary is also helpful. For example, one might hold a person's arm and say "up" instead of "lift your arm." Use of gesture and facial expression will also aid comprehension. If a person does not appear to understand, rephrase the message using different words and accompany it with a demonstration. Even guiding a person through a task manually in combination with the verbal message often facilitates comprehension. Use of written directions, even a single word, can also be helpful to some aphasic patients. Consult the speech-language pathologist who is familiar with an aphasic patient's level of comprehension and the most useful facilitating techniques for workable approaches for individual patients. It is critical to know what the aphasic patient's best input level is and tailor directions and requests accordingly.

When aphasia is described as global, there is a poor prognosis for recovery because there is severe impairment of both the production and comprehension of language. The individual may be incapable of any meaningful expressive speech.

In terms of prognosis, although aphasic patients can improve their communication skills with speech-language pathology treatment, most will never regain their premorbid levels of communication. Complete recovery occurs in few aphasic patients. Global aphasia and Wernicke's aphasia have poorer prognoses than Broca's aphasia. Recovery rates are highest during the initial three months during spontaneous recovery. Significant recovery occurs as well in the next three months, slows after six months, and reaches a plateau after a year or more post onset.[19] Variables that predict better improvement are younger age, good health prior to onset of aphasia, early speech and language therapy intervention, less impaired auditory comprehension along with overall less severe initial symptoms.[22]

A mild impairment may involve few overt symptoms, yet the aphasic person may feel a restricted verbal output, compared with the previous level of functioning, and could benefit from speech-language pathology treatment. Persons with moderately involved aphasia can make significant changes in their communication skills with treatment.[19] Severely impaired aphasic patients can benefit from speech-language treatment and/or augmented communication aids, such as language boards and gesture systems, even if the verbal system cannot be restored to a functional degree.

Dysarthria

Dysarthria describes a collection of motor speech disorders caused by damage in the central or peripheral nervous system. Dysarthria can be a symptom of neurologic disorders such as Parkinsonism, multiple sclerosis, amyotrophic lateral sclerosis, and Bulbar palsy or can result from stroke, tumor, or head trauma. Although young people may suffer from dysarthria, it is more common among older people.

Symptoms may involve respiration, phonation (voice), resonation, articulation, and prosody (the melody of speech).[23] Each dysarthric person's speech will be different, depending upon the speech system/systems affected and the severity of the disorder. The symptoms of dysarthria can range from mild, in which speech is intelligible but sounds bizarre, to speech that is completely unintelligible. Specific systems and symptoms are discussed below.

When the system of respiration is affected, the person's speech can be rushed or choppy because of attempts to fit the intended message into the available breath. In addition, sufficient loudness is often a problem and patients may tire from speaking for any length of time. In treatment, posturing exercises to build subglottal air pressure and visual monitoring of air pressure on an oscilloscope are a few techniques employed to improve the respiration component of speech.

If a dysarthric person's voice is affected, the phonation system is involved. Several types of vocal symptoms may emerge: The voice may be deep and gravelly, the pitch may be difficult to control, or the voice may sound strangled and harsh. Restricted elasticity of the vocal cords can lead to monotonous-sounding pitch. Breathy speech and hoarse voice may also occur.

Insufficient loudness and vocal fatigue are difficulties related to phonatory disorders also. Exercises to increase phonation time and to improve quality are successful with many dysarthric patients.

Resonance difficulties are frequently affected by a degree of hypernasality. Nasality is the sound of talking through one's nose. In dysarthria, because of a weakness of the soft palate, hypernasality is the resonance disorder that typically occurs. In the disorder, sounds that are usually emitted through the mouth pass through the nasopharynx because of weak palatal musculature or structural insufficiency. This can result in insufficient build-up of air pressure to produce some of the consonant sounds, especially b, p, s, sh, ch, and z. These speech sounds will emerge as a burst of air through the nose and sound like a nasal snort. The result will be a dramatic reduction of intelligibility. This symptom can often be ameliorated in some individuals by a palatal lift prosthesis which improves the closure of the nasopharynx.

Articulation—which involves the precise, coordinated movement of tongue, teeth, lips, and jaw to form specific speech sounds in rapid sequence—can also be affected by dysarthria, resulting in a reduction of the clarity of speech. Speech sounds may be produced in a slurred manner. Or one speech sound may be substituted for another, for example, "tupper" for "supper." There also may be speech sound omissions, for example, "top" for "stop." When the listener becomes familiar with the pattern of errors, which are generally consistent in dysarthria, it is easier to understand the speaker. The goal of treatment is to maximize compensated intelligibility and communication efficiency. Correct production of phonemes as well as normalizing prosody are main considerations at the level of articulation. Improvement can be made by establishing an optimum rate/intelligibility relationship; by use of pacing boards; use of limited vocabulary; and, in severe cases, training of the communication partner.

Clinically, six main types of dysarthria have been identified: flaccid, spastic, mixed, ataxic, hypokinetic, and hyperkinetic.[23] These can be associated with areas of neurologic site, speech symptom clusters, and disease types. For example, hypokinetic dysarthria occurs when there is damage to the extrapyramidal tract. It is characterized by slowness, limited range of motion of the articulators, and limited muscle force. Parkinsonism is typical of this type. The speech of Parkinsonism is characterized by monopitch, monoloudness, reduced stress, imprecise consonants, inappropriate silences, short rushes of speech, and a harsh breathy voice.[23]

In speech-language pathology treatment, the dysarthric patient learns to do purposefully what was once accomplished automatically in speech. The specific treatment depends upon the system or systems involved in the disorder. For example, a person with weak vocal cords can strengthen the voice by pushing while voicing. People with nasality can learn to discriminate a nasal voice from a denasal voice and to make certain articulatory compensations to produce less nasal consonants. When the articulation system is involved, tongue, lip, and jaw exercises that involve specific placement strategies and overarticulation techniques improve intelligibility. In addition, stress is placed on identifying errors and manipulating the rate of speech for maximal intelligibility. When dysarthric persons speak slowly and in syllables, their speech usually becomes more intelligible; when intelligibility is maintained, rate is increased to normalize speech.

The physical mechanism in conjunction with the ear and feedback system automatically compensates for many physical and functional differences. There is a great deal of compensation in dysarthric speech, some adaptive and some less so. Speech-language pathology treatment involves maximizing these positive adaptive compensations. Prognosis for improved intelligibility is often good, depending on the degree and type of impairment.

When the dysarthria is a symptom of a progressive neurologic disease, treatment is adjusted to the course of the disease. The progression of amyotrophic lateral sclerosis does not lend itself to a good prognosis because the disease is progressive. However, some speech conservation techniques can assist the maintenance of a functional communication level for a longer period of time and can prepare for an alternative system, such as gesture language or eye blinks. These dysarthric patients can also learn to maximize breath and to minimize unneces-

PHYSICAL ASPECTS OF AGING

sary wording to convey only the most important elements of a message. Use of the word "toilet" is more efficient than "I would like to go to the bathroom." Dysarthric persons who need to learn conservation measures can also be taught phrasing to ensure maximum intelligibility. It is important that compensatory techniques be developed as early as possible during the progression of these neurologic diseases.[23]

The person speaking in a slurred unintelligible manner can feel very self-conscious about his or her speech. This person is not only highly frustrated by not being understood but can be embarrassed about the way he or she sounds, for dysarthric speech can sound like drugged or drunken speech. These feelings are factors in whether or not the person is willing to talk and to whom he or she will talk.

In general, the remedial programs for the dysarthric person can be assisted by others. Most dysarthric people need to be encouraged to slow their rate of speech, to use a syllable-by-syllable approach to words, and to exaggerate consonants. With respect to phonation, cues can be provided regarding the adequacy of volume. Dysarthric patients should be encouraged to speak in phrase lengths that are compatible with meaning and breath support. Staff can be most supportive by providing honest feedback regarding the intelligibility of the speech. If dysarthria is accompanied by aphasia, the impaired language system of the patient must also be considered while conversing with the individual.

Apraxia

Apraxia is a motor planning disorder of articulation and prosody owing to brain damage. It is characterized by impaired capacity to program the position of speech musculature and the sequence of respiration, phonation, and articulation for the volitional production of phonemes. The usual cause of apraxia is cerebrovascular accident and other neurologic disorders and diseases such as brain tumor and head injury. Apraxia can range from a mild problem that sounds like slight, inconsistent articulation difficulty to severe difficulty that consists of a few effortful, misarticulated utterances produced after lengthy struggle. The experience of recovered apraxic persons who are able to verbalize about the disorder indicate that it is like not being able to remember how to begin to move any part of the speech mechanism to produce a particular word or speech sound. The disorder is exacerbated by stress and by increased length of words and message.

Speech-language treatment might take several forms. The goal of treatment is to help the apraxic person regain voluntary accurate control over the speech mechanism and to produce intelligible speech sounds and words.[45] A well-described treatment program is Rosenbek's light step task continuum, consisting of a hierarchy of auditory-visual stimulation and imitation.[21] Treatment may vary from articulation training of the placement and movement of the speech mechanism to using melody and gesture to aid in word production. In general, prognosis for improvement of apraxia mirrors that of prognosis for aphasia, which often accompanies apraxia.[19] When usual treatment methods do not result in improved speaking, it is possible for a speech-language pathologist to teach the apraxic person to benefit from augmented means of communication, such as gesture language or a communication board/book.

When one is talking to an apraxic individual, it is important to have time and patience. If the disorder is moderate to severe, the person will be slow to verbalize and the difficulty will increase under pressure or stress. One can structure questions so that the answers required are "yes" and "no" or just one word in length. Speech can sometimes be started by using automatic responses and carrier phrases ("I want a _____"). If there is an overlay of aphasia, one will also have to structure conversation with consideration of other language problems. Although apraxia can lead to markedly diminished verbal output, it does not affect comprehension.

Apraxia can be confusing to the listener at times, because of the inconsistency of the speech difficulty. Sometimes the apraxic person speaks with islands of fluent speech. For example, many can respond to overused social exchanges adequately. Even some of the most severely impaired have stereotyped expressions available to them; often they can curse fluently and participate in social niceties. However, when this conversational level becomes more purposeful and less automatic, their real difficulty in production emerges. In general, apraxic speech is marked by equal and excessive stress and effortful, groping, repetitive attempts to produce a sound correctly.

Right Hemisphere Communication Syndrome

Aphasia occurs when the brain damage is in the dominant hemisphere of the brain, usually the left. When the damage occurs in the right hemisphere, the nondominant side of the brain, a different set of communication behaviors, described as right hemisphere communication syndrome, emerge. A person with right hemisphere communication disorder has difficulty organizing information in an efficient, meaningful manner. These persons have difficulty distinguishing between what is important and what is not; they have problems in assimilating and using contextual cues; there is a tendency to overpersonalize external events; and literal interpretation is given to figurative language. There is generally a reduced sensitivity to what is expected in a particular communication situation. The right hemisphere disordered person often is not aware of extralinguistic features, such as body language, affect, gesture, and tone of voice, which are significant factors in communication.[24]

These types of communication deficits are often overlooked by an untrained observer, but they are generally evident to the family of the person or to those interacting with the person on a regular basis. When asked questions, they respond conversationally but with related tangential information. They address the question but do not answer it. They have real difficulty organizing information when asked an open question. The following is an example of an exchange between a therapist and a person with right hemisphere communication syndrome.

> Question: What do you see as your most major problem since your stroke? What bothers you?
>
> Response: Major ones? I—new difficulty for me.... I did many things.... I doctor switched me from a blood thinner, anticoagulant. I was taking aspirin—two aspirin once a day. Our little secrets. I had difficulty walking. I played golf. First, last January, I played golf . . . was painful. My friend was a doctor. Pediatrician. He said—we know him many, many, many years. Went to high school together. I hate to tell you how many years, hum?[24]

In order to help a person with this type of language difficulty it is useful to structure less open-ended questions and to cue to the relevant details. For example, rather than ask, "Tell me one thing that bothers you since your stroke," it would be better to ask, "Does your speech bother you?" Provide the patient with direct answers and meaningful feedback, especially if the patient does not answer your questions. Provide structured rather than unstructured activities. Keep distracting stimuli to a minimum; the person has enough internal stimuli to inhibit. It is important to make optimum use of the person's residual functions. For example, a person may be able to verbalize a strategy prior to accomplishing a task or to talk through the sequence of a task, which will enable him or her to carry it out.

It is critical to be aware that the person may not be able to understand complex instructions. Without talking down to the person, provide repetitions as needed. The person may have difficulty understanding implied or intended meaning and may be less sensitive to the overall context of the message. Often these people have diminished emotional affect, both receptively and expressively, and this can reduce their social competence.[24] Because those who are suffering from right hemisphere communication disorders tend to deny or to minimize their difficulties, it may be necessary to help them recognize their problems.

Dementia

Organic brain syndrome (OBS), or dementia, is another disease of the aging brain having a language component. This is a devastating, irreversible disease caused by diffuse central nervous system deterioration. Onset is slow and insidious. It is a disorder of ideation affecting memory, intellect, and communication. Organic brain syndrome affects 15 percent of Americans 65 years of age or older; another 11 percent have a mild involvement.[25] There are several types of dementia which result from disorders such as Parkinsonism, Huntington's chorea, Pick's disease, multi-infarct dementia, and Korsakoff syndrome.

Language impairment is a significant component of dementia.[26] Language characteristics include preserved articulation and syntax, with a deterioration of semantic function. Conversational ability is maintained until the later stages. Speech is verbally fluent, but content erodes gradually and clichés and use of concrete language pervades.[26] There is a reduction in all aspects of language capability, a loss of ability to think, and a decrease in verbal and performance intelligence. These people do not, as a rule, express frustration over their inability to communicate, as do aphasic persons. They may attempt to conceal deficiencies by repeating what has already been said, blaming others for misunderstandings, and dismissing a task as trivial. Memory problems are universal, and there is difficulty forming new memories. Disorientation increases along with reduced awareness of others. The degree of language impairment is proportional to the level of mental function, but articulation and intelligibility are generally spared in classic dementias of the Alzheimer's type. There is poor articulation and reduced intelligibility (dysarthria) in secondary dementias, such as those types accompanying Parkinsonism or Huntington's disease.[25] Language is a particularly sensitive predictor of mortality in dementia, more so than the degree of cerebral atrophy as apparent on a computerized axial tomography (CAT) scan.[26]

In the advanced stages of dementia, language may consist only of nonsensical utterances; some people become mute, and others may produce jargon. These people attempt to repeat word sequences they have not understood but for which they have retained a sensory image. They are generally unable to generate a sequence of meaningfully related utterances. They no longer recognize family and friends or form new durable memories.[26]

In terms of management in the later phases, it would be helpful for family to know that although a demented person talks, this person does not understand most that is not cliché. Long anecdotes and lengthy discourse are impossible for the person to follow; word retrieval may be a problem; many words no longer have their accepted meanings. Therefore, eliminate the use of long complex sentences; be concrete, direct, and brief in exchanges with demented people. Avoid long discourse; give multimodal input, such as a combination of visual-auditory-kinesthetic stimuli. Avoid open-ended questions and instead give choices.[25] For example, avoid "What do you want for breakfast?" Instead, use "Do you want eggs or cereal for breakfast?" The person is more likely to handle this successfully and it is also more likely to be productive for the listener. Indirect daily orientation sessions and memory aids (name bracelets, reminder signs, calendars, clocks) might improve the person's daily functioning. As the dementia progresses, the overall prognosis for improving language function is poor and aimed more toward functional management. There is no doubt that these are among the most difficult people with whom to communicate.

Laryngectomy

There are approximately 9000 laryngectomies annually; the average age of a person having a laryngectomy is 62.[27] A laryngectomy is the surgical removal of the larynx owing to cancer. After a laryngectomy, the individual has no voice with which to communicate; the person even laughs and cries silently. Persons with laryngectomies can communicate by gesture, by mouthing words, by using exaggerated facial expressions, or by writing; but with the help of a professional they can also be taught the use of speech again. This can be accomplished through the use of an artificial larynx, a portable device that is placed on the neck or inside the mouth to provide a source of sound, which is then modified in the normal manner by the articulators. The artificial larynx produces a mechanical-sounding voice which is reasonably intelligible when used correctly. The artificial larynx is relatively simple to learn to use and when introduced provides an immediate means of communication for some laryngectomees. Esophageal speech is another technique for developing voice, but it is far more difficult to learn. With esophageal speech air is swallowed into the esophagus and emitted in a controlled belch which can be shaped into intelligible speech. About half of the elderly people with laryngectomies develop adequate, dependable esophageal speech for oral communication.[20] There are also surgically implanted prostheses, such as the Blom-Singer artificial larynx, which serve as sound sources and which require minimal instruction for successful use.

There are some special rehabilitation considerations for the persons with laryngectomies. They may feel both mutilated by the operation and frightened by the cancer and therefore need additional emotional support. Health professionals working with these people can become an extremely valuable resource and support system. Another difficulty that can compound communicating with a laryngectomy patient is hearing loss, for esophageal speech is more difficult to hear than normal voice. A female laryngectomy patient has to adjust to the use of a more "male" voice.

When communicating with a laryngectomy patient, one should not be afraid to ask for repetitions if the message is not understood. Sometimes esophageal speech is difficult for a listener to get accustomed to. Try not to be discouraged, because these patients can be quite intelligible when given the opportunity. Comprehension by these persons is not impaired in any manner. It is easiest to listen to a laryngectomy patient in a quiet environment. The use of facial expression, gesture, and context will aid understanding.

If a patient uses writing or gesture as the chief means of communication, referral to a speech-language pathologist provides an opportunity to learn more natural methods of communicating. In treatment, an artificial larynx, esophageal speech, or a Blom-Singer type of prosthesis will be explored. Prognosis for use of some alternative voice system is excellent.

Chronic Obstructive Pulmonary Disorder

The incidence of chronic obstructive pulmonary disorder (COPD) increases in aging individuals.[5] These people are likely to have voice problems, including restricted loudness and pitch range. Chronic hoarseness, easy tiring, and inability to talk and to walk simultaneously are common complaints. Treatment procedures incorporate diaphragmatic breathing and pacing strategies during speech. A common goal for people with COPD is the use of fewer syllables per breath. When involved in physical activities and therapies requiring exercise, it is important to remember the person's limited speech capability, especially during physical exertion. Staff can reinforce the idea of short utterances. Phrases like "slow down and take your time" are appropriate with this type of disorder.

SUMMARY OF STRATEGIES FOR IMPROVING COMMUNICATION

Normal Aging Person

1. Do not pretend to understand what is said. This only gives a false sense of communicative competence.
2. Request a repetition if message is not understood.
3. If a person is speaking too loudly, tell the person that you can hear at a lower loudness level.
4. Communication is easiest in a quiet environment.
5. When an older person exhibits some comprehension difficulty, use shorter sentences and a slower rate of speech.
6. Give the person plenty of time to respond.
7. If there are word-finding difficulties, give the person time to think of the word, then politely suggest a possibility. Also, one could provide the category or topic to help cue the person to the word.
8. If the person goes off on a tangent while speaking, bring the person back to the topic at hand.

Hearing Loss

1. Early detection can be accomplished through routine annual screenings.
2. Communicate in a quiet, well-lighted environment free of distraction.

3. Secure the person's attention by calling the person's name, touching the person, or making eye contact prior to speaking.
4. Speak at eye level to facilitate speech reading.
5. Speak in a moderately loud voice, in a normal rate and tone.
6. Rephrase what was said if it is not understood the first time.
7. Introduce conversation and topic transitions with an orienting topic statement to cue listener to what will be discussed.
8. Check hearing-aid batteries regularly.
9. Person should wear glasses, if prescribed, for communication.
10. Persist in communication, and let the person experience success.

Aphasia

1. Give the person time to respond.
2. Let the person know that you have understood the message by repeating it back conversationally.
3. Use concrete, familiar vocabulary in short, clear sentences.
4. Use gesture and facial expression to augment what is said.
5. Phrase questions for short responses, multiple choice, or yes or no responses.
6. Rephrase a message if not understood initially.
7. Provide written and visual cues.
8. Be familiar with the person's level of comprehension and adjust rate, length, and complexity of speech to a level at which the person can respond with success.

Dysarthria

1. Provide honest feedback about the intelligibility of the message.
2. Encourage the person to speak at a slower rate.
3. Have the person exaggerate production of consonants and syllabilize words in speech.
4. Have person use shorter utterances compatible with breath supply.
5. Give the person appropriate feedback about loudness level.
6. Communicate in a quiet, nondistracting environment.
7. Use letter cueing or language boards in severe cases.

Apraxia

1. Give the person plenty of time to respond.
2. Be patient.
3. Ask questions requiring one- or two-word responses.

    4. Reduce stress.

    5. Engage in familiar social exchanges so that the person can experience some communication success.

Right Hemisphere Communication Syndrome

1. Provide structured activities and speech opportunities.
2. Help person structure responses by giving cues with relevant details.
3. This person may not understand lengthy complex directions, so repeat and rephrase to assure understanding.
4. Be concrete and direct in language; avoid figurative language and sarcasm.
5. Provide honest feedback and help the person recognize his or her difficulties.

Dementia

1. Although these patients talk, they understand very little that is not cliché.
2. Use short, direct, concrete input.
3. Use sensory input, both visual and touch, to enhance comprehension.
4. Communication should occur in brief exchanges.
5. Avoid conflict or arguments.
6. Provide external memory aids, such as name bracelets, reminder signs, and calendars.
7. Provide orientation sessions.

Laryngectomy

1. Talk in a quiet environment.
2. Ask the person to repeat if a message is not understood.
3. Provide support and encouragement for use of the new voice.

Chronic Obstructive Pulmonary Disorder

1. Encourage short utterances compatible with breath supply.
2. Don't engage in conversation while the person is involved in physical activity.

Both normal and pathologic communication changes in the aging population have been described. The effects of speech, language, and hearing disorders on individuals as well as on the people with whom they communicate can be devastating. A hearing loss, acquired gradually over time, can confuse the aged person and irritate the family. Slurred, unintelligible speech can be frustrating for both the listener and the speaker. It can become an ordeal to share simple information or to express a need. A language disorder, such as aphasia, can significantly disrupt communication and have impact on family life in a variety of ways. It can force role changes, alter spousal relationships, and lead to isolation. Cognitive language disorders, such as those accompanying organic brain syndrome, can be difficult for families as communication capabilities erode. Fortunately, there are means to improve and to facilitate communication to some degree in all disorders. This chapter has outlined some techniques and treatment available for the person with communication disorders. Management strategies for those who interact with communicatively impaired persons have been described. Communication is a human behavior that enriches life by enabling people to exchange ideas, information, and feelings regardless of their age. To ensure efficient, effective communication for the aged it is necessary to be aware of potential difficulties and to be prompt to identify, to treat, and to remediate their communication disorders.

REFERENCES

1.   Wood, KS: *Terminology and nomenclature.* In Travis, LD (ed): *Handbook of Speech Pathology and Audiology.* Appleton-Century-Crofts, New York, 1971.

2.   Hutchinson, JS and Beasley, DS: *Speech and language functioning among the aging.* In Oyer, HO and Oyer, JE (eds): *Aging and Communication.* University Park Press, Baltimore, 1980.

3.   Saul, S: *Aging: An Album of People Growing Old.* John Wiley & Sons, New York, 1974.

4.   Luchsinger, R and Arnold, GE: *Voice-Speech-Language.* Wadsworth, Belmont, CA, 1965.

5.   Brody, H: *Neuroanatomy and neuropathology of aging.* In Busse, EW and Blazer, DG (eds): *Handbook of Geriatric Psychiatry.* Van Nostrand Reinhold, New York, 1980.

6.   Tierney, J: *The aging body.* Esquire 87:5, 1982.

7.   Ryan, WJ and Hutchinson, JM: *Conversation: The aging speaker.* ASHA Magazine 22:6, 1980.

8.   Clifford, S and Gregg, JB: *Considerations for the laryngectomized elderly patient.* Seminars in Speech, Language, and Hearing 2:3, 1981.

9.   Diggs, C: *ASHA recognizes needs of older persons.* ASHA Magazine 22:6, 1980.

10.   Kasten, RW: *The impact of aging on auditory perception.* Seminars in Speech, Language, and Hearing 2:3, 1981.

11.   Maurer, J: *Auditory impairment and aging.* In Jacobs, B (ed): *Working with the Impaired Elderly.* National Council on the Aging, Washington, DC, 1976.

12.   HELLER, B AND GAYNOR, E: *Hearing loss and aural rehabilitation of the elderly.* Clinical Nursing 3:1, 1981.

13.   *Tuning in on hearing aids.* In *FDA Consumer.* Department of Health and Human Services, 80–4024, 1981.

14.   *Communication Disorders and Aging.* ASHA, Rockville, MD.

15.   SANDERS, D: *Aural Rehabilitation: A Management Model.* Prentice-Hall, Englewood Cliffs, NJ, 1982.

16.   RONCH, JL: *Drugs/medication: Their impact on communication and the elderly's response to treatment.* Seminars in Speech, Language, and Hearing 2:3, 1981.

17.   MEYER, L: *Depression in the old.* Washington Post, November 29, 1982.

18.   GROHER, ME: *Neurologically based disorders of speech and language among older adults.* Seminars in Speech, Language, and Hearing 2:3, 1981.

19.   KERTEZ, A: *Aphasia and Associated Disorders: Taxonomy, Localization and Recovery.* Grune & Stratton, New York, 1979.

20.   ADAIR, M: *Communicative problems in older persons.* In JACOBS, B (ED): *Working with the Impaired Elderly.* National Council on the Aging, Washington, DC, 1976.

21.   ROSENBEK, J: *Treating apraxia of speech.* In JOHNS, DF (ED): *Clinical Management of Neurogenic Communication Disorders.* Little, Brown & Co, Boston, 1978.

22.   MARSHALL, R: *Prognosis in aphasia.* Short Course Presentation, ASHA Convention, Toronto, Canada, 1983.

23.   DARLEY, F, ARONSON, AE, BROWN, JR: *Motor Speech Disorders.* WB Saunders, Philadelphia, 1975.

24.   MEYER, P: Right hemisphere communication syndrome. Submitted for publication.

25.   BAYLESS, K: *Language and dementia.* Short Course Presentation, ASHA Convention, Los Angeles, 1981.

26.   BAYLESS, K AND BOONE, D: *The potential of language tasks for identification of senile dementia.* J Speech Hear Disord 47:2, 1982.

27.   HULL, RH: *Demography and characteristics of the communicatively impaired elderly in the United States.* Seminars in Speech, Language, and Hearing 2:3, 1981.

CHAPTER 5

LEISURE SKILLS

JEROME F. SINGLETON, M.T.R.S., Ph.D.

BEHAVIORAL OBJECTIVES

Upon completion of this chapter, the reader will be able to
1. Identify and explain the effect an institution has on an elderly individual.
2. Discuss the roles of work and leisure in an elderly person's life.
3. Summarize the planning process.
4. Identify and explain what should be encouraged in a recreation program.
5. Identify and explain the activity analysis process.
6. Discuss how volunteers can be used to deliver leisure services in an institution.

The elderly who reside in institutions relinquish many of their opportunities to make decisions concerning daily activities. Leisure opportunities should not superimpose further limitations upon the individual. The elderly should be given the opportunity to control one area of their life in the institution. They should be able to choose their own leisure activities. Leisure opportunities should be planned with, not for, the individual, thus allowing the individual to feel that he or she is controlling his or her leisure choices. This chapter will illustrate how leisure services can accomplish this goal through environmental factors, development of leisure patterns, planning for the elderly, activity analyses, and volunteers.

ENVIRONMENTAL FACTORS

The majority of the elderly reside in the community; but, with increased life expectancy, more individuals may be residing in long-term care facilities, owing to the normal physiologic aging process of the mind and body. When individuals reside in the community, they can decide when or where they will participate in recreational activities. Participation will depend upon finances, accessibility, transportation, time available, health status, and previous exposure to the activity. The elderly residing in the community have access to a variety of recreational programs such as the YMCA, YWCA, community recreation centers, theaters, pubs, shows, and social clubs.

The extent to which an individual has control over his or her environment is dependent upon several components: (a) the time the individual has at his or her disposal; (b) the resources the individual has available, and the financial opportunities available; and (c) the individual's physical and psychologic abilities (Fig. 5-1). An individual who retires increases the time available, but there may be a decrease in one or both of the other areas. These variables affect an individual's perception of the control over his or her lifestyle.

When an elderly person enters a long-term care facility, his or her life becomes regimented around the routine of the institution. An individual loses control of alternatives because of physical limitations or enforced institutional regulations. Goffman[1] states that an individual "comes into the establishment with a concept of himself made possible by certain stable social arrangements in his own world. Upon entrance he is immediately stripped of the support provided by these arrangements." As a result, large institutions often initiate and hasten a process of depersonalization in which the individual is made to conform to the regimentation and tyrannization of the institution.[1]

The environment (the institution) controls the lifestyle of an individual. The institutional routine (breakfast, lunch, dinner, therapy hours, and so forth) forces the individual to conform to a specific lifestyle—one determined by the institution. Goffman[1] defines a total institution "as a place of residence and work for a large number of like-situated individuals, cut off from the wider society for an appreciable period of time, [who] together lead an enclosed, formally administered round of life." Hirsch[2] states that "nursing homes for the aged are being criticized for operating on a pathology model of aging, viewing the individual in terms of medical management factors instead of the overall human needs of the person." Langer and Rodin[3] believe that many of the debilitating conditions of those found in an institution were partially the results of the decision-free environment they resided in. They found that the opportunity to make meaningful decisions about one's life imparts the feeling of mastery over one's environment.

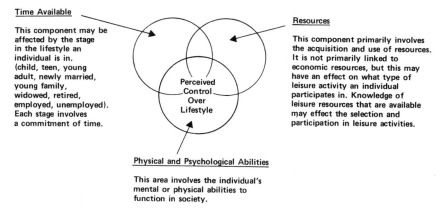

Time Available

This component may be affected by the stage in the lifestyle an individual is in. (child, teen, young adult, newly married, young family, widowed, retired, employed, unemployed). Each stage involves a commitment of time.

Resources

This component primarily involves the acquisition and use of resources. It is not primarily linked to economic resources, but this may have an effect on what type of leisure activity an individual participates in. Knowledge of leisure resources that are available may effect the selection and participation in leisure activities.

Perceived Control Over Lifestyle

Physical and Psychological Abilities

This area involves the individual's mental or physical abilities to function in society.

Figure 5-1. This schematic drawing illustrates the extent to which an individual has control over his or her environment.

The institutional environment that the elderly enters fosters dependence, not independence; routine, not spontaneity; and restrictions, thus leaving the elderly individual with a narrow spectrum of leisure opportunities to select from.

These environmental factors need to be taken into consideration by recreation and health professionals in delivering leisure services to the elderly in long-term care facilities. McGuire[4] states that "the environmentalist's role becomes more important when older individuals are involved and the need for assistance in manipulating the environment to either eliminate or mitigate factors constraining leisure become more necessary with increasing age." Iso Ahola[5] indicates that "it is not the recreational activity in itself that is crucial, but the extent to which such activity induces a sense of control and responsibility over one's behavior, environment and entire life."

DEVELOPMENT OF LEISURE PATTERNS

As the elderly move from the community into the long-term care facility, they are bringing with them a perception of their leisure time and their past participation patterns in recreational activities. Participation in leisure activities in adulthood is dependent upon past experience in work and in leisure, finances, and the individual's retirement situation (physiologic and/or psychologic).

Prior to retirement, work is a major focus of one's life. It has priority for time allotment during the waking hours, and, as a result, daily activities are planned around the work schedule. In addition, vacations, social engagements, and family interactions are all dependent on the time apart from one's work commitment.

Work also becomes a resource providing an income to establish financial security for life's basic needs (food, shelter, clothing). In establishing financial security through work, one develops a sense of purpose, usefulness, and self-respect. A man's work establishes his identity and his role in society. Kaplan[6] notes, "Work gives order to life ... through work, man finds his own level ... the house in which we live and all its conveniences ... the food we eat and the clothes we wear ... these and infinitely more, do we receive and give through a common bond, work."

The Puritan work ethic has had an effect on society and the perception of leisure. Kaplan[7] identifies the following aspects of American life that have contributed to the interpretation of leisure:

> American leisure patterns reflect the history of a nation that grew up without a rigid carryover of the European or feudal principles or systems.
>
> Leisure patterns in America have been related to the heterogeneity of our population—a factor that, in turn, is a part of the immigrant waves.
>
> It was as hard workers that our immigrants came to this country.
>
> The rise in mass literacy ... becomes a ... key element in the leisure of this country.
>
> The social class levels of participants in community transformation are undergoing radical changes creating new areas of significant leisure involvement.
>
> The private business sector ... has become a more and more important factor in ... activities, attitudes, and tastes for leisure.
>
> The public sector has also grown as a major instrument for leisure.
>
> A growth has been evident in the artistic life of America.

These variables have affected the way an individual interprets what leisure is; in addition, the period of history an individual lives through affects that individual's perception of leisure and work.

Different professions require different amounts of one's time. The development of leisure activities will depend not only on the time available after the workday but also on interest, finances, health status, family involvement, and energy level after completion of work.

As stated previously, individuals have traditionally found a feeling of purpose, usefulness, and self-respect in work. The individual who retires needs to find another vehicle to fulfill these needs as well as to fill the time that has suddenly become available. The retiree has lost the center of identity—work—through retirement. This brings about a change in one's lifestyle by changing the focus of one's life from the occupation to the meaningful use of one's leisure time. The retired person is a victim of enforced leisure—unobligated time an individual neither seeks nor asks for.

Kaplan[7] feels that leisure is the social role in retirement that could provide unique opportunities for the individual to enhance self-worth in society. "Like the roles of a child, which are to play and [to] learn, the new leisure roles of the elderly retirees are to play and to teach."[7] This can be accomplished through involvement in various activities, such as hobbies, clubs, senior centers, and organizations such as Vista, the Peace Corps for Action. The task of the elderly in relation to leisure is easier than that required of the young person in finding a job, for at the retirement stage, one has a lifetime of developed tasks, varied experiences upon which to draw.[7] It is the individual's past participation in leisure activities that will determine the types of activities he or she will participate in once he or she retires.[8]

Past recreation participation patterns will carry over once the elderly individual enters a long-term care facility. Therefore, the job of recreators and health professionals is not to find substitutes for work but to build upon the nonwork complex, called leisure, to help the elderly maintain current recreation participation patterns and to explore new activities through which they may demonstrate their skills and tastes and meet their needs. This will allow the elderly individual the opportunity to develop an interest in a leisure activity that he or she can participate in.

Has the leisure profession allowed this to occur? Gunn[9] states that, "ironically old people and young people face many of the same crises. Neither [are] taken seriously, and both are often beset by seemingly benevolent despots intent on running programs resembling qualified playpens." Guadagnolo[10] further elaborates when he says, "Through acts of commission and omission, we have witnessed a selection process which, in the final analysis, permits a very narrow spectrum of elderly with both the opportunity and ability to engage in public sponsored leisure services."

The aged are stereotyped in certain activities in recreation. Recreationists perpetuate myths of the elderly by offering passive activities. Verhoven[8] observed that

> There have been many studies on how aging persons use their leisure. The most often mentioned leisure activities of the aged include reading, watching television, visiting, working around the yard, and going pleasure driving. These activities are strikingly similar types of leisure activities participated in by other groups. To continue to perpetuate stereotyped activities and label them "senior citizens" activities is a gross injustice.

This was verified in other studies on leisure activities participated in by the elderly.[11-15] For example, in the study of the outdoor recreation participation patterns of the elderly, Singleton[16] found that "nonelderly" (18–54) "young-old" (55–74) and "old-old" (75 and above) participated in 10 similar outdoor recreation activities. They did differ in the frequency of participation in outdoor recreation activities; the nonelderly participated in 39 activities, the young-old participated in 27 activities, and the old-old participated in 17 activities. Thus there is a gradual decline in outdoor recreation participation as one grows older. The activities the young-old and old-old did not participate in (sledding, scuba diving, surfing, rock climbing, downhill skiing, cross-country skiing, gliding, skateboarding, snowmobiling, ice skating) may be the result of lack of exposure to the activity or the opportunity to participate in them. Less than 1 percent of the nonelderly participated in these activities, indicating that the nonelderly participate less frequently in these activities as well. This may be due to the fact that the majority of these activities are vigorous activities with a degree of risk involved and thus attract specific individuals who are interested in these types of activities.

In addition, it was found that the social economic variables of occupation, education, income, race, and sex appear to have a stronger association than age with the outdoor recreation activities in which the elderly participated. This finding may indicate that recreation programming in the future may need to be based on more than age alone. Programs for the elderly should be planned activities based not upon age but on interests as criteria.

The following is a list of some activities an older individual could participate in.

Recreation Activities

Sports
Volleyball
Swimming
Tennis
Golf
Badminton
Jogging
Bowling
Skating
Bicycling
Softball
Downhill skiing
Cross-country skiing
Racquetball
Squash

Games
Chess
Checkers
Bridge
Euchre
Solo
Poker
Other card games
Pool, billiards
Horseshoes
Shuffleboard
Board games

Nature Activities
Hiking
Sailing
Birdwatching
Walking in parks
Boating
Hunting
Fishing

Crafts and Hobbies
Sewing
Knitting
Macrame
Carpentry
Crocheting
Car repair
Models
Weaving
Pottery
Rug making
Candle making

Arts
Painting
Photography
Sculpturing
Creative writing
Ceramics
Dancing
Drama
Playing a musical instrument
Singing

Collections	Entertainment
Coins	Watching television
Stamps	Going to museums
Antiques	Reading for pleasure
Cars	Going to parks
Records	Going to parties
Pictures	Dining out
	Home entertainment
Volunteer Services	Attending church
Member of community club	Going to movies
(e.g., Kiwanis, Rotary)	Listening to radio
Member of church club	

The individual's participation in the above activities will be limited only by their abilities, not by where the individual resides (home or institution) or by age. Individuals who are frail and are residing in the community will probably participate in activities similar to those participated in by individuals residing in an institution.

PLANNING FOR THE ELDERLY

Iso Ahola[17] indicates that recreation professionals need to let elderly individuals plan for themselves. Seleen[18] verifies this when she states, "If older people could spend their time as they wish, this could contribute to higher life satisfaction." Therefore, recreation opportunities should be designed to allow the individual to feel in control of leisure choices.

This can be accomplished through the following ways:

1. Utilize a leisure inventory scale to assess the individual's leisure interests. Current assessment tools that may be utilized are primarily checklists asking the individual about past, present, and future recreational participation patterns or needs. Instruments that are currently being used are the Mirenda Leisure Interest Finder,[19] the Self Leisure Interest Profile (SLIP),[20] the Leisure Activities Blank,[21,22] and the Avocational Activities Inventory.[23]
2. Interview the incoming individual to determine the individual's leisure preference using one of the above leisure inventory scales. A process that could facilitate this is leisure counselling. Gunn and Peterson[24] define leisure counselling as "a helping process that utilizes verbal facilitation techniques to promote self-awareness; awareness of leisure attitudes, values and feelings; and the development of decision-making and problem-solving skills related to leisure participation with self, others and the environment."

3. Form a committee of elderly individuals at the long-term care facility to plan their leisure activities. This would allow consumer input into the types of programs to be offered in the facility. Leisure services for the elderly in the long-term care facilities should be planned in cooperation with other health professionals (occupational therapists, physical therapists, nurses, social workers, psychologists, health educators, doctors). This method would provide a comprehensive leisure program for the elderly based on their abilities. The leisure delivery process is a component of the total team process, dependent on, not independent of, other health professionals. Cooperation, coordination, and communication are necessary requirements between the professions to provide comprehensive leisure services to the elderly.[25]

A recreation program for an older individual needs to encourage the individual to attain the following goals:

1. an increase or maintenance of the level of independence by allowing decisions regarding the recreation program,
2. participation in new recreation activities,
3. participation in current or past recreation patterns,
4. socialization, not isolation, through environments that encourage socialization,
5. use of physical abilities,
6. development of positive self-esteem and self-concept,
7. recognition of the benefits of participating in recreation activity (that is, physiologic, social, emotional),
8. continued community involvement.

Programming based upon the continuity theory of aging may be appropriate to accomplish these goals. The continuity theory of aging holds that "as an individual grows older, [he or she is] predisposed towards maintaining continuity of habits, associations, preferences and so on."[26] Davis and Teaff[27] state that "a leisure programmer, through an assessment of the older person's biological and physiological capabilities, personal preferences and experiences, can construct situational opportunities for an individual to maintain continuity of habits, associations and preferences into later life." This is an important concept in planning recreational activities for the elderly once they enter the long-term care facility.

A model program developed at the Byer Activity Center, Dallas Home for Jewish Aged, Dallas, Texas, was based upon the above theory. As a result of an interview with each new resident, a role was created for that individual to participate in a leisure activity. Some of the roles created are described below.

"The Hostess" greets and welcomes guests for a party, serves on the welcoming committee, plans refreshments for the tea, helps make decorations in the craft group for a luau. All these activities allow the continuance of the preference for hostessing.

"The Salesman" helps with the raffle for the women's group, helps run the gift shop, organizes flea markets, white elephant sales, the annual bazaar, serves on the committee for fund-raising projects.

"The Organizer" serves as president of the council, helps on the program committee, brings helpful hints and ideas from all newspaper sources, helps call for activities, and sets up games such as bridge.

"The Entertainer" who has always enjoyed the limelight is the bingo caller, tells jokes at social gatherings, helps provide entertainment for parties, is a member of the drama club, and is the master of ceremonies for talent shows and grandchildren's day.

"The Humanitarian" helps with service projects, cancer society bandages, crocheting for shut-ins, knitting for babies, friendly visiting with the sick, phone calling, helping with the sunshine committee, sending get-well cards, and reporting on human interest stories at the current events groups.

"The Motherer" has always had a preference for caring for others. She enjoys those activities in which she can lend a hand and take a mothering role. She bakes for others as well as for many activities and lunches. She helps with the cooking group, suggests recipes for the recipe book, and adds helpful hints to the center newsletter. She also participates in the tutoring program and children's storytelling.

"The Reporter" knows lots of information on a variety of subjects. The activities of the reporter involve announcing community events, acting as a secretary of the resident council, and interviewing members for the "mystery resident."

"The Musician" helps with all music endeavors, acts as a link to community resources for performers, helps with the choral group, plays the piano, assembles sing-a-long books, and participates actively in music listening and music appreciation groups.

Other roles that have emerged include "The Family Man," "The Artist," "The Complainer," "The Signmaker," "The Receptionist," "The Pastor." Members may have a single role or a variety of roles within the framework of the activity program. Not all members will have an active role, since some may perform the role of observer or visitor.[27]

As a result of these roles, individuals were socialized into an environment based upon predisposed activity patterns and situational opportunities. This is one method of assisting an individual to adjust to a new environment in a non-threatening manner.

ACTIVITY ANALYSIS

A process that would provide a recreator in an institution with knowledge regarding the inherent tasks that need to be accomplished in an activity is an activity analysis. This step is necessary since individuals possess different levels of ability and skills in performing an activity. Activity analysis enables one to reduce the activity to its component parts prior to instruction.[28-30] Once the activity is reduced to its component parts, a recreator would know which part of the activity the individual has difficulty in mastering. Activity analysis has four components: assessment, planning, implementation, and evaluation.

Assessment

Assessment can be broken into the following steps:

1. Determine the activity that the individual is interested in. It is easier to implement such an activity than one the individual is not interested in.
2. After determining the activity, break it into its component parts. Place these components in sequential order.
   a. What does the person need to know first in the activity?
   b. What does the person need to know next in the activity?
   Keep asking the above until the activity is reduced to its component parts.
3. Assess the individual for the basic physical skills required for the activity. This would include adequate strength, flexibility, balance, endurance, agility, speed, and coordination. Physical limitations of the elderly need to be considered for planning the activity (for example, is the individual confined to a wheelchair, does he or she walk with the aid of canes, does he or she have arthritis?). Does the individual have a health condition that would affect participation in an activity (for example, paralysis, paresis, heart condition)? Other health professionals should have input into the assessment procedure to ensure that a realistic and accurate assessment is achieved to assure safe and successful participation.

Planning

Planning the activity consists of determining if the activity needs adaptations or modifications and reducing the activity to sequential tasks or steps that may be taught to the individual. Activities can be adapted or modified by changing the mobility factor, changing the body position, changing boundaries or space requirements, changing weight and size of implements, and changing duration of the activity. The activity should progress from simple skills to complex skills. Planning should also include progressive increments for exercise or physical activity. Reducing an activity to its component parts consists of analyzing each step needed to perform the activity. Each task should build upon the previous task until the activity is complete. When the activity has been reduced to its component parts, then you need to select an appropriate teaching method. Three methods are listed below.

1. Present the entire activity from beginning to end to the consumer (forward chaining).
2. Present the entire activity from the last step and gradually work toward the first step (backward chaining).
3. Present the entire activity. Future trials are used to refine the activity.[28-30]

Implementation

Before the activity is performed, the elderly individual should be aware of (or educated to) his or her exercise tolerance, limitations, and emotional stress threshold. The activity can be implemented utilizing the determined adaptations and sequential tasks.

Evaluation

The evaluation process will determine if additional modifications are required or additional steps are needed. The elderly person's successful mastery of the activity will form the basis of the evaluation. Activity analysis enables an individual to determine the component of the activity that has not been mastered by the individual. Evaluation is a continual process for all activities to enhance the recreational participation of the elderly.

Activity Analysis Using Bowling as an Example

ASSESSMENT

Strength: Does client have strength in upper body to lift standard (10 to 16 pounds) bowling ball and deliver the ball? Does client have strength in hand and fingers to grasp the ball with one hand, with two hands?
Flexibility: Does client have flexibility in shoulder to deliver the ball? (full range of motion for pendulum swing of the ball).
Balance: Does client have adequate balance for walking/slide approach?
Coordination: Can the client coordinate the approach with the delivery of the ball?
Endurance: Does client have adequate endurance to participate (bowl 10 frames, one game)?
Physical Limitations: Does the client have any disability that requires adaptations or modifications?

PLANNING

Adaptations, Modifications

1. If the patient has difficulty grasping balls, adaptors can be used which provide for bar grip.
2. Problems with coordination, flexibility, and strength can be aided by the use of a ball ramp.
3. Balance problems can be aided by the use of a rail such as those used by visually impaired patients.
4. Games can be shortened to five frames for those with limited endurance.
5. Bowling can be performed by the disabled with the aid of grip adaptors and ball ramps.

SEQUENTIAL STEPS FOR BALL DELIVERY

1. Approach ball ramp.
2. Grasp ball, place second and third fingers and thumb in holes, extend first and fourth finger along contour of ball.
3. Take beginning stance facing the pins approximately four and one half walking steps from the foul line.
4. Begin four-step approach to foul line with a simultaneous push-away forward motion of ball and the first step.
5. Continue approach by coordinating the next three steps with the pendulum swing. Walk straight toward the foul line.
6. The last step, executed as a slide, will be coordinated with the forward swing of the ball.
7. Release the ball by letting it roll off the palm and fingers out over the foul line.
8. Continue to lift hand for the follow through and hold pose.

Tasks can be reduced further to include different grips, different stances, different approaches, and different releases. Suggestions are listed below.

Grips:	conventional, semifingertip, fingertip
Stances:	different starting positions of ball and feet
Approaches:	three-, four-, and five-step approaches
Releases:	hook, straight, backup deliveries

Modified Activities

Additional instructions can also be added to improve techniques of an individual once the basic skills of any activity have been mastered. Several activities and some modifications that can be made to them are listed below.

ACTIVITY	MODIFICATION
Reading	enlarged print books
Sewing	enlarged print pattern
Cards	braille cards, large print cards, cardholders
Swimming	floatation devices
Bowling	ramps, rails, grip adaptors
Exercises	chair exercises, graduated increments
Volleyball	lower net, balloon, nerf volleyball
Dance	wheelchair dances

The modifications of the activity will depend on the abilities of the individual. Thus modifications of each activity will vary according to the individual's abilities.

Once the mastery of this process has been accomplished, one can apply it to any of the following activity areas: arts, dance, drama, literature, self-improvement, sports, outdoor recreation hobbies, social recreation, volunteer services, and travel and tourism.[31] The activity analysis process allows the professional to document the individual's development in the activity that that person has selected, no matter what his or her level of ability. The development of the program should be based upon the individual's interest, not upon the therapist's interest. It allows the individual the opportunity to decide what he or she wants to do in an environment that often lacks this phenomenon. Owing to budget constraints resulting in higher staff/consumer ratio, it is often difficult to implement individual attention. Volunteers may be the solution to this problem in a long-term care facility.

VOLUNTEERS

Volunteers have been used to deliver recreation programs to the elderly in long-term care facilities. There are many benefits and drawbacks in using volunteers. If a long-term care facility chooses to use volunteer services to deliver recreation services, the agency should be prepared to select, to train, and to retain volunteers just as they would full-time employees. Koh[32] states that "screening is the quality control factor for effective volunteers." There is a need to interview volunteers just as you would an individual for any other type of a job in the agency. Through the interview, the long-term care agency can find out where the applicant has previously worked, establish initial rapport, enforce criteria for selection, and reach a mutual decision with the applicant regarding whether he or she is suited for the agency.

Once the volunteers have been selected, an agency needs to establish a training program for them. Banes[33] indicates that during the training process "the roles, responsibilities, and parameters of authority are the most important subjects a volunteer should know, understand, and accept. That same understanding and acceptance are necessary for the professionals and the elected officials involved. Too often it is assumed volunteers know what is expected, know what their limitations are and know how to act."

If volunteers are to be a viable component to deliver services in a long-term care facility, they need to be properly oriented and trained. Schindler-Rainmann[34] indicates that the following steps may be used in training volunteers:

1. Preservice training; that is, training of a volunteer beginning work.
2. Start up support, that is, assistance to the volunteers as they begin their volunteer work.
3. Maintenance of effort training. Throughout the volunteer's period of service, regular times are needed for asking questions and gaining additional job-related knowledge.
4. Periodic review and feedback.
5. Transition training. Volunteers have a need to grow and to assume more responsibility.

The development of a volunteer handbook may aid in the training of volunteers because it should outline the responsibilities of the volunteer as well as those of the agency. The handbook should include such items as a brief history of the agency, the agency program policies, the evaluation procedure used for volunteers, volunteer rights, physical aspects of aging, sexuality, and death and dying.

SUMMARY

If the elderly are to retain a degree of control of their leisure choices, the institution may need to establish the following to achieve this goal:

1. A practicum experience with students in health-related fields (occupational therapy, physical therapy, health education, recreation) at nearby universities. This will provide the institution with individuals who are interested in elderly individuals. Also it would allow for more one-to-one interaction between the elderly and the staff.
2. An advisory committee of patients to plan leisure activities in the institution.
3. A volunteer program that would properly select, train, and retain volunteers. Volunteers could be a benefit or a liability, depending on how well they are trained.
4. The use of existing community facilities for leisure opportunities. This will allow individuals to remain active in a community that is not *age* segregated.
5. Health professionals' awareness of existing programs in the community for the elderly, as well as programs that provide activities for all ages. This ensures that the elderly people will not be segregated into one type

of activity but given the opportunity to participate in a variety of programs regardless of age. The only criterion should be ability.

6. Use of the activity analysis process to develop programs based upon the patient's interest, not upon the staff's interest.
7. Plans that are concerned with, not for, older individuals. These encourage control of one area of individuals' lives in the institution.
8. Encouragement of the maintenance of past recreation practices and of new leisure opportunities.
9. Activities based on interest, not age, categories.
10. Modified activities based on the abilities of the individual, not on his or her disability.
11. Modified living environment so that it encourages social interaction, not isolation, of the individual.
12. Communication, cooperation, and coordination of activities with other members of the health team to deliver a comprehensive program.
13. The use of the activity analysis process to determine modifications necessary for activities that are suggested by the patients.
14. Evaluation of individuals' accomplishments based on the activity analysis process, not subjective criteria.

Through the establishing of these brief points, the elderly may begin to feel control of their leisure lifestyle.

Leviton and Campanelli[35] state that

1. Leisure activities may contribute significantly to the older person's life satisfaction meaning given to life.
2. Leisure activities may serve as "healthy" stressors, mediators of stress, or responses to stress.
3. Empirical and scientific data offer a firm basis for the development of gerontologically oriented leisure service.

Thus health professionals working with the elderly should plan *with* the elderly, rather than *for* them. If health professionals who work with the elderly do not plan *with* the elderly in providing leisure services, they are contributing to further devaluation of the individual in the institution.

This chapter is based on the premise that an elderly individual surrenders too many rights once he or she enters a long-term care facility. The individual enters an environment that encourages dependence instead of independence via such mechanisms as institutional routine (for example, meals at specific times) and administrative policies (for example, permission to attend community events). How does one resolve this issue? One method could be based on the process outlined in this chapter. This would allow an individual some control over one component of his or her lifestyle in the institution, the choice and enjoyment of leisure activities.

REFERENCES

1. GOFFMAN, E: *Asylums*. Doubleday & Co, New York, 1961.

2. HIRSCH, C: *Integrating the nursing home resident into a senior citizens center*. Gerontologist 17:277, 1977.

3. LANGER, EJ AND RODIN, J: *The effects of choice and enhanced personal responsibilities for the aged. A field experiment in an institution*. J Pers Soc Psychol (34):191, 1976.

4. McGUIRE, A: *Constraints and leisure involvement in advanced adulthood*. In ROBERT, RO (ED): *Leisure and Aging*. University of Wisconsin, Madison, 1979, p 78.

5. ISO AHOLA, E: *Perceived control and responsibility as mediators of the effects of therapeutic recreation on the institutionalized aged*. Therapeutic Recreation Journal, Vol XIV, First Quarter, 1980, No. 1, p 38.

6. KAPLAN, M: *Leisure: Theory and Policy*, John Wiley & Sons, New York, 1975, p 278.

7. KAPLAN, M: *Leisure: Lifestyle and Lifespan Perspective for Gerontology*. WB Saunders, Philadelphia, 1979.

8. VERHOVEN, J: *Recreation and the aging*. In STEIN, AT AND SESSOMS, HD: *Recreation and Special Populations*. Allyn and Bacon, Boston, 1977.

9. GUNN, LS: *Labels that limit life*. Leisure Today, Journal of Physical Education and Recreation, October, 1977, p 27.

10. GUADAGNOLO, B: *1000 handmade ashtrays—meaningful leisure*. Leisure Today, Journal of Physical Education and Recreation, October, 1977, p 5.

11. EKERDT, DJ, ET AL: *Longitudinal change in preferred age of retirement*. Journal of Occupational Psychology 49:161, 1976.

12. KELLY, RJ: *Recreation Prediction by Age and Family Cycle*. The Third Nationwide Outdoor Recreation Plan, Appendix II, Survey, Technical Report 4, 1978.

13. BALEY, JA: *Recreation and the aging process*. Res Q Exerc Sport 26:1, March, 1955.

14. COWGILL, DO AND BALCH, BN: *The use of leisure time by old people*. J Gerontol 17:302, July, 1962.

15. FORD, MP: An analysis of leisure time activities and interests of aged residents in Indiana. Unpublished Ph.D. dissertation, Indiana University, 1962.

16. SINGLETON, J: A profile of the outdoor recreation participation patterns of the elderly. Unpublished Ph.D. dissertation, University of Maryland, 1981.

17. ISO AHOLA, E: *Perceived control and responsibility as mediators of the effects of therapeutic recreation on institutionalized aged*. Therapeutic Recreation Journal, Vol XIV, First Quarter, No 1, 1980, p 36.

18. SELEEN, RD: *Life satisfaction and the congruence between actual and desired participation in activity by older adults*. In ROBERT, RO (ED): *Leisure and Aging*. University of Wisconsin, Madison, 1979, p 57.

19. MIRENDA, JJ: *Mirenda leisure finder*. In EPPERSON, JA, ET AL (EDS): *Leisure Counseling Kit*. American Alliance for Health, Physical Education and Recreation, Washington, DC, 1973.

20. McDOWELL, CF: *Toward a health leisure mode: Leisure counselling*. Therapeutic Recreation Journal 8(3):96, 1974.

21. McKechnie, GE: *Manual for Leisure Activities Blank*. Consulting Psychology Press, Palo Alto, CA, not dated.

22. McKechnie, GE: *Psychological foundations of leisure counseling. An empirical strategy.* Therapeutic Recreation Journal 8(1):4, 1974.

23. Overs, RP: *A model for avocational counseling.* Journal of Health, Physical Education and Recreation 41(2):28, 1970.

24. Gunn, LS and Peterson AC: *Therapeutic Recreation Program Design Principles and Procedures.* Prentice-Hall, Englewood Cliffs, NJ, 1978, p 214.

25. Humphrey, F: *Communication, Cooperation, Coordination.* Proceedings, Volunteer Venture, Connecticut, Department of Health, 1969, p 6.

26. Atchley, R: *The Social Forces in Later Life: An Introduction to Social Gerontology.* Wadsworth Publishing, Belmont, CA, 1977, p 27.

27. Davis, BN and Teaff, DJ: *Facilitating role continuity of the elderly through leisure programming.* Therapeutic Recreation Journal, Second Quarter, 1980.

28. Gold, WM and Scott, KG: *Discrimination tearing.* In Stephens, WB (ed): *Training the Developmentally Young.* John Day, New York, 1971.

29. Gold, WM: *Task analysis of a complex assembly by retarded blind.* Except Child 43:2, 1976.

30. Gold, WM: *Vocational training.* In Wortis, J (ed): *Mental Retardation and Developmental Disabilities.* Bruner/Nazel, New York, 1975.

31. Edginton, RC and Williams, GJ: *Productive Management of Leisure Service Organizations: A Behavioral Approach.* John Wiley & Sons, Toronto, 1978.

32. Koh, M: *Effective use of volunteers in therapeutic recreation settings.* Therapeutic Recreation Journal, Vol VI, No 1, 1972, p 23.

33. Banes, ER: *Maximizing Human Resources.* Parks and Recreation, December, 1975, p 27.

34. Schindler-Rainmann, E: *The Volunteer Community Creative Use of Human Resources.* Learning Resources Corporation, Fairfax, Virginia, 1975, p 75.

35. Leviton, D and Campanelli, L: *Health, Physical Education, Recreation and Dance for the Older Adult: A Modular Approach.* American Alliance for Health, Physical Education and Dance, Reston, Virginia, 1980, p 220.

CHAPTER 6

THE CHANGING REALM OF THE SENSES

GAIL HILLS MAGUIRE, Ph.D., O.T.R.

BEHAVIORAL OBJECTIVES

Upon completion of this chapter, the reader will be able to
1. Identify common sensory deficits in the elderly.
2. Describe compensation techniques for problems in vision, hearing, taste, smell, touch, and communication.
3. List modifications of the clinical environment to assist elderly patients with impaired hearing and vision.
4. Discuss the effects of sensory deficits on rehabilitation potential.
5. Recognize sensory deficits in the elderly.
6. Recommend modifications for the personal and physical environments of older persons.

An individual's potential for interaction with the environment is highly dependent on his or her capacity to receive and to respond to information obtained through the senses. The senses that will be discussed here are what are commonly referred to as the five senses and include sight (vision), hearing (auditory), taste (gustatory), smell (olfactory), and touch (tactile). Each of these senses contributes a specific type of information necessary for a person to adapt and to adjust to the environment. Limitations in sensory input associated with aging can affect an individual's safety, functional ability, self-image, and interaction with others. Health professionals must be sensitive to the potential effects of sensory deficits to the total rehabilitation program and be prepared to modify the environment as needed.

Fortunately, a young individual usually has sensory acuities far in excess of what is needed for normal activities. As a person ages there is a gradual decline in the senses, and the sensory threshold levels increase. Threshold refers to the minimal degree of stimulus needed to activate the system. A higher threshold means that stronger stimuli are required to activate the sensory receptors, for example, brighter lights, louder sounds, stronger tastes and smells. Initial sensory losses are often unnoticed because of the ample margin of surplus available before normal function is affected and because of unconscious compensation techniques. However, at a certain point, depreciation of the sensory processes can become critical and seriously affect behavioral or psychologic functioning.[1]

An individual sensory process deteriorates to a greater degree over time the more it possesses one or several of the following characteristics: high specialization, greater complexity, higher discrimination, and increased articulation with other bodily systems.[1] However, this is a generalization, and aging occurs in all systems of the same and different individuals at varying rates. Each aged individual must be approached as a unique person.

VISION

The aged person may maintain nearly normal sight until well into old age. Nevertheless, the aging eye is subject to various changes and pathologies.

Visual changes can be congenital or can occur throughout the life cycle. In the normal (emmetropic) eye (Fig. 6-1), the eye muscles (ciliary) are relaxed, and

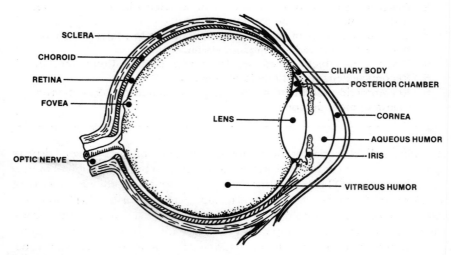

Figure 6-1. Shown here are the complex parts of the eye.

parallel light rays from distant objects are in sharp focus directly on the retina. Divergent rays from near objects require contraction of the ciliary muscles to increase the curvature of the lens so that the focal point will still fall on the retina.[2]

Common Refractive Problems

The refractive power of the eye is the ability of the lens to bend light rays. Myopia, hyperopia, and astigmatism are some of the common refractive defects of the eye that can occur at any age.

MYOPIA

Myopia (nearsightedness) occurs when parallel light rays from distant objects focus before the retinal surface rather than on it (Fig. 6-2) when the ciliary muscles are relaxed. This can occur when the eyeball is too long, or, less commonly, when the lens system is too strong. Only objects that are less than 20 feet from the subject are in focus. All objects beyond this distance appear blurred.[2,3,4]

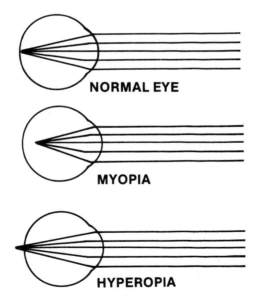

Figure 6-2. Parallel light rays focus on the retina in the normal eye, in front of the retina in myopia, and behind the retina in hyperopia. (Adapted from Guyton, AC: *Textbook of Medical Physiology*. WB Saunders, 1981, p 730.)

HYPEROPIA

Hyperopia (farsightedness) occurs when parallel light rays from distant objects are not refracted sufficiently by the lens system to come into focus by the time they reach the retina when the ciliary muscles are relaxed. The point of focus is beyond the retinal surface. This is due to an eyeball that is too short or a lens system that is too weak (see Figure 6-2). Objects less than 20 feet from the subject are blurred, and objects beyond 20 feet are also blurred; in the earlier years of the developmental cycle the lens of the eye can usually accommodate by focusing. In later years the lens is less capable of making this accommodation, particularly with near objects.[2,3]

ASTIGMATISM

Astigmatism is a refractive error of the lens system caused by irregularities in the curvature of the cornea or the lens. Curvature of the astigmatic lens along either the vertical or horizontal plane is less than curvature along the other plane. There will be less convergence owing to less refractive power, and the focal point of one plane will be farther from the lens than the focal point of the other plane. Rays of light are not focused equally, and both distant and near objects appear blurred.[2-4]

Age-Related Changes in Vision

PRESBYOPIA

Presbyopia (old sight) is associated with the aging process. The lens loses its elastic nature and becomes more rigid. The ciliary muscles that hold the lens in position may become weaker, lose tone, and decrease in ability to accommodate rapidly from far to near distance (and vice versa). Once the lens becomes unaccommodating, the eye remains permanently focused at an almost constant distance. This distance varies with individuals. In order for an older person to be able to see both near and far objects, he or she must wear bifocal glasses. The upper segment focuses for distant objects, and the lower segment focuses for near objects, such as printed material.[2,3]

Visual acuity as well as accommodation decreases with age. Normal vision is described as 20/20. Vision of 20/30 means that a person can identify objects at 20 feet or less that a person with normal vision can identify at 30 feet or less. Vision levels of 20/40 can still be quite functional; a person can drive a car and do most activities. However, when vision reaches 20/50 or worse, driving is not permitted in many states. Serious problems arise at vision levels of 20/70 and less. Recognition of objects and people becomes difficult, including reading, and seeing television, bus numerals, and signs. Roughly one third of individuals over age 80 have vision of 20/50 or less.[5,6]

Strong reading glasses, magnifying glasses, and low vision aids are available, but the individual's tolerance for aids affects how well he or she will adapt.

TEAR FLOW

The research of Furukawa and Polse[7] suggests that a 40 percent reduction in tear secretion accompanies aging. The symptoms and signs, such as dryness commonly observed in older individuals, seem to be caused by altered tear chemistry and insufficient tear secretion. This condition, as all others, should be followed through regular eye examinations and treatment. Medication is available to relieve the symptoms.

GLAUCOMA

Glaucoma is one of the leading causes of blindness in individuals over 35 years of age and is especially prevalent in the elderly. Ninety-five to ninety-eight percent of this blindness is preventable. It is due to pathologically high intraocular pressure. It occurs principally in two forms: open-angle glaucoma and closed-angle glaucoma. Open-angle glaucoma, the most common, affects approximately 2 percent of those over age 40. It is painless and asymptomatic until major damage and visual loss have occurred. It is insidious because the initial loss of peripheral vision is usually not noticed by the victim. Therefore, screening examinations are an important preventive measure. Acute closed-angle glaucoma is usually very sudden and painful. The entire chamber is occluded by a pushed-forward iris, leading to a rapid rise in intraocular pressure. If the pressure is not reduced, compression of the retinal artery can result in retinal atrophy and blindness. Treatment with topical eyedrops can control the disease in most cases, but surgical intervention may be necessary. Early diagnosis is important; the earlier in the course of the disease treatment is begun, the easier it is to control the process. Older people need to have an eye examination at least once a year and more often if indicated;[2,5] it is the only way to diagnose the condition.

CATARACTS

Cataracts, the most common visual problem of old age, are a developmental or a degenerative opacity of the lens of the eye causing obstruction of the passage of light rays to the retina. Central vision is restricted first, with gradual involvement of the peripheral field (the opposite process of glaucoma). The person is bothered by glare from bright lights reflected on shiny surfaces, a gradual darkening of vision, and loss of acuity.

Myopia can develop in the early stages of nuclear cataracts so that a presbyopic individual may be able to read without glasses for a period of time. Pain is absent unless the cataract swells and produces secondary glaucoma.

People will vary greatly as to when they seek treatment, depending on how critical vision is to their daily activities.

Removal of the cataract (lens) is the only treatment and creates aphakia. The aphakic eye has no focusing mechanism, and so corrected lenses in eyeglasses and/or contacts are prescribed. Cataract eyeglasses are less than a satisfactory substitute for the normal eye lens. Glasses cause confusing magnification of images.[8,9] The increase in the magnification makes objects appear much larger and closer than they actually are. This can cause difficulties with self-care, ambulation, and household tasks.[10] For example, a person may underestimate the distance one's hand is from a table and thus drop and break a glass or, when descending stairs, one may stumble and fall owing to misjudging the distance of the steps.

Objects in the periphery are distorted, making driving a car or walking in unfamiliar surroundings frightening and hazardous if the person does not learn to accommodate. Because of the lack of focusing ability, distorted visual images occur when the person moves his or her eyes back and forth. This results in a momentary sense of disorientation and confusion. The health profession must take these conditions into account when working with a person who wears cataract glasses and allow sufficient time for the individual to visually adjust to body movements.[10]

Better vision is obtained with contact lenses. They greatly reduce the distortions and are preferred to glasses whenever possible. However, not everyone can wear contact lenses, and no one wears them exclusively. Hard lenses are worn about eight to ten hours per day, but soft lenses can be tolerated about twelve hours per day. The elderly person may have less tolerance for contact lenses when he or she is tired or ill.[10]

Intraocular lens implants are also being used but have not been fully evaluated over long periods of time. They are generally recommended for older patients.[2,6,8,9]

MACULAR DEGENERATION

This third major source of visual disability is more serious than cataracts or glaucoma because it is the least treatable at present. It is a pigmentary change of the macular area of the retina caused by small hemorrhages. Individuals see a gray shadow in the center of vision but can see well at the outer border. This condition is often seen in the elderly but rarely results in total blindness. Compensation techniques can include wearing sun visors because vision is less acute in bright light, looking to the side to utilize peripheral vision, and the use of magnifiers. Many older individuals find such compensation techniques quite frustrating, especially because the loss of sharp central vision makes reading, watching television, and hand activities difficult.[2,6,8]

RETINITIS PIGMENTOSA

Retinitis pigmentosa is a progressive pigmentary degeneration of the retina. It is more common in men than in women and is usually bilateral. Night blindness is one of the first symptoms because, unlike macular degeneration, the peripheral retina, where the rods are located, is involved first. When the person reaches 50 or 60 years of age, only three to five degrees of central vision may remain. However, the residual central vision is often sufficient for reading until the patient reaches 70 or 80 years old.[2,8,11]

DIABETIC RETINOPATHY

Diabetic retinopathy has become the leading cause of blindness in the United States, above even glaucoma, owing to the increased lifespan of diabetics. The condition can occur whether or not diabetic control is good and usually takes two forms. The majority of the cases are simple diabetic retinopathy, in which microaneurysms and hemorrhages coagulate and obstruct light rays to the retina as well as damage the retina itself. Damage is bilateral and similar in both eyes. Treatment is very difficult and unsatisfactory. Diabetes tends to have remissions and exacerbations, and therefore the course of the visual impairment may also fluctuate. Sudden changes in the eye are not uncommon. For example, the refractive status may change several diopters when changes in the blood sugar level affect hydration of the lens. Proliferate diabetic retinopathy, the second type, may be superimposed on the simple type. Large recurrent hemorrhages and retinal detachment can result in blindness.[2,5,8,11]

RETINAL DETACHMENT

Complete or partial detachment of the retina can occur as a result of trauma as well as of diabetes. Loss of vision occurs wherever the retina is detached. Flickering flashes of light in the peripheral visual field and a sudden increase in floating specks are common symptoms, followed by a blotting out of vision if the retina becomes completely detached. The retina can often be reattached if treatment is initiated soon after it occurs. However, once detachment has progressed, extensive surgical intervention becomes necessary. The risk of reoccurrence of retinal detachment owing to strain is high.[2,5,8]

LEGAL BLINDNESS

Any of the former conditions can lead to sufficient visual impairment for the individual to be classified as legally blind. Legal blindness does not necessarily mean total blindness. Over 90 percent of individuals in this classification have some residual sight. The definition of legal blindness includes (1) central visual acuity of 20/200 or less with the better eye with corrective lenses; the individual can identify objects at only 20 feet or less that a person with normal vision can identify at 200 feet; and (2) if the peripheral vision is restricted to a 20° angle or less; the person sees no more than what an individual with normal vision might see through a tube or tunnel.[8]

Visual Care

Good preventive care begins with regular professional eye examinations. As a person ages, the need for such care increases. Everyone over age 70 needs at least yearly professional care to correct or to prevent visual problems. Yet it is estimated that the normal length of time between eye checkups for residents of nursing homes is from five to seven years.[12]

As part of initial evaluations, the nurse or therapist should check to see whether patients wear glasses and how long it has been since their last opthalmologic examination. If it has been longer than a year, a referral should be made. In the meantime, quick screening of vision can be done with the Snellen chart. This is the common eye chart with rows of diminishing size E's, beginning with a large letter E at the top. Visual acuity is recorded in the form of a fraction. The numerator (20) is the distance from the patient's eyes to the chart. The denominator is the different size of the test number recorded from each line on the Snellen chart. The subject is positioned 20 feet from the chart, and vision of each eye is measured separately while vision of the opposite eye is occluded. Vision with eyeglasses is checked in a similar manner. This gives an indication of visual acuity with and without eyeglasses. A gross check of peripheral vision can be done by having the subject sit and face the evaluator. The subject is asked to fix his or her gaze on the evaluator's nose. Holding a pencil in his or her hand, the evaluator positions it behind and to the side of the patient's head. It is gradually moved into the subject's peripheral visual field. The subject is asked to indicate by word or gesture as soon as he or she first sees the pencil. The subject must maintain eye fixation during this procedure. The same process is repeated for the opposite side. It is desirable to have two evaluators, one to sit in front of the subject to be sure the subject looks straight ahead and one to move the pencil from the side. Since this is often not possible, the method described can be used.

If the visual field is imagined as a half circle around the front of the subject's head from the sides of the eyes, the potential visual field would be 180°. Imagine you divide this into two equal 90° triangles, with 90° at the side of the eyes and 0° directly in front of the eyes. The subject should see the pencil on both sides of the eyes at 90°. As the pencil moves toward the center of the semicircle, the number of degrees of the visual deficit (loss) on each side can be estimated by plotting from 90° toward the center. For example, if the pencil is halfway from the sides of the eyes (90°) to the front (0°) on both sides, the remaining degrees would be 45° on each side. If you add the remaining degrees on both sides (45° + 45°), the resulting peripheral vision is only 90°. In legal blindness, the peripheral vision is 20° or less. This means a residual vision of 10° bilaterally or combined vision of 20° (10° + 10° = 20°). This is a gross test that is reliable only to indicate the difference between eyes or monocular problems.

Poor vision that is not corrected can interfere with a total rehabilitation program. For instance, a person's difficulty with daily chores and ambulation may be greatly influenced by visual deficits.

Compensation Techniques for Visual Problems*

The following suggestions include things that can be done to compensate for visual changes associated with age or illness.[13]

1. Provide adequate light. Persons with visual problems need much more light than the average person.
2. Reduce glare. Avoid shiny surfaces which will reflect light. Window shades, blinds, sunglasses, visors or hats with brims may reduce the glare from sunlight.
3. Avoid color coding when safety is a factor. Pastel colors, blues, greens, and very dark colors may all look alike to the elderly. Color coding should not be used for pills, markings on appliances, etc. Colors used for identification and location should be strongly contrasting, such as yellow and blue.
4. Avoid abrupt changes in light. The older eye takes more time to accommodate to sudden changes. Lights should be strategically arranged, and some lights should be kept on at night in hazardous locations. For example, night lights can be left on in the bedroom, hall, and bath so there is an even distribution of light.
5. Use large print on all signs, directions, labels, etc. Large print is easier for everyone to see.
6. People with cataract lenses may need assistance crossing streets or wherever depth perception is a safety factor.
7. Low vision aids, such as large print books, magnifying glasses, etc., may be of assistance.
8. Touching can be used in communication when vision is limited. A pat on the hand can let someone know you are listening.
9. Verbally describe a new room or situation to a visually impaired person. Help him or her to locate hazards, furniture, and who is in the room. Stay with him or her until he or she is comfortably oriented.

HEARING

The following brief discussion will emphasize hearing problems as part of total sensory loss.

A review of the literature suggests that there is no general agreement on the specific effects of aging on the auditory system. However, there does seem to be a general concensus that (1) auditory acuity decreases with age, and (2) the speech discrimination skills of the elderly are poorer than would be expected based on their pure tone loss.[14] Some hearing loss is usually present by 30 years of age, and the rate of loss increases as age increases.[15]

A 10-year study by Bergman and associates[16] found a noticeable decline in speech discrimination in the fifth decade of life, with a much steeper decline in the seventh decade. The reason for a greater decrement in speech discrimination

---

*From Maguire,[2] p 28, with permission.

scores for older listeners as compared with younger listeners in difficult situations is not understood. It may be due to a greater distortion of auditory signals.

Research is still needed on auditory problems of the elderly, particularly on measures to analyze and to distinguish among peripheral and central (neural) losses. Unfortunately, most past studies did not make such distinctions and lumped all conditions under the label presbycusis.[14]

Peripheral Losses

A variety of factors can interfere with the conduction of sound waves to the inner ear, which is why such defects are often called *conduction* problems.

Peripheral problems can include external ear diseases and acute or chronic diseases of the middle ear.[17]

Otitis media, or inflammation of the middle ear, is one of the most common problems. In most cases the infection results from microorganisms from the nasopharynx which enter via the eustachian tube. It is treated with medication but can result in permanent ear damage and hearing loss.[15]

Otosclerosis is a genetic condition characterized by a spongy bone formation around the oval window, resulting in ankylosis of the stapes. It is usually treatable with surgery, so the major problem is one of diagnosis and referral.[15]

Treatment for peripheral problems includes lowering the frequency of the sound, including the pitch of the speaking voice, and amplification through sound systems and hearing aids. People with hearing difficulties may have a very small range between the decibel (loudness) level necessary for them to hear a sound and the decibel level that may be painful or irritating. This can make adjustments of a hearing aid very difficult.[2]

A loss of hearing may interfere with receiving danger signals from the environment, such as horns or sirens, which may impede safety.[2]

Sensorineural Losses

Central, or neural, losses in the elderly have been attributed to degeneration or changes in the neural receptors in the cochlea, the eighth nerve, the central auditory nervous system, or the central nervous system in general.

Excessive noise is a common cause of hearing loss, with the most pronounced loss in the higher frequencies. Discrimination of consonants, particularly S, Z, T, F, and G, is more difficult than for vowels.[2,13]

Neural losses are usually permanent, and compensatory techniques such as lipreading may be advised.

PRESBYCUSIS

Presbycusis is an inner ear loss of auditory acuity associated with aging (see Chapter 4). Previously it was thought to be a normal part of aging but now is seen as having a major genetic component. It varies tremendously in the time of onset and intensity of loss.[2,15] Presbycusis may represent any one of several different types of disorders at various sites in the auditory system or a combination of these disorders. Presently there is no battery of tests that can make distinctions between the relative contributions of disease at the various neural sites. Therefore clear-cut distinctions about pathology are difficult. It is usually characterized by a gradual bilateral symmetrical perceptive hearing loss occurring with old age. Loss of hearing is usually greater in the higher frequencies.[2,9,15]

TINNITUS

A wide variety of "ear noises" are grouped under the general term tinnitus. A small percentage of the elderly suffer from this condition to varying degrees. Commonly reported noises including hissing, ringing, and buzzing. Tinnitus may be constant or intermittent and is very annoying. The condition may be due to various diseases, allergies, obstruction of the ear canal, and other causes and is often accompanied by hearing loss. Treatment of the primary etiology is essential, but many times it is unsuccessful. If relief is not obtained, stress to the elderly person can be great, and tranquilizers may help, as well as patience and consideration on the part of others.

Assessment of Hearing Loss

Assessment of hearing loss is done with audiometric and nonaudiometric evaluation. Nonaudiometric assessment may include a physical exam, testing with a tuning fork, interviewing the patient and family, and self-reporting by the patient. An examination by the physician can determine if there is any evidence of structural changes or diseases of the ear. A physician will often check for hearing loss with a tuning fork as part of the exam. However, it can be done by other health professionals as a screening device, especially when medical treatment has been infrequent. The Rinne test is performed by striking the tuning fork and then placing the handle to the mastoid process (behind the ear). The patient is asked to indicate when he or she can no longer hear the sound. When this point is reached, the vibrating head of the tuning fork is immediately placed next to the external ear. The patient should continue to hear the sound because air conduction is normally greater than bone conduction. If the patient continues to hear the sound, the test is recorded as a positive Rinne test, showing air conduction (AC) is greater than bone conduction (BC): (AC) > (BC). If the patient does not continue to hear the sound, then a conduction loss is present.

Questioning the patient concerning possible problems is also helpful. (See Ebersole and Hess[18] for a comprehensive interview scale, p 217.) Older people may report no difficulties because the change is very gradual or because they are sensitive about admitting losses. It is, therefore, also important to observe behavior carefully. Common behaviors which indicate hearing loss include inattentiveness, loud speech, inappropriate responses, frequent requests to repeat conversation, and consistently turning one ear to the speaker (see discussion in Chapter 4). If a hearing loss is suspected, it is best to recommend a referral to an otologist or otolaryngologist to identify any medical conditions and then to an audiologist for an evaluation, which will include audiometric testing. Physical examination, interview, self-assessment, and audiometric findings are all essential to evaluate an older person's hearing fully. This is especially true with presbycusis because the hearing loss involves confusion and jumbling of the auditory signal and not just diminution in auditory sensitivity. Treatment usually involves counselling the patient and family in communication techniques and training in the use of a hearing aid, if indicated.

Compensation Techniques for Hearing Problems*

The following points include ways to compensate for hearing changes associated with age or illness.[13]

1. Speak slowly and clearly but do not shout.
2. Face the person at eye level so he or she can read your lips.
3. Lower the pitch of your voice if the hearing loss is in the high frequencies.
4. Adjust electronic or audio system so that the base or lower tones are predominant.
5. Avoid background noise whenever possible. Choose a quiet environment.
6. Check to see if the person's hearing aid is on and adjusted properly.
7. Use nonverbal communication in your conversations, such as smiles, waving, pointing, etc., to emphasize your "message."
8. Write a message that needs clarification.
9. Share in activities that require less pressure to communicate, such as cards, bowling, etc.
10. Orient the person about the topics of conversations which he or she cannot hear. This reduces the tendency to become paranoid or withdrawn.
11. Recognize that a hearing aid does not work for all people.
12. Remember that what appears to be "selective hearing" may actually be due to factors such as high frequency, fatigue, and environmental distractions.

MODIFICATION OF THE CLINICAL SETTING FOR HEARING AND VISION PROBLEMS

Simple adaptations in the clinical environment can effectively reduce certain common problems associated with reduced hearing and vision.

1. Accoustic material such as tiles, drapes, and carpeting can be used near noisy traffic areas.

---

*From Maguire,[2] p 31, with permission.

2. Locations of meetings, recreation, and treatment rooms should be away from noisy equipment, such as fans, air conditioners, and appliances.
3. Noise and traffic in treatment areas should be controlled. Treatment of several people close together on a mat or in curtained cubicles can cause distracting noise and should be regulated.
4. Speak slowly in low distinct tones when giving directions.
5. Glare from unfiltered sunlight, highly waxed floors, and shiny surfaces should be avoided.
6. Floors, railings, steps, handles on walkers, and parallel bars can be marked in a high contrast color, such as bright yellow.

TASTE AND SMELL*

Not all studies agree, but evidence suggests that the thresholds for taste and smell increase with age.[19,20] This means that food which seems tasteless will be less appealing and may discourage the elderly from eating. This can lead to poor nutrition and a difficulty recognizing food which is starting to spoil. There is also the potential hazard that an aged person will not smell leaking gas from a stove or furnace.

Compensation Techniques*

The following are possible ways to compensate for decreases in taste and smell associated with illness or age.[13]

1. The choice of foods should emphasize appearance (for those with good sight) and texture for their appeal.
2. Desirable temperatures of foods should be maintained whenever possible.
3. Condiments other than salt or restricted items should be used liberally to enhance flavor.
4. The social aspects of mealtime including the table settings, lighting, and pleasant company should be emphasized whenever possible.
5. Older people themselves and their family and friends should be encouraged to check pilot lights, stored food, etc., to detect any safety problems.

TOUCH

The sense of touch, or tactile sensation, has had limited study in relation to aging. There does seem to be evidence that tactile sensation also decreases with age, although this varies individually.[21] The related sense of kinesthesia is the

---

*From Maguire,[2] p 32, with permission.

person's awareness of his or her body in space. Information comes from receptors in muscles, joints, and the inner ear which aid movement, touch, and positioning. Decreased kinesthetic sensitivity in the elderly person results in postural instability and difficulty in reacting to bodily changes in space. Dizziness and vertigo, associated with a fluid imbalance in the semicircular canals of the inner ear, are common problems with people over age 50. When combined with dysfunction in kinesthetic and tactile senses, they increase aged individuals' vulnerability to accidental falls.[22]

Health professionals should note behaviors such as exaggerated body sway, a wide-based gait, and difficulty with balance, especially during fast movement. These may indicate compensation techniques for age-related changes in vestibular and kinesthetic senses or be symptomatic of neurologic disease.

Compensation Techniques

1. Use touch as a means of communication and orientation.
2. Consider sitting closer to an elderly individual when communicating. This makes physical contact easier as well as input from the other senses, such as sight and hearing.
3. Avoid sudden unexpected changes in body position in space.
4. Allow the individual sufficient time after he or she changes position, for example, standing from a sitting position, before beginning to walk, and so forth.
5. Incorporate sensory stimulation into all aspects of the rehabilitation program.

SUMMARY

The impact of the senses on the quality of life of an individual cannot be overemphasized. The senses are important sources of input from one's environment. When these receptors are broken or impaired, sensory deprivation may result. This can lead to confusion, disorientation, social isolation, and the appearance of senility. Rehabilitation of the total person must include evaluation of the degree and effect of sensory impairment before planning and implementing a treatment program.

REFERENCES

1. HENDRICKS, J AND HENDRICKS, CD: *Aging in Mass Society*. Winthrop, Cambridge, MA, 1977.
2. MAGUIRE, GH: *An Introduction to Aging—Module I*. Howard University, Washington, DC, 1982.

3. GUYTON, AC: *Textbook of Medical Physiology.* WB Saunders, Philadelphia, 1976.

4. SAXON, SV AND ETTEN, MJ: *Physical Change and Aging: A Guide for the Helping Professions.* Tiresian Press, New York, 1978.

5. WUEST, FC, ET AL: *The aging eye.* Minn Med 59:540, 1976.

6. MARMOR, MF: *The eye and vision.* Geriatrics 32:63, 1977.

7. FURUKAWA, RE AND POLSE, KA: *Changes in tearflow accompanying aging.* Am J Optom Physiol Opt 55:69, 1978.

8. *Caring for the Visually Impaired Older Person.* Minneapolis Society for the Blind, Minneapolis, 1973.

9. HOLVEY, DN (ED): *The Merk Manual.* Merk & Co, Rahway, NJ, 1972.

10. DOWALIBY, M: *Geriatric ophthalmic dispensing.* Am J Optom Physiol Opt 52:422, 1975.

11. CHALKELY, T: *Your Eyes: A Book for Paramedical Personnel and the Lay Reader.* Charles C Thomas, Springfield, IL, 1974.

12. SLAUGHTER, T: *Vision care for the elderly.* Mod Health Care 4(5):47, 1975.

13. CARROLL, K (ED): *Compensating for Changes and Losses.* Ebenezer Center for Aging and Human Development, Minneapolis, 1978.

14. MARSHALL, L: *Auditory processing in aging listeners.* J Speech Hear Disord 46:226, 1981.

15. VERNON, M, GRIFFIN, D, YOKEN, C: *Hearing loss.* J Fam Pract 12:1053, 1981.

16. BERGMAN, M, ET AL: *Age-related decrement in hearing for speech: Sampling and longitudinal studies.* J Gerontol 31:533, 1976.

17. KEIM, RJ: *How aging affects the ear.* Geriatrics 32:97, 1977.

18. EBERSOLE, P AND HESS, P: *Toward Health Aging: Human Needs and Nursing Response.* CV Mosby, St Louis, 1981.

19. RILEY, M AND FONER, A: *Aging and Society,* vol 1. Trinity, New York, 1968.

20. SCHIFFMAN, SS, MOSS, J, ERICKSON, RP: *Thresholds of food odors in the elderly.* Exp Aging Res 2:389, 1976.

21. THORNBURY, JM AND MISTRETTA, CM: *Tactile sensitivity as a function of age.* J Gerontol 36:34, 1981.

22. WANTZ, MS AND GAY, JE: *The Aging Process: A Health Perspective.* Winthrop, Cambridge, MA, 1981.

BIBLIOGRAPHY

ALLEN, HF: *Insight into the aging eye. Part 1: Cataracts: Functional disability is important in determining the clinical significance.* Geriatrics 30:47, 1975.

ARENBERG, D: *Differences and changes with age in the Benton visual retention test.* J Gerontol 33:534, 1978.

CANETTA, R: *Decline in oral perception from 20 to 70 years.* Percept Mot Skills 45:1028, 1977.

CELESIA, GG AND DALY, RF: *Effects of aging on visual evoked responses.* Arch Neurol 34:403, 1977.

COHEN, S: *Programmed instruction: Sensory changes in the elderly.* Am J Nurs 81(10):1851, 1981.

DEVANEY, LO AND JOHNSON, HA: *Neuron loss in the aging visual cortex of man.* J Gerontol 35:836, 1980.

EDZALL, JO AND MILLER, LA: *Relationship between loss of auditory and visual acuity and social disengagement in an aged population.* Nurs Res (27)5:296, 1978.

ELIAS, JW AND ELIAS, MF: *Matching of successive auditory stimuli as a function of age and ear of presentation.* J Gerontol 3:164, 1976.

GORIN, G: *Glaucoma in elderly.* NY State J Med 78:938, 1978.

GRANICK, S, KLEBAN, MH, WEISS, AD: *Relationships between hearing loss and cognition in normally hearing aged persons.* J Gerontol 31:434, 1976.

HOPKINS, HL AND SMITH, HD (EDS): *Willard and Spackman's occupational therapy.* JB Lippincott, Philadelphia, 1978.

HUGHES, PC AND NEER, RM: *Lighting for the elderly: A psychological approach to lighting.* Hum Factors 23:65, 1981.

HUTMAN, LP AND SEKULER, R: *Spatial vision and aging II: Criterion effects.* J Gerontol 35:70, 1980.

KLINE, DW AND ORME-ROGERS, C: *Examination of stimulus persistence as the basis for superior visual identification performance among older adults.* J Gerontol 33:76, 1978.

KLINE, DW AND SCHIEBER, F: *What are the age differences in visual sensory memory?* J Gerontol 36:86, 1981.

LEDEN, HV: *Speech and hearing problems in the geriatric patient.* J Am Geriatr Soc 25:422, 1977.

LEWIS, SC: *The Mature Years.* Charles B. Slack, Thorofare, NJ, 1979.

NEWMAN, HF: *Palatal sensitivity to touch: Correlation with age.* J Am Geriatr Soc 27:319, 1979.

OSTER, C: *Sensory deprivation in geriatric patients.* J Am Geriatr Soc 24:461, 1976.

SEKULER, R AND HUTMAN, LP: *Contrast sensitivity.* J Gerontol 35:692, 1980.

SHAVER, K AND VERNON, M: *Genetics and hearing loss: An overview for professionals.* American Rehabilitation 4:6, 1978.

WOO, G AND BADER, D: *Age and its effect on vision.* Can J Public Health 69 (Suppl 1):29, 1978.

CHAPTER 7

CLINICAL IMPLICATIONS OF MUSCULOSKELETAL CHANGES WITH AGE

CAROLE BERNSTEIN LEWIS, R.P.T., M.S.G., M.P.A., Ph.D.

BEHAVIORAL OBJECTIVES

Upon completion of this chapter, the reader will be able to
1. Define hypokinesis.
2. List three normal and pathologic causes for changes in strength, flexibility, posture, and gait.
3. Identify limitations a geriatric patient may have in a musculoskeletal rehabilitation program.
4. Suggest specific treatment modification for musculoskeletal problems encountered by older patients.
5. Describe how older patients may differ from younger patients in musculoskeletal parameters.
6. Design a treatment protocol for a geriatric patient with a musculoskeletal disability.

Emily Gordon, a fragile-looking woman in her eighties, fractured her hip one week ago. She is sitting in your office for evaluation and treatment. Next to her is Rachel Spencer, a twenty-year-old athletic-looking woman. Rachel also has a week-old hip fracture.

Their diagnoses are the same. Both have had this injury for the same period of time. Both are women, and they are waiting for you to provide them with the best rehabilitation program. However, they are very different.

If we were to look inside each of them, we would see different musculoskeletal pictures. Rachel is at the point in life when bone density in humans is the greatest, between the ages of 20 and 30 years.[1] After the age of 30 a gradual decrease in bone density occurs (this decrease is greater for women than for men). A general name for this decrease in bone mass is osteoporosis. Characteristic of osteoporosis is a decrease in total skeletal mass; however, the shape, morphology, and composition of the bone are normal.[1] Emily is a candidate for osteoporosis simply because she is a woman over 50. Other contributing factors to this general bone condition are hormonal, nutritional, and circulatory. Women, after menopause, lose large amounts of bone. This is linked to the decrease in hormonal levels.[2] The older person who has a history of poor nutrition will also be a prime candidate for osteoporosis. Finally, decreased circulation as a result of bedrest has been shown to cause osteoporosis in even young and healthy populations.[3] Osteoporosis is usually asymptomatic. However, it can be the major cause of pain, fractures, and posture changes.[4]

Therefore, a general look inside at Emily and Rachel reveals a distinct biologic difference in their seemingly similar bone structure. This difference in bone structure alone can be the cause of orthopedic problems with age.

On the surface, the way Emily and Rachel appear and act focuses on their outward differences. The differences you see are results from biologic, functional, or pathologic causes, or a combination of these causes.

Emily reaches slowly and with much effort for a magazine, but Rachel easily stretches across the table for a journal. You note the difference in their flexibility.

The changes in strength become apparent when Rachel jumps from her chair to the upright posture in the parallel bars. Meanwhile, Emily methodically, cautiously, and with tremendous effort pushes intently on her arms to stand upright in the parallel bars.

Looking back and forth at the parallel bars from Emily to Rachel, you notice the variation in postures.

The two women begin their jaunt down the parallel bars for your examination. Rachel's steps are long and sure. Emily walks in a hesitating and shuffling manner.

As the two pass in the adjacent parallel bars, they discuss the pain they are experiencing. Even in the area of pain they have different outcomes and perceptions.

Flexibility, strength, posture, gait, and pain are functional criteria for independence in daily living. Yet all these criteria change considerably with age.

The change in flexibility, strength, posture, gait, and pain are influenced internally by biologic aging and disease. In addition, functional changes in the lifestyles of the older person can also influence flexibility, strength, posture, gait, and pain. Emily demonstrated large differences in these criteria upon simple observation. Exploring these criteria in detail as to biologic, functional, and pathologic causes, along with modifications for evaluation and treatment, will provide us with the tools to design the best rehabilitation program for someone like Emily Gordon.

LOSS OF FLEXIBILITY

The first difference we noticed in our observation of Rachel and Emily was flexibility.

The change in flexibility as one ages can be the result of the change in collagen, the effects of arthritis, hypokinesis (decreased activity), or a combination of these. The loss of flexibility compounds problems such as difficulty in walking, difficulties in daily activities, pain, and the ability to improve strength.

Collagen—A Biological Cause

Collagen is defined as "the main supportive protein in skin, tendon, bone, cartilage, and connective tissue."[5] These fibers become irregular in shape owing to cross-linking, which increases as one ages.[6] The fibers are less likely to be in a uniform parallel formation in the elderly than they are in younger individuals. This closer meshing and decreased linear pull relationship in the collagen tissue is one reason for the decreased mobility in the body's tissues.[7] Muscles, skin, and tendon are not as flexible and mobile in older persons. In addition, the spine is less flexible owing to collagen changes in the annulus and decreased water content of nucleus pulposa. This results in a decrease in the disk size and a more inflexible spine.

Time is an important treatment consideration in working with tightness caused by collagenous adhesions. Collagen in older persons is less mobile and slower to respond to stretch, but with time it does stretch. The older person can gain flexibility with some compensation for time, just as the younger person can.[8] An effective treatment modification is to provide slow, prolonged stretching activities, either individually or in group exercise classes.

An example of an individual program for stretching a knee flexion contracture caused by collagenous adhesions is to have the person lie prone with a weight on his or her ankle or stump. The person can lie comfortably for 20 minutes. This same type of activity can be done in a group on a large mat. The individuals can face each other and work on fine hand movements, such as picture puzzles. Once the stretch has been held for at least 20 minutes, the group or individual should be encouraged to pursue functional activities with the lengthened limb for as long a period as possible. The nursing staff and family should also be encouraged to participate in the stretching activities.

Elderly people with flexibility decrements require longer rehabilitation programs than do younger patients; however, this is not always possible. An older person with a frozen shoulder, for example, can usually gain full functional range of motion given enough time to slowly progress through an exercise program. Insurance companies will not always recognize needs for this longer period of time for rehabilitation and will limit reimbursement for services. Therefore, the basic treatment strategy should emphasize home exercises from the beginning, thus limiting the need for lengthy clinic treatment care.

Functional exercises and functional ways of measuring improvement should be the core of the home exercise program. An example of this is having the elderly person with shoulder limitations work on reaching objects in the cupboard. The method of evaluating improvement for this person would be comparing heights of objects reached. Elderly persons can also perform daily tasks that encourage their functional motion. As in the case of shoulder limitations, as a person is able to reach for light switches or to dust cabinets, these activities can be given as exercises.

Hypokinesis—A Functional Cause

Hypokinesis, or decreased activity, also can cause an older individual to become less flexible. Elderly people generally sit for longer periods of time than do younger people. This increase in sitting time can cause the older person to have tightness in many of the body's flexor muscles. These flexor muscles, when put into a shortened position for long periods of time, may develop the previously mentioned collagenous adhesions more easily.[9] The hip and knee flexor muscles are commonly tight in the older person. The rotators of the hip also may become tighter because of decreased use in functional activities.

Many times older persons are thought to "naturally" lose range of motion in various joints, such as the shoulders and hips. However, on closer examination these joints reveal a very adequate *functional* range of motion. This then raises the question of which joints are losing flexibility and need rehabilitation intervention. The answer is to consider functional independence in the older person and not to strive for "normal" range of motion as one would for a younger patient.

An assessment of the person's daily activities and how these relate to flexibility should be noted. Although the older person may appear independent and display muscular flexibility, there may be a tightness problem that is manifesting itself in another way. A tightness in the hip rotators may be reflected in the older person's gait pattern or hip stabilization. Therefore, when these problems are seen, a simple range of motion test should be done. Gait difficulties and "daily inertia" problems may relate directly to tight knee and hip flexors, because of the extra strength needed to overcome the tightness.

Decreased flexibility occurs along any muscle that is put in its shortened state for a long period of time. The treatment for this is simply to break up the periods during which the muscles are in a shortened state. Older people need to be encouraged to stand up, to walk around, to lift their arms, to rotate their hips, and to turn and to straighten their legs a minimum of three times a day.

The decreased flexibility displayed by the older person that is clearly a result of hypokinetics does not require intense rehabilitation measures. The rehabilitation professional should act as a consultant to activity programs that will help change the hypokinetic older person into a more active individual. Instruction to members of the health care team and family about flexibility and exercise can be a starting point for daily programs encouraging increased movement. One excellent way to encourage increased motion for home patients is to instruct patients to stand, to stretch, and to shift weight with every television commercial.

Finally, prevention of tightness through activity needs to be encouraged with the older person. Involvement in activities at frequent intervals in the day to maintain range of motion, along with education about the deleterious effects of a sedentary lifestyle on muscular flexibility, provides important tools for intervention in this area.

Arthritis—Pathologic Cause

There are numerous forms of arthritis that can affect any age group. Osteoarthritis, rheumatoid arthritis, and polymyalgia rheumatica are discussed here because they can frequently cause limitations in the elderly.

Osteoarthritis is defined as "an extremely common, noninflammatory, progressive disorder of movable joints, particularly weight-bearing joints, and is characterized pathologically by deterioration of articular cartilage and by formation of new bone in the subchondral areas and at the margins of the joint."[10] The areas most involved in older persons that affect functions are the knees, hips, and the distal interphalangeal joints.[11]

The limitations in motion observed with osteoarthritis may be caused by an acute synovitis caused by minute fragments of articular cartilage that appear in the synovial fluid or by the inability of joint surfaces to slide smoothly owing to deterioration of this articular cartilage. Muscle spasms secondary to pain can also cause limitations of motion. The physical presence of osteophytes that form at joint margins may cause limitations. These structures may also cause pain because they stretch the periosteum, which in turn limits motion. Weakness of muscles owing to disuse may also inhibit a joint's full motion.[11,12]

The treatment modifications for limitation in motion owing to osteoarthritis are first to identify the source of limitation (that is, pain, weakness, or physical limitation). Pain and weakness can easily be identified with the administration of a pain questionnaire and a muscle test.

A physical limitation caused by an osteophyte can be identified by a bony end feel at the point of limitation and by looking at x-ray films.

The appropriate treatment modifications for what has been described above are proper individualized exercise instruction and programming. Exercise is extremely important and should be taught to the patient with care. Frequency of exercises rather than large numbers of repetitions are important to teach to the older person. An average program of instruction should include taking the limited joint through the range of motion two to three times a session three times a day.

Analyzing the cause of flexibility changes as one ages and then using effective treatment planning can improve a situation that may be interfering with an older person's independent functioning. Carefully searching for the biologic, pathologic, or functional cause may reveal a very simple intervention that can provide someone like Emily Gordon more independence in reaching for objects or walking with a more stable step.

LOSS OF STRENGTH

Of course, the inability to move a joint through its range of motion is a factor in independence, but strength is also necessary to perform motion.

Biologic Causes

The obvious decrease in muscular hypertrophy and change in muscular function which occur in the elderly are a result of complex interactions between a variety of factors. These include the reduced ability of the cardiovascular system to deliver raw materials to the working muscles and alterations in the chemical composition of the muscle fibers.[13]

The cardiovascular system does lose some of its efficiency with age.[14] As a consequence, important elements, such as various proteins, are not delivered to the muscle tissues in the same quantity as with younger persons. Glycoproteins are small molecules that produce an osmotic force important in maintaining the fluid content of the tissues. The reduction of this molecule (as in aging) results in an increased difficulty for the tissues to retain their normal fluid content.[15] This results directly in muscle hypertrophy differences in older persons.

In a study of younger and older men in a strength-training program of the quadricep muscle, it was found after two months that both groups had increased in strength to the same level. The interesting point is that the older group increased in girth only by 1 percent to 2 percent, whereas the younger group increased by 12 percent.[16]

The clinical implications of this concept are twofold. First, the physical and occupational therapists need to be aware that the older person does have the potential to significantly increase in strength as a result of treatment intervention. Secondly, in the elderly, increasing girth measurement is not a good indicator of improved muscle strengths. Assessment of an individual's ability to carry out functional activities without muscle fatigue or evaluation of workload achieved in an exercise program (that is, measuring increase in weight per exercise) is a better indicator of the older person's performance.

Chemically, the greatest change with age is a decrease in efficiency of the muscle cells' selectively permeable membrane.[17] Certain chemicals, particularly potassium, magnesium, and phosphate ions, are in high concentration in the sarcoplasm, but other materials, such as sodium, chloride, and bicarbonate ions, are largely prevented from entering the cell under resting conditions. A characteristic feature of senescent muscle is a shift from this normal pattern. In particular, the concentration of potassium is reduced. Lack of potassium ions in aging muscle reduces the maximum force of contraction the muscle is capable of generating. Complaints of tiredness and lethargy by elderly persons result from reduction of potassium ion contents in the tissue. The clinical implication of this is to check for potassium deficiencies if a patient complains of excessive tiredness or lethargy. Attempting exercises with someone who has a potassium depletion will only fatigue the patient more. Therefore, it is imperative to check the tired person's electrolytes prior to beginning exercises.

Pathologic Causes

Numerous strength-altering diseases affect all segments of the population. These causes for muscle weakness may contribute to an older person's loss of strength. One strength-altering disease singular to older persons that has no neurologic basis, can be detected easily, and can be treated effectively is polymyalgia rheumatica.

Polymyalgia rheumatica is a syndrome occurring in older individuals and is characterized by pain, weakness, and stiffness in proximal muscle groups along with fever, malaise, weight loss, and very rapid erythrocyte sedimentation rate. The areas most affected in these persons are the neck, back, pelvis, and shoulder girdle.[18]

The origin is not known, and it affects both men and women, mostly over 65 years of age. The most important aspect of this disease is that it responds dramatically and almost completely to cortocosteroid therapy.[19] Therefore this is not only the best treatment modality but also a diagnostic tool.

The rehabilitation professional should be aware of this disease as a possible cause for weakness, limitation, and pain in the older person. The professional also should realize that the most and only effective treatment is cortisone in the acute phases. Stretching and strengthening exercises may be useful later, along with heat (after the acute phase), if the older person has any residual weakness or limitation.

Functional Causes

Numerous studies show the decline in strength as one ages, especially after the age of 60. Some studies have shown a loss of up to 40 percent of maximum force by the age of 65 years, whereas others indicate a loss of up to 18 percent to 20 percent.[20] The populations of older persons used in these studies have a direct bearing on the results stated. Most older people are less active than when they were younger and therefore will have less strength. A decrease in activity can affect not only flexibility but strength. The subsequent loss of strength will be seen in the muscles that are being used less. The muscles that continue to be used in everyday activities may not have any loss of strength with age. In a study of the abductor muscles of the thumb, it was found that no significant decrease in strength was apparent across age groups. This was due to the continued use of this muscle in daily activities by the older person.[21]

The areas most likely to show a decrease in muscle strength are the active antigravity muscles, such as the quadriceps, hip extensors, ankle dorsiflexors, latissimus dorsi, and triceps.[22] These muscles are used frequently in daily activity; however, they are used to a much greater extent when a person is engaging in vigorous work or athletic-related activities. The older person may no longer engage in these strenuous activities and, therefore, may have less maximum strength, comparatively, in these muscles.

An effective approach to evaluating the functional limitations caused by a decrease in strength is to evaluate the person in a situation that closely resembles the difficult functional activity.[23] The muscles involved can then be strengthened in a close resemblance to the functional activity. Specificity of exercise for functionally strength training an older person is extremely important because, in many older persons, tolerance for activity is decreased. It is imperative not to waste on meaningless exercises the older person's ability to improve in strength.

The following is an example of how to evalute and to train functionally for strength in an older person. If the person has difficulty getting up from a chair, he or she should be evaluated through the stages it requires to achieve that task successfully. In the evaluation, the phase that is most difficult should be noted. The treatment then works on that particular stage and integrates it into the entire activity. Coming up from a chair is broken up into its stages, and each stage is practiced separately. Then the whole activity is practiced with some modifications. The seat levels, for example, can be raised and lowered, or the person can be asked to hold and to resist at various points up and down in the process. This approach would be more beneficial than having the person on a restorator to work on quadricep strength. This approach also requires very little extra equipment.

POOR POSTURE

A decline in strength and flexibility will lead to poor posture. One of the most noticeable orthopedic changes with age is in the area of posture. Normal or good posture traverses a plumb line of the individual in the standing position[24] (Fig 7-1). The lateral view of normal posture has the ear, acromion, greater trochanter, posterior patella, and lateral malleolus in a straight line. In an older person these landmarks and various body curves change their position around this line (Fig 7-

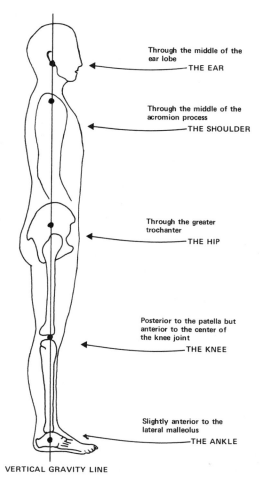

Through the middle of the
ear lobe
THE EAR

Through the middle of the
acromion process
THE SHOULDER

Through the greater
trochanter
THE HIP

Posterior to the patella but
anterior to the center of
the knee joint
THE KNEE

Slightly anterior to the
lateral malleolus
THE ANKLE

VERTICAL GRAVITY LINE

Figure 7-1.   This drawing illustrates proper posture.

2). The older person's head tends to be more forward, shoulders may be rounded, and the upper back will have a slight kyphosis. Populations of older persons who tend to sit for longer periods of time overall have flatter lumbar spines. The lordotic curve may be flatter or more accentuated. The knees and hips will be in slight flexion. There are two major reasons for these changes: One is the changing structure of the intervertebral disk (IVD), and the other is hypokinetics.[25]

Biologic Causes

The IVD is composed of two parts, the anulus fibrosis and the nucleus pulposus. The nucleus pulposus is composed mainly of water. In the sixth and seventh

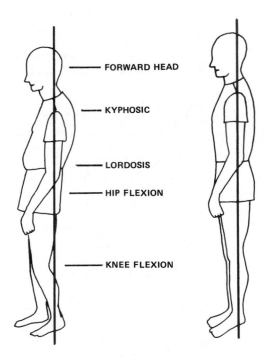

Figure 7-2. This drawing illustrates posture changes with age.

FORWARD HEAD

KYPHOSIC

LORDOSIS

HIP FLEXION

KNEE FLEXION

decades, intracellular water is decreased by 30 percent.[26] The anulus is composed of collagen, which becomes less elastic as one ages. The decreased water in the nucleus and the increased fibrousness of the anulus cause the older person to have a flatter and less resilient disk. This structurally different disk can cause the spine's natural curves to become accentuated or more flexed. This is due to this less-resistant disk succumbing to the continued forces of gravity and muscle pull on the spine, along with the osteoporetic vertebra crumbling, owing to this pressure.

The easiest method of evaluating posture is the use of a plumb line (mentioned earlier). Key points and curves can be noted and measured. The number of centimeters from the ear to the plumb line is an objective and useful measurement. The number of inches from the curve apexes to the plumb line in both the cervical and lumbar areas should be noted.[27] The degree of flexion of the hip and knees while standing can be obtained by goniometry.

The treatment modifications for improving posture in the older person are based on exercise and education. The older person must learn the components of good posture. The patient should then receive information on how his or her posture deviates from this model. Simple stretching exercises can be given along with instruction in adaption of daily activity for improved posture. A simple exercise for a forward head is neck flats (Fig 7-3). These exercises should be en-

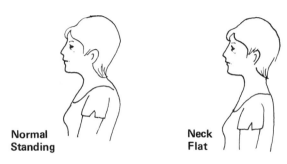

Figure 7-3. Neck flats. Instructions: Standing up straight, tuck the chin in and pull the upper back part of the head toward the ceiling. Hold 10 seconds, breathing normally. Repeat five times.

couraged to be done three to five times twice daily. The Williams exercises can be done for an increased lordosis.

Hyperextension exercises can be tried for a decrease in lordosis. Because the elderly population spends so much time in flexed positions, resulting in kyphotic or decreased lordotic curves, these exercises may prove beneficial (Fig 7-4). For the wheelchair-bound person, a towel roll in the lumbar area or a McKenzie pillow can help restore the lumbar curve and decrease pain.[28] Pectoral stretches can also be very beneficial in stretching muscles commonly tight in the older person (Fig 7-5).

Recreation classes should encourage good posture in their exercise programs. Rehabilitation professionals should not assume that recreational therapists or activity directors understand the components of good posture. Often a rehabilitation professional can visit these classes as a guest lecturer on the topic of good posture.

Functional Causes

Hypokinesis affects posture. Older persons sit for longer periods of time, whether in job situations or during leisure-time activities. The body's flexor muscles will shorten because sitting requires bent hip and knees, decreased lordosis, and increased kyphosis.[29]

Treatment considerations are obvious. Increased activity in positions other than sitting are mandatory. The suggestions for hypokinesis presented in both the strength and flexibility sections can be implemented here.

Pathologic Causes

Any neurologic disease, arthritic involvement, or cardiopulmonary decrement may affect posture. Muscle imbalance caused by neurologic disease can be evaluated and treated. Pain and joint limitation caused by arthritis can be evaluated

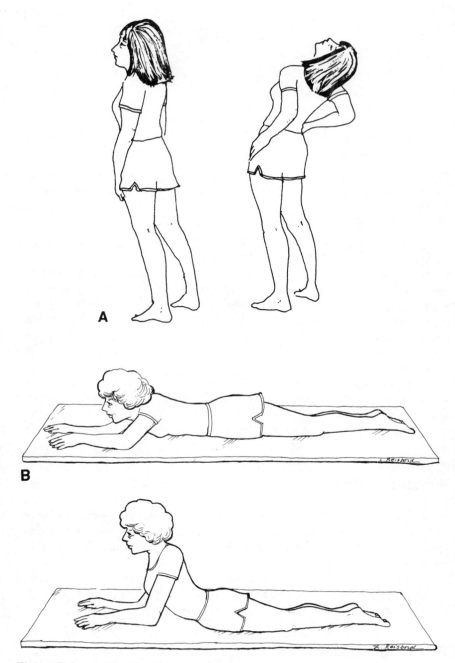

Figure 7-4. A, Place hands in the small of the back and gently bend backward from the waist. Hold 10 seconds and stand up straight. Repeat five times. B, Lying on the stomach, slowly raise the trunk and head and prop on the elbows. Hold 10 seconds. Repeat five times.

METHOD A

METHOD B

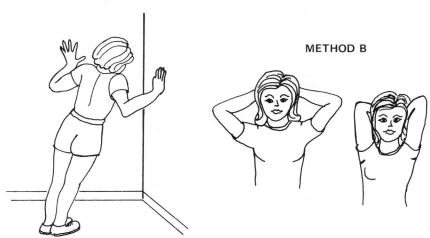

Figure 7-5. Instructions for a pectoral muscle stretch follow. *A*, 1. Stand facing a corner. 2. Hold arms at shoulder level (at shoulder width). 3. Place palm of each hand on each wall. Tighten abdominal muscles. 4. Slowly let the weight of your body fall forward. Do not bend at the waist but move your chest closer to corner. You should feel a "pulling" sensation on the upper part of your chest near the arm. 5. Hold for count of 10. 6. Return to starting position. 7. Do 3 times. Remember to keep the line from the ankles to the hips to the shoulders a straight line. *B*, 1. Lie on your back with your hands behind your head, knees bent, feet flat on mat. 2. Try to touch your elbows to the surface you are lying on (no pillow under head). 3. Be sure not to arch your back. 4. Hold for count of 10. 5. Return to starting position. Relax. 6. Do 3 times.

and treated, as well as chest cavity limitations caused by cardiopulmonary complications. Any disease entity may cause a postural change in the older person, therefore contributing factors of multiple disease should be analyzed and corrected.

Even though poor posture may not directly impede an older person's functional activity, it is worth the small effort required for evaluation, instruction, and treatment intervention. The approach of decreasing postural abnormalities not only has the possibility of preventing increased disability but also encourages improved self-image, body awareness, and body language.

The human body is most efficient in its upright state, allowing maximum length and contraction of its muscles and joints.

CHANGES IN GAIT

The functional application of motion is gait. Just as balance, strength, and flexibility provide for proper posture, so do these three elements provide the background to insure adequate walking in a person of any age.

Figure 7-6 depicts the normal gait cycle. Within this cycle are numerous changes with age. The following is a list of these changes:

1. Mild rigidity, proximal greater than distal (There will be less body motion.)
2. Fewer automatic movements, decreased in amplitude and speed (For example, arm swing will be less.)
3. Less able to use gravity, thus increasing muscle work
4. Less accuracy and speed, especially seen in the hip muscles
5. Shorter steps, to insure safety
6. Stride width broader for a more stable base, to insure safety
7. Decrease in swing-to-stance ratio (This, too, improves safety by allowing more time in the phase of double support.)
8. Decrease in vertical displacement (This is usually secondary to stiffness.)
9. Increase in toe-to-floor clearance (A slight steppage gait may be the result of this.)
10. Decrease in excursion of leg during swing phase (The free leg extends to a much smaller degree.)
11. Decrease in heel-to-floor angle (This may be due to the lack of flexibility of the plantar flexor muscles.)
12. Slower cadence (A slower gait is also another assurance of safety.)
13. Decrease in rotation of the hip and shoulders (This person appears to have a very stiff, unidimensional gait.)
14. Decrease in velocity of limb motions (Arms and legs move at a slower rate when walking.)[30]

Gait is simply the loss and recovery of balance. Inertia and the use of gravity are important aspects of effective, effortless walking. Many of the gait problems of the elderly relate to the inability to maximize inertia and the use of gravity.

Biologic Causes

A combination of the biologic causes of flexibility, strength, and posture limitations are involved in gait changes with age. Stiffness caused by decreased collagen mobility in joints and muscles will cause shorter strides, decreased ancillary limb movements, and less efficient use of gravity and inertia. Decreased strength caused by chemical or circulatory deficiencies will cause a shuffling gait with a dangerously decreased heel-to-floor angle that may cause an older person to fall and thus to sustain a fracture.

Poor posture caused by changes in the internal structure of the bones or disks enhances the decreased vertical displacement as well as the slower cadence.

These biologic changes can be treated by stretching, strengthening, and positioning techniques that closely resemble the deficient phase of gait. For example,

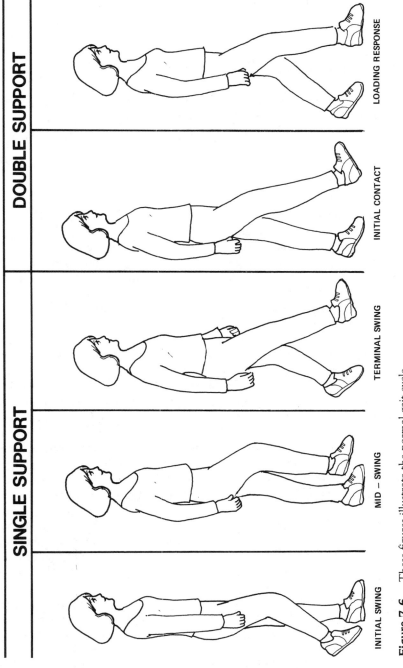

Figure 7-6. These figures illustrate the normal gait cycle.

standing someone with shortened hip flexors in a position of exaggerated hip extension will help increase the range of hip extension in the push-off phase of the gait cycle.

Functional Causes

Functional causes directly relate to hypokinesis. Tightness and weakness in the flexor muscles compound the inefficient gait of the elderly.

Daily routines of exaggerated hip extension, hip rotation, and arm movements practiced regularly will enhance the gait pattern.

Pathologic Causes

"By supporting a newborn infant on his feet, steppage movements can be elicited; however, the mechanism of antigravity support, postural function, and control of equilibrium takes time to develop. These responses depend on the integrity of many interrelated neurological mechanisms and final integration at the cerebral cortical level. Therefore it is not surprising that performance in this area deteriorates with age and that this deterioration is accelerated by pathology changes."[31] (For specific information on nervous and sensory effects on gait, see Chapter 8.)

The particular disease manifestation that will be discussed here is the geriatric amputee. The geriatric amputee is considered to be an amputee over 55 years of age. These special patients stand out because they are more likely than their younger counterparts to have complications or associated problems. Some common complications are stump contractures, atrophy, skin breakdown, and difficulties with the other leg. Some problems the geriatric amputee may have to cope with are financial problems, general weakness, arteriosclerosis, diabetes, cardiovascular and neurologic deficits, in addition to decreased sensory input, difficulty with balance, and a change in posture. This type of patient poses tremendous challenge and is a prime candidate for continuous evaluation and prevention measures.

Ninety percent of people over 55 years of age that have had an amputation had it as a result of a disease.[32] Seventy percent of the same population are amputees as a result of arterial disease.[32] These statistics point out how important it is in the rehabilitation process to consider the entire person with all the concurrent diagnoses and intervening variables.

The following are some treatment modifications for working with someone who is older and has had an amputation. If you are lucky and are able to see the patient before surgery, an evaluation should be done to establish a baseline. The patient should not be allowed to drop below this baseline after surgery. The person should be checked in this evaluation and taught transfer skills and three-point ambulation with the walker in preparation for postoperative programming.[32]

In prosthetic fitting there are several rules to follow. The therapist should be careful of any belts or straps because of the possibility of rubbing on various scars or pressure areas. The older person's skin is more fragile, especially if the patient is diabetic, and breaks down quickly. Remember also that, owing to the older person's decreased reporting of pain, the patient may not report the pain until a sore has already developed.[32]

The prothesis itself should be easy to manuever in gait and application. Many times arthritis of the hands can lead to difficulties with buckles and straps. Therefore, alternative methods of fastening, such as velcro or a suction socket, may be needed. The prosthesis should be as light as possible because of the decreased strength found in the older population; however, this should not be at the risk of security.

It has been found that the most critical phase for the geriatric amputee in the gait cycle is at the point of heel contact and immediately following. This relates directly to the stability of the knee. There are two factors that can cause instability of the knee in a prosthesis. One is the loss of extensor power. This can be compensated for by

1. exercises to increase the quadriceps strength
2. redesigning the prosthesis
3. changing the body alignment
4. attaching elastic to help pull the knee into extension
5. using a knee lock.[32]

The second factor causing instability at heel contact is too much plantar flexion. This can be alleviated by using a soft-sach heel or a single-axis heel.

The energy expenditure in using a prosthesis for the older persons is also an important variable. It has been shown that the energy expenditures required for an elderly patient to walk with an above-knee prosthesis is 55 percent greater than for a normal elderly person.[33] It is also important to remember that a large portion of this energy is being expended by the upper extremities. Any time the upper extremities are used in an activity, there is a tendency for systolic blood pressure to rise.[31] If the patient already has difficulty with cardiovascular compromise, an upper extremity stress test should be done to evaluate the person's ability to ambulate successfully with the prosthesis.

Finally, in working with the geriatric amputee it is extremely important to have a team approach. Encourage frequent and intensive followups and define success of prosthetic wear in terms of its functional usage and psychosocial support for the older person. Ideally, the internist should be part of the rehabilitation process because of the numerous complications the geriatric amputee may face. The team is extremely useful if it can encourage and perpetuate on-going patient groups. There are numerous psychologic and social problems that are faced by an amputee at any age. The ability to participate, to learn, and to share with others who may have similar problems can be very helpful. Frequent and intensive followups are very important in this population because of the continual change in status. Such problems as arthritis, cerebrovascular accidents, weight change, and vascular problems can cause severe complications if not assessed frequently.

The success of the prosthesis must be judged not only in terms of functional ambulation but also in terms of quality of life. If wearing the prosthesis while in the wheelchair enhances the person's self-esteem and social participation, it is not only functional but, in the long run, cost effective. In many instances, because the person has "two legs," he or she will do his or her own dressing, feeding, and daily hygiene without fears of social rejection. This independent functioning instead of using costly personnel to help in these endeavors can be very cost effective. It is obvious that providing a prosthetic device to someone without adequate mentality, motivation, or vigor is inappropriate; however, if the person can appreciate how this device improves the quality of life, its worth is unquestionable.

The geriatric amputee is a very special patient and requires very special care. Modifying the evaluation procedure to include specific aging variables, along with altering the treatment programs to fit the pace and complications commonly seen in these older persons, is essential. The most important aspect treatment, however, is a team approach that probes and encourages individual maximum functional independence.

PAIN

In all the functional criteria previously mentioned, pain can be a limiting factor of each or the cause for functional limitations themselves.

Biologic Causes

There are two major causes for pain differences in the older person. One is the difficulty an older person has in localizing pain.[34] Clinically, this should alert the practitioner to be very specific when asking the older person about pain. The elderly person should also be encouraged to point to the exact location of the pain.

The second difficulty involves the pain pathways. Associated with the pathway that sends most of the chronic pain messages, the spinothalamic pathway, are a number of cells that secrete enkephalin. Enkephalins are the body's own opiates, or pain killers. In older subjects, the production and liberation of enkephalin is reduced, and chronic discomfort becomes more of a problem.[34]

Clinically, techniques for relieving chronic pain should be attempted rather than many of the acute interventions. Such programs as visual imagery, relaxation, and biofeedback transcutaneous electric nerve stimulation can be very effective with older clients in the treatment of chronic pain.[35]

Functional Causes

The primary functional differences in pain between younger and older clients is of a social origin. The older person does not want to complain about pain. Older people as well as younger people hold the stereotype of "the complaining old crock." To avoid fitting into this mold they tend not to report pain as often as their younger counterparts.

Any complaints of pain expressed by an older person should receive very serious attention from the health professional. Knowing that the older person complains of pain less should encourage the practitioner to solicit responses from the older person about his or her feelings of pain through specific questioning techniques.

Pathologic Causes

The two most common disease-induced causes of pain in elderly persons are fractures and arthritis. Fractures in the older person are more common for a number of reasons. On the physiologic level, the osteoporotic bone will fracture with significantly less force. The older person's equilibrium as well as vision may be poorer. These decrements make older people less safe in daily activities and more likely candidates for falls.[36]

The most common areas for fractures in the older person are the hip and wrist.[36] The increased incidence in these areas are directly related to falls. The wrist fracture occurs because the older person attempts to catch himself or herself on the extended wrist. The increased incidence of hip fractures occurs because of the position of the fall and the less efficient kinesiologic leverage at the hip joint.

A fracture in an older person differs from one in a younger person for several reasons. First, the older person heals more slowly. Second, the older person is more prone to complications during the healing process. Some common complications are pneumonia, osteoporosis, decubiti, and mental status complications. The older person may also have fewer support systems to aid in the rehabilitation process (that is, family and friends).[34]

The evaluation of an elderly person with a hip fracture should include very specific questions about complaints of pain. The evaluation should also include assessment of the person's equilibrium, five senses, strength, flexibility, posture, and gait.

Pain in a fractured hip should subside in a few days, or at the most in a week. If the person still complains of pain, the problem should receive additional consideration to determine the source of the pain. Pain in a fractured hip could be nonunion, osteomyelitis, aseptic necrosis, displaced fixation device, bursitis, referred pain from the hip or spine, or fibrositis.[37] This list has specific implications for modifications of treatment.[38] For example, the person may need an additional modality treatment for bursitis that developed as a result of a new gait compensation.[39] It is important that the underlying cause of pain be found and treated so that the person can resume exercise and ambulation activities.

Stress fractures can occur easily with daily activities. The signs of stress fractures are

1. unusual complaints of pain after an exercise,
2. local tenderness,
3. local swelling.[37]

In working with an older person who is suspected of having a stress fracture, encourage activity as long as it doesn't cause pain from the suspected fracture site. It is important that the older person stay as active as possible to avoid future complications. Caution must be taken, however, in any activity to avoid any undue strain on the possible fracture site. In other words, the elderly person can exercise as long as no pain is elicited from the suspected fracture site. (This last bit of information may be very helpful for persons working in facilities that seem to take forever to get the needed physician services.)

Arthritis can cause pain by the presence of osteophytes which stretch the periosteum and may stretch, pinch, or wear nerve endings. Finally, muscle spasms can compound the effects of this pain.[18]

Modalities for the treatment of osteoarthritis begin by incorporating some of the drugs prescribed by the physician. These do not cure osteoarthritis, but they can relieve the symptoms. The modalities that can be used by the older person in a home program with instruction from a rehabilitation professional are heat, cold, and exercise. Heat can be applied in the most simple forms for relief of pain and relaxation. Caution should be stressed in checking for burns. Heat pads should never be turned above low for home use. The older person should be warned about the dangers of sleeping with heat on a body part. Bandages may be advantageous as a form of superficial heat. They are easy for an older person to apply and keep in the body heat. The bandages should be checked to assure enough looseness so that there is no restriction of motion or compromise of the venous system. Many older persons also use linaments as a form of heat. This practice need not be discouraged if the person receives benefit. Many times linaments act as a counterirritant and may work as well as more expensive treatment modalities. If the older person can tolerate its application, cold works to decrease pain and in many cases allows better joint mobilization than heat.

When exercise is treated as a modality, it can do more than just increase range of motion. Increasing strength around a weight-bearing joint can help decrease the shock on that joint during weight bearing. A study done by Radin found that active contraction of a muscle against tension can absorb tremendous amounts of stress.[25] Therefore, strengthening programs are very important, especially in the weight-bearing joints, to aid in relieving stress and improving function.

Mobilization techniques can be used with the older person who has osteoarthritis; however, care should be used. There should be careful consideration of the person's ability to assess and to report pain accurately. Inaccurate reporting of pain can lead to possible damage of fragile joint structures during a mobilization technique.

Some additional treatment comments on osteoarthritis are specific to the different body parts. Osteoarthritis of the shoulder in the older person is usually rare.[18] There is not much degeneration in the shoulder joint, but there is frequently degeneration of the rotator cuff muscles and capsulitis, which may be the cause of pain and limitation. These pathologies respond extremely well to a program of ultrasound, exercise, and mobilization.

The problem of hip pain should instantly alert the rehabilitation professional to make a thorough investigation of the person's daily activities. Too often older people don't complain of their hip pain and continue to walk beyond their pain limits. This actually aggravates the pain, degeneration, and limitation associated with osteoarthritis. The person is putting more stress on an already stressed joint and should be instructed in an incremental ambulation program along with non-weight-bearing exercises. Older persons also can be victims of bursitis. The intertrochanteric bursa is a very common place for inflammation. Many times bursitis around the hips mimics deep joint pain; therefore, careful assessment is needed. Hip bursitis responds well to a decrease in usage along with heat, ultrasound, and/or cold applications.

Osteoarthritis in the knee relates strongly to a person's past or present weight and occupation. It is usually very localized. Ultrasound and cold applications for 20 minutes three times a day, along with exercises to strengthen muscles and decrease stress, may be very helpful. Weight reduction is imperative to help decrease the stress on the knee joint.[40] Again, non-weight-bearing exercises are extremely beneficial in providing the shock-absorbing mechanism discussed earlier.[25]

The cervical area in the older person presents quite an enigma in many instances. Maitland claims that there is no such thing as disk herniation in the older person, and yet there are frequent reports of older persons complaining of radiculitis.[26] Because osteoarthritis of the cervical spine is a continuous process beginning at maturity, it is common to see osteophyte formation at the apophysial joints that may impinge on the intervertebral foramina or any other pain-sensitive structure in the cervical spine. There may also be hyperostosis at the vertebral margins, especially at C-5 and C-6, which may cause neurologic involvement (Fig. 7-7). Any of the above schemas can be exacerbated by a recent injury, such as whiplash. A recent trauma may also bring out an asymptomatic spondylosis in the cervical spine. If the person's pain relates to an acute incident, then rest, positioning, and the use of a collar are indicated until the acute episode subsides. Once the person has received some mild relief or is in a chronic stage, such modalities as heat, ultrasound, traction (beginning gently), and slow range of motion exercises are indicated. When the older person finally has little or no pain, a strengthening and posture program done regularly and gradually should be taught before discharge. The strengthening exercises will aid in providing strong muscles to prevent future injuries and complications. The hyperostosis in the cervical area needs special mention in a very common problem in

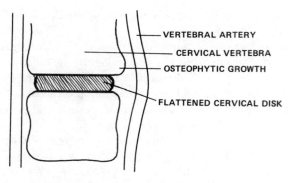

Figure 7-7. This drawing illustrates hyperostosis in the cervical area.

the elderly—falling. Because the disks are smaller and the vertebral margins are larger, owing to the hyperostosis, the vertebral arteries begin to pursue a very torturous path. These arteries can be compromised by even a simple motion, such as neck extension or rotation. One of these motions with its effect on the artery can cause a momentary decrease of blood flow to the brain, and a person may fall or become dizzy. A simple form of treatment for this problem is to limit these motions, and there is hardly a better way than a cervical collar.

CONCLUSION

Looking back on our meeting of Emily Gordon and Rachel Spencer, you now see two patients at varying stages of aging. We now understand how and where they differ on some functional criteria. Now we not only can modify our treatment and evaluation strategies accordingly, but also we can become more adept at outlining the best plan of care for the geriatric patient.

REFERENCES

1. VILLAVERDE, M: *Ailments of Aging From Symptom to Treatment.* Reinhold, New York, 1980.
2. STEINBERG, F: *Cowdry's The Care of the Geriatric Patient.* CV Mosby, St Louis, 1976.
3. CURETON, T: *The Physiological Effects of Exercise Programs on Adults.* Charles C Thomas, Springfield, IL, 1969.
4. SHEPARD, R: *Physical Activity and Aging.* Yearbook Medical Publishers, Chicago, IL, 1978.
5. AGNEW, L: *Dorland's Illustrated Medical Dictionary,* ed 24. WB Saunders, Philadelphia, 1965.

6. SMITH, E AND SERFASS, R: *Exercise and Aging: The Scientific Basis.* Enslow Publishers, Hillside, NJ, 1981.

7. BICK, EM: *Aging in the connective tissues of the human musculoskeletal system.* Geriatrics 11:445, 1971.

8. LESLIE, D AND FREKANEY, G: *Effects of an exercise program on selected flexibility measurements of senior citizens.* Gerontologist 15:182, 1975.

9. HARRIS, R: *Guide to Fitness after Fifty.* Plenum Press, NY, 1977.

10. RODMAN, G: *Primer on the Rheumatic Diseases.* J Am Geriatr Soc 224:5, April 30, 1973.

11. RANEY, B AND BRASHEAR, R: *Shand's Handbook of Orthopaedic Surgery.* CV Mosby, St Louis, 1971.

12. FUDEL'-OSIPOVA, SI AND GRISHKO, FE: *The electromyogram in voluntary contraction of the muscles in old age.* Bulletin of Experimental Biology and Medicine 53:251, 1962.

13. MITOLO, M: *Electromyography on aging.* Gerontolgie, 14:54, 1968.

14. FRANTZELL, A AND INGELMARK, BE: *Occurrence and distribution of fat in human muscles at various age levels: A morphologic and roentgenologic investigation.* Acta Societatis Medicorum Upsaliensis 56:59, 1951.

15. CARLSON, KE, ALSTON, W, FELDMAN, DJ: *Electromyographic study of aging in skeletal muscle.* Am J Phys Med 43:141, 1964.

16. SACCO, G, BUCHTHAL, F, ROSENFALCK, P: *Motor unit potentials at different ages.* Arch Neurol 6:366, 1962.

17. GUTMANN, E AND HANZLIKOVA, V: *Fast and slow motor units in aging.* Gerontology 22:280, 1976.

18. STECHER, R: *Osteoarthritis and old age.* Geriatrics 16(4):167, 1961.

19. DEVAS, M: *Geriatric Orthopedics.* Academic Press, New York, 1977.

20. MURRAY, P: *Strength of isometric and isokinetic contractions in knee muscles of men aged 20 to 86.* Phys Ther, Vol 60, No 4, April, 1980.

21. KAUFMAN, T: *Strength training in the aged* (unpublished master's thesis, 1979).

22. BROWSE, N: *The Physiology and Pathology of Bed Rest.* Charles C Thomas, Springfield, IL, 1965.

23. KAUFMAN, T: *Association between hip extension strength and stand-up ability in geriatric patients* (unpublished manuscript, 1980).

24. KENDALL, H AND KENDALL, F: *Posture and Pain.* Williams & Wilkins, Baltimore, 1980.

25. RADIN, E: *Mechanical effects of osteoarthritis.* Bull Rheum Dis 26:7, 1976.

26. MAYNE, I: *Examination of the back in the geriatric patient.* J Am Geriatr Soc 25:559, 1977.

27. KENDALL, H: *Normal flexibility according to age groups.* J Bone Joint Surg 39(390):694, 1948.

28. MCKENZIE, R: *The Lumbar Spine.* Spinal Publication, Waekanae, New Zealand, 1981.

29. CHERRY, D: *Review of physical therapy alternatives for reducing muscles contracture.* Journal of the American Physical Therapy Association, Vol 60, No 7, July, 1980.

30. IMNS, F AND EDHOLM, F: *The assessment of gait and mobility in the elderly*. Age Aging 8:261, 1979.

31. ADAMS, G: *Essentials of Geriatric Medicine*. Oxford University Press, New York, 1977.

32. PEDERSEN, H: *The Geriatric Amputee: Principles of Management*. Printing and Publishing Office, Washington, DC, 1971.

33. EBERHART, H: *The Geriatric Amputee*. National Academy of Science—National Research Council, Washington, DC, 1961.

34. KATZMAN, R AND TERRY, R: *The Neurology of Aging*. FA Davis, Philadelphia, 1982.

35. ZIEBELL, B: *Wellness: An Arthritis Reality*. Kendall/Hunt Publishing, Dubusque, IO, 1981.

36. KALCHTHALER, T, BASCON, R, AND QUINTOS, V: *Falls in the institutional elderly*. J Am Geriatr Soc 26:424, 1978.

37. SWEEZY, R: *Pseudo-radiculopathy in subacute trochantive bursites of subgluteus maximus bursa*. Arch Phys Med Rehabil 57:387, August, 1976.

38. ADAMS, P, EYRE, H, MUIR, H: *Biochemical aspects of development and aging of human lumbar intervertebral disks*. Rheumatol Rehabil 16:22, 1979.

39. VERNON-ROBERTS, S, AND PIRIE, OJ: *Degeneratuve changes in the intervertebral disk of the lumbar spine and their sequelae*. Rheumatol Rehabil 16:13, 1977.

40. STEINBERG, F: *Gait disorders in the aged*. J Am Geriatr Soc 20:537, 1972.

CHAPTER 8

CLINICAL IMPLICATIONS OF NEUROLOGIC CHANGES WITH AGE

CAROLE BERNSTEIN LEWIS, R.P.T., M.S.G., M.P.A., Ph.D.
KAREN S. JORDAN, O.T.R.

BEHAVIORAL OBJECTIVES

Upon completion of this chapter, the reader will be able to
1. Identify the changes that occur with age in the nervous system.
2. Discuss the opposing theories of nervous system changes with age.
3. Identify precaution in treating the elderly patient with neurologic disabilities.
4. Recognize diseases that will influence the neurologic functioning of the geriatric patient.
5. Understand oromotor dysfunction and design an appropriate feeding therapy program.
6. Apply neurodevelopmental treatment techniques to the geriatric hemiplegic patient.
7. Analyze perceptual motor and self-care dysfunction and understand compensatory and treatment techniques to improve activities of daily living skills.
8. Assess abnormal muscle tone and provide appropriate positioning techniques for the elderly hemiplegic patient.

The nervous system may be thought of as the communication system of the body, the relayer of information. If there is a breakdown or a slowing of this communication system, then the depending structure (the body) will slow and work less efficiently. Picturing the nervous system in this way helps us realize the importance of degenerative effects on the body by an aging nervous system. One of the facts of aging is the decline in neuromuscular function. This decline can be seen as changes in coordination, strength, and speed of movement. Looking more closely at these changes in terms of morphologic, electrochemical, and metabolic changes in the aging nervous system will build a foundation for examining the functional impact of these changes on the elderly individual. This chapter will explore cellular and systemic level changes in the nervous system, as well as subsequent pathologic conditions that may be present. The final portions of this chapter will discuss evaluation and functional approaches to neurologic disabilities.

One of the most widely known facts of the aging nervous system is that there is a loss of neurons.[1] This is due to the fact that neurons are postmitotic cells and do not duplicate themselves.[2] In many other systems of the human body the cells replicate themselves to keep a constant number as various other cells die. This lack of replication makes the neuron very vulnerable to wear and tear. Associated with this loss is the decrease in brain weight as one ages, which can be 10 percent to 12 percent.[3] The gross effects of these losses are narrowing of the convolutions and widening of the sulci. There is much controversy in the literature on aging about the overquoting of neuron loss. First of all, it must be realized that neurons are lost in only certain areas; others show no change.[4] A few of the areas that show the greatest loss of neurons are the frontal lobe (which is the main area for cognition), superior portion of the temporal lobe (which is the main auditory area), occipital lobe (visual area), and prefrontal gyrus (sensory-motor area).[4] If we equate loss of neurons with a decrease in function, we can see where the rehabilitation of an older person may be affected by these changes. The rehabilitation professional may have to compensate for cognitive hearing and visual decrements in the treatment program. The area of sensory-motor decline is also important in expectations and goal setting. Goals that are set by taking into consideration a possible decline in this area and working within these limits may be more realistic to the older person than goals that are set for all different ages, without consideration of possible cognitive impairments.

Another problem in quoting a loss of cells with age is the types of cells that are lost. Recent studies indicate that the greatest loss of cells occurs in those that appear latest and function as associational cells. These cells bear the burden of integrating higher-level activity in the brain.[4] This, too, can emphasize the importance of a health professional's role in simplifying the environment. If the older person has difficulties in integrating, sensory input, and motor activity, then single-step responses and simple commands can be very helpful and assuring.

The final problem in quoting neuron loss in aging is that this process is on a continuum and that there is not a sudden loss with age. Researchers have suggested that there is a continual loss of neurons that does not increase with old age but, rather, is greatest in childhood.[5] This should cue the health professional to begin early intervention of encouragement of all ages to work on various sensory and cognitive enrichment and training activities.

The loss of neurons has also received a counter theory suggested by Marion Diamond.[6] She suggests that plasticity or increase in the branching of nerve cells occurs in all ages; however, it has been found to be at a slower rate in the elderly. She found that animals exposed to a richer environment display more plasticity or branching than animals in a less stimulating environment. This concept can be crucial to the rehabilitation professional. It encourages programs that will provide stimulation to enhance branching of neurons in the central nervous system. What better group to design stimulating environments and programs than health professionals trained in programs that encourage repetition and high-level sensory motor integration?

The inner structure of the nerve cell also changes. This is usually characterized by the accumulation of lipofuscins and neurofibral tangles. Lipofuscins are yellow, insoluble granular material that are thought to be the undegraded waste from partly broken-down membranes and other cell components. These wastes can fill up the cytoplasm and cause the cell to work less effectively.[5] Lipofuscins don't accumulate to the same degree in all nerve cells. They are found more frequently in cells that are less functionally active (or less frequently fired). The vagus nerve that is constantly working to help control the parasympathetic system shows no lipofuscins pigment, whereas the trigeminal nerve that provides sensory and some motor activity to the face and jaw shows the earliest signs of accumulation. On the other hand, neurofibral tangles, which are abnormal neurofibers that are present in large amounts in all different cell bodies, are found only in humans and are present to a much smaller extent in active elderly persons. These tangles are also seen to a greater degree in Down syndrome and Parkinsonism.[7] These cell changes in the elderly appear to point to the importance of continual use of all the different components of the nervous system. This can be done by a well-designed and well-rounded sensory-motor program that would involve exercises of coordination, sensory integration, and repetition for all parts of the body.

The older brain shows some significant electrochemical changes when compared with the younger brain. There is a documented decrease in sulfur and nitrogen in the brain and an increase in sodium.[8] The sulfur and nitrogen are important elements in protein systhesis, and the sodium affects the action potential of nerve impulses. On a larger scale, what is seen is a decrease in nerve conduction velocity.[9] Nerve conduction velocity in the ulnar nerve in an infant is 30 meters per second, in an adult it is 60, and in the elderly person it is 50.[9] Therefore, what is seen is a slight decrease in conduction velocity but not enough to cause the slowing commonly associated with the older person. There is also no difference in velocity from dominant to nondominant side. This probably means that the nerve conduction velocity is unaffected by function. The health professional should be aware of this slight slowing because it may have an effect when tied in with all the other neurologic variables.

Neurotransmitters in the brain of an older person show varied and somewhat inconclusive changes. Because many researchers feel that this is the key to aging, the breakthroughs in neurologic rehabilitation may come in this area. The literature states that there are some decreases in different areas of the central nervous system in the availability of various neurotransmitters (that is, dopamine, noradrenalin, and so forth). However, certain cells with age become more sensitive to these neurotransmitters, and the seemingly serious neurologic deficit that would occur is lessened.[5]

The metabolic changes in the nervous system can be reflected in the oxygen mechanisms of the brain and the microenvironment of the neurons. In the brain there is a decrease in cerebral blood flow and an increase in cerebral vascular resistance as well as a decrease in cerebral oxygen consumption with age[10] (Figs. 8-1 and 8-2). The question is whether the decrease in cerebral metabolism comes from a decrease in cerebral blood flow or if a decreased metabolic rate causes a decrease in oxygen demands. It appears that the decreased metabolic demands are the cause, because animals that do not develop arteriosclerosis still show nerve cell death.[4] In addition, there is a closer arrangement of neurons and capillaries in older persons to compensate for this oxygen decrease. The microenvironment of neurons is changed in the aged in their ability to transport ions and metabolites. The extracellular space is decreased in size by half, along with a decrease in energy metabolism.[8] Glycolysis has an increasing role with age in maintaining the membrane potential of the cell. A fall in this intensity of energy metabolism in the neurons will result in a slowing of the outflow of sodium from the cell and a slowing of the inflow of potassium into it. This is important to the health professional because this can limit the potential and the capacity of the nerve cell for prolonged activity and thus lead to a more rapid development of fatigue.

Finally, all these changes can be integrated, and the older person as a whole entity can be examined neurologically. A few of the aging changes affected by the nervous system that can be seen are in the areas of strength, speed, motor coordination skills, and gait.

Muscle strength is defined by the rate of motor unit firing, the number and frequency of motor unit recruitment, and the cross-sectional diameter of the

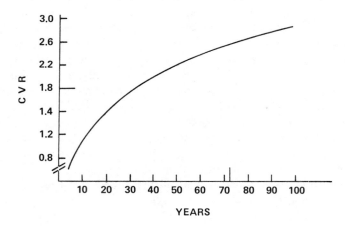

Figure 8-1. Human cerebrovascular resistance changes with age (adapted from Kety[10]).

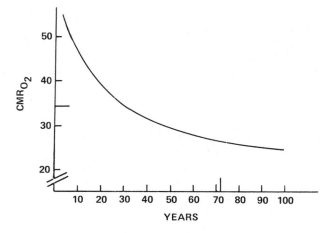

Figure 8-2. Human cerebral oxygen consumption changes with age (adapted from Kety[10]).

muscle.[11] From studies dating back as far as 1835, strength has been shown to peak in the third decade of life and to decline thereafter.[12] This information is based on an average, and there is a great variability in strength decline. This variability depends largely on the activity levels of the persons tested. Therefore, despite the obvious relationship the cellular level neuromuscular changes have to strength decline, disuse, or hypokinesis, plays a very important role in determining the extent of strength decline seen in many older persons. Although the literature quotes the loss of strength with age, new studies are challenging this. One example was a rat study that showed no change in muscle fiber in active old rat diaphragm muscles.[13]

Speed of movement changes are also supported by the earlier cited findings as well as being supported by effects of hypokinesis, or disuse. Generally speaking, older persons are slower on reaction time tasks; however, reaction time tasks measure a complex response pattern. A reaction time task involves different pathways, central processing, afferent pathways, and the effector organ. Sensory stimuli and cognitive functioning become involved in the reaction time task. Therefore, despite effects of other variables, reaction time is a valid assessment of speed of movement.

Coordination motor skills have been shown to decline as early as age 40.[13] In numerous studies there are significant differences between the young and old on varied tests of coordination and fine motor skills. In addition, older persons also display a larger "sway area."[14] In other words, the older person has a diminished ability to maintain balance and requires a larger base area to do this. Even coordination declines with age have been shown to be less with active older persons than with sedentary older persons.[15]

Chapter 7 specifically discusses changes that occur with age in the gait pattern. In addition, the decrease in nerve conduction velocity, as well as the effects of impaired sensory input with age, lead to a sensory motor deficit which can cause or compound the gait changes noted in Chapter 7.

In the neurologic assessment of the older person there are also three other factors that are very important. These are the environment, psychologic forces, and pathology. The environment can affect the older person by decreasing his or her ability to interact with it. If a person interacts less and becomes less active, he or she sends fewer messages up the nervous pathways, which contributes to neurologic atrophy.[16] Psychologic studies have shown that in rats there are some drive changes with age. The example of "unspecific motor drive" or moving or searching without purpose is seen clearly in young rats and is extinct in older rats.[17] Does this happen naturally in the human species also? Is this tied to a lack of biologic drive? This is an interesting question to ponder as one watches an older person in a wheelchair who receives all his or her food and daily care without any motivation to work or even to move for it.

This lack of movement or drive on one side of the continuum can be juxtaposed to fitness on the other side. Fitness is the result of adaptation to repeated motor activity. When a person is fit, the decrements in strength, endurance, and coordination are minimal. The health professional should attempt to encourage a fitness of the older person to the environment by repeated activities that may be broken down into simpler tasks. These simple tasks can then be added together until the older person is "fit" at the entire task and has thus adapted. Although there are changes in the nervous system with age, it appears from more recent research that a few of these changes can be slowed by continued activity throughout life.

Another influencing factor is the effects of pathology on the nervous system of the elderly. There are numerous disorders, such as Parkinsonism, neoplasms, strokes, and vertebral artery syndrome, that are more prevalent in the elderly and can cause extensive damage to the nervous system.[18] It is important for the health professional to remember that these pathologies are not "normal aging" and that in a rehabilitation program these pathologies combine with the previously mentioned age changes in the nervous system.

Parkinsonism is a neurologic disease characterized by the following signs and symptoms:[16]

1. Appearance and attitude:
   (a) unnatural immobility of facial muscles; impassive expression;
   (b) wide palpebral fissures; diminished blinking and eye movements;
   (c) slight or moderate flexion of the head or shoulders, thorax, and pelvis;
   (d) flexion and adduction of limbs at proximal joints;
   (e) slight extension of wrists; fingers flexed at metacarpophalangeal joints and extended peripherally with thumb adducted and extended;
   (f) equino-varus deformity of feet in late stages.
2. Voluntary movement:
   (a) slowness, more conspicuous than weakness, especially of small muscles, i.e., affecting eye movements (poor convergence), mastication, swallowing, articulation (monotonous slurred speech), and fine movements of fingers (writing, dressing, sewing, piano-playing);

(b) associated and synergic movements impaired (arm-swinging in walking, gestures with speech);

(c) paroxysms of akinesia (inability to initiate voluntary movement) complicate the variable state of bradykinesia (slowness of movements).

3. Muscular rigidity:
    (a) agonists and antagonists uniformly affected, but distribution usually unequal on the two sides at onset;
    (b) characteristically "lead pipe" (plastic) unless tremor is evident when it becomes "cog-wheel";
    (c) full range of movements can be elicited until contractures develop.

4. Gait:
    (a) akinesia may make it difficult to start walking;
    (b) bradykinesia creates a shuffling walk of short steps which becomes "festinant" when increasing flexion and diminishing control of equilibrium oblige the patient to catch up with his centre of gravity as it falls forward (or backwards).

5. Tremor:
    (a) most conspicuous at rest;
    (b) rhythmical, 4–6 per second;
    (c) begins unilaterally, usually in an arm, and spreads to affect limbs and trunk, seldom the head;
    (d) associated always with bradykinesia and extrapyramidal rigidity;
    (e) increased by emotional upset;
    (f) suppressed by voluntary movement; by conscious effort and during sleep.

6. Autonomic disturbances:
    (a) uncomfortable flushing, sweating, and seborrhoea;
    (b) excessive salivation;
    (c) tolerance of cold better than of heat.

7. Mental changes:
    (a) irritability;
    (b) depression;
    (c) delirium;
    (d) dementia.

There are no sensory or reflex changes other than difficulty in getting a tendon jerk as muscular rigidity increases.[16]

Parkinsonism is a slow, progressive, degenerating disease. Treatment is aimed at relieving symptoms and increasing or maintaining function. Levadopa is the major medication used for this purpose. Rehabilitation therapists play a role in providing instruction and training in activities of daily living such as feeding, dressing, and ambulating (feeding and dressing are addressed later in this chapter).

Ambulation ideas for improving gait patterns for patients with Parkinsonism are as follows:

1. Footsteps
    (a) assess patient's footstep pattern by lightly painting bottom of patient's shoes with water-soluble paint and asking patient to walk on

shelf paper; show patient his or her gait pattern and then compare it with a normal pattern;

    (b) place cut-out footprints on floor with larger, broader steps for patient to follow.

2. Use reciprocal canes to encourage appropriate arm motion. Have patient hold the ends of two canes while the therapist holds the other ends. The therapist gently moves the canes back and forth while the patient ambulates. This encourages appropriate arm motion.
3. Have patient ambulate in front of a mirror to encourage better posture and gait pattern.

Any age group can be affected by meningiomas or neurofibromas. Neuropathy in older persons may be the first signs of neoplasms. Many growths are slowed by the aging process, so metastasis may be worth removing if it produces a significant neurologic deficit or pain in an older person. Rehabilitation professionals must be aware that neoplasms can affect neurologic responses of the older person.

Patients with cerebrovascular accidents (CVA) comprise a large number of the patients seen by rehabilitation. The older stroke victim has the additional complication of an aging nervous system. This person may be slightly weaker, less coordinated, and slow. Exercises should begin slower, with adequate warm-up and cool-down sessions that last from 5 to 10 minutes before and after an exercise or ambulation session. Special emphasis on coordination exercises is also helpful and can be used as either the warm-up or cool-down activity. Balance exercises for the elderly CVA patient are also very important and can be started as soon as the person can sit with moderate assistance. Balance activities should be continued even if the patient is independent in ambulation. Daily hip circles and weight shifts will ensure the patient's continued proprioceptive realization of the hip joint. Intensive rehabilitation techniques should be encouraged in rehabilitation of the older CVA patient; however, they may have to be broken up into shorter, more tolerable, treatment sessions. Cautions for the use of intensive rehabilitation techniques, such as proprioceptive neuromuscular facilitation, Bobath, Brunnstrom and Rood, are as follows:

1. Be aware of osteoporosis and the possibility of fracturing a bone.
    (a) Avoid positions that place undue stress on the bones.
    (b) Avoid hand placements that place excessive stress on a bone.
    (c) Listen for complaints of unusual pain or tenderness at a specific site after an exercise. Have this checked for a fracture.
    (d) Avoid weight bearing on extremities that have not been actively exercised or where no muscle tone exists. This may cause a stress fracture.
2. Avoid having patient strain when resisting an exercise (avoid Valsalva maneuver).
3. Gently and slowly stretch tight muscles. Allow longer treatment sessions for an older person with tight muscles.

4. Check to be sure that the patient can keep up. Monitor heart rate and allow frequent rests.

The vertebral artery syndrome (VAS) is a blockage or lessening of blood supply in one or both of the vertebral arteries.[19] The vertebral artery syndrome is becoming more well known in rehabilitation owing to the growing interest in mobilization. One of the classic tests in mobilization is to check the blood flow of the vertebral artery. This is done by having the person lie supine while the tester extends, laterally flexes, and rotates the head to the opposite side. If the person being tested has VAS, the person may become dizzy, have blurred vision, or even black out. Similar signs can occur with an older person who has VAS; however, the older person may elicit these signs by simply turning the head. To picture what is occurring, see Fig. 7-7.

From this diagram it is easy to see that the blood supply can be cut off and the person will probably have a "drop attack" and find himself or herself on the floor. To check for this syndrome, simply have the person turn the head to each side. If he or she experience dizziness, nystagmus, or blurred vision, this may be positive for VAS. One easy method of temporary, or in some cases permanent, treatment is to wear a soft cervical collar that does not permit rotation, extension, and lateral flexion of the cervical spine.

Before examining functional approaches to neurologic disabilities, the area of falls must be addressed. Falls are the second leading cause of accidental deaths in the United States, and almost 75 percent of all falls occur in the aged.[20]

Some of the major physiologic reasons for falls among the elderly are

1. decreased cerebral circulation
2. decreased sensory input
3. decreased coordination and balance
4. musculoskeletal changes.[21]

Decreased cerebral circulation can be a result of the vertebral artery syndrome, mentioned earlier, or orthostatic hypotension, which occurs from pooling of blood in lower extremities owing to less muscle mass pushing the blood up the legs and causing dizziness when the person rises suddenly. The elderly person should be instructed to rise slowly, to sit at the edge of the bed before walking, and to take time before walking about after eating a large meal.

Decreased sensory input can cause an older person to miss a step, not to see a rug, or not to hear an on-coming bicycle. Any of these can cause the person to fall. As mentioned in Chapter 6, modifications to enhance the sensory input will aid in preventing falls.

Coordination and balance have already been discussed in this chapter.

Some musculoskeletal changes that may affect stance stability are the occurrence of bunions, hammertoes, corns, and painful arthritic joints. A person who possesses these musculoskeletal changes may ambulate with a different, less steady, gait and hence may fall more easily.

Total rehabilitation of an older person requires checking for the person's safety at all times. Simple shoe modification, exercises, and activity of daily living protocols can help the older person be safer in all environments.

In addition to modifying the environment and treatment programs, rehabilitation professionals working with neurologically impaired older adults can provide effective treatment by initiating functional approaches to the treatment of neurologic disabilities. Common functional problems seen in the older adult with neurologic disability are difficulties in swallowing and performing self-care as well as changes in perceptual motor activities and normal movement.

FUNCTIONAL APPROACHES TO NEUROLOGIC DISABILITIES

Dysphagia

Coughing during eating and aspiration, drooling, and difficulty swallowing are common symptoms of dysphagia. Dysphagic problems need immediate intervention so that feeding therapy may be given to facilitate nutritional intake, to prevent dehydration, and to activate movement of the oromotor structures.

When evaluating a dysphagic patient, the first step is to test for a gag reflex by placing a cotton swab on either side of the uvula (Fig. 8-3). When a gag reflex is absent, it is not feasible to begin oral intake because the patient has no means to prevent aspiration. To facilitate a gag, the therapist places gloved index and middle fingers midway back on the tongue and vibrates it 1 to 2 minutes until a gag reflex occurs. Caution: Do not attempt this technique with a patient who has a bite reflex.

The therapist observes the patient's positioning during feeding. The preferred position to avoid aspiration and facilitate a normal swallowing pattern is to have

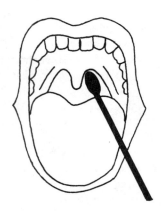

Figure 8-3. Procedure for testing gag reflex.

the patient sit upright in a chair and lean forward (see Figures 8-9 to 8-12). The therapist should be sitting at the patient's eye level or lower so that the patient will keep the head in good alignment and prevent the chances of food going into the trachea and causing aspiration.

The therapist encourages the patient to chew because chewing activates facial musculature contraction and is an activity that helps decrease facial droop and improve speech. If the patient wears dentures or other oral prostheses, immediately place them in the patient's mouth. Ignoring the placement of the patient's dentures causes shrinkage of the gums and results in ill-fitting dentures.

Oromotor assessment includes asking the patient to open and to close the jaw; observe lip closure and lip purse. Sucking ability can be seen by having the patient suck liquid up with a straw. Neuromuscular facilitation of sucking is carried out by use of a facial vibrator for stimulation to the orbicularis oris muscle[22] (Fig. 8-4). Follow by manually pressing the lips to familiarize the patient with the lip-pursing motion. To activate contraction of the orbicularis oris during feeding, care should be taken not to scrape the food off the teeth; active or assistive movement is used to facilitate independence with lip closure over the spoon (Fig. 8-5).

Tongue mobility is evaluated by asking the patient to lick the lips. During this oromotor examination, a graduation of tongue mobility can be documented as follows:

		none	minimal	fair	normal
Protusion					
Depression					
Lateralization	left				
	right				
Evaluation					

Check the appropriate strength.

To increase tongue mobility, paint the lips and the area around the lips with grape jelly, then ask the patient to lick the jelly off. Use a mirror for a visual cue.

Internal tongue lateralization is seen when food is transferred from midline to molars, resulting in chewing. If this motion is weak or absent, food is not chewed or is left in midline. Food should be placed on the molars for stimulation of chewing and for acting as a sensory cue, which facilitates tongue lateralization.

Weakness of tongue-palate motion can be palpated by placing the therapist's gloved index and middle fingers on the tongue and asking the patient to push

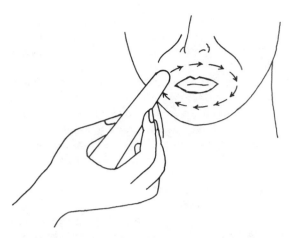

Figure 8-4. Stimulation of the orbicularis oris muscle (adapted from *Sensorimotor Evaluation and Treatment Procedures for Allied Health Personnel*, The Indiana University Foundation, Bloomington, IN, 1974).

the tongue up against the fingers. Tongue-palate evaluation also can be graded on a spectrum of none, minimal, fair, and normal. Strengthening exercises consist of placing a frozen pop between the tongue and roof of the mouth, then instructing the patient to push up against the frozen pop.[23] Frozen pops can be made from lemonade or cranberry juice in a 1 ounce cup that is used for distributing medicine. A tongue blade is used for a holding stick.

Check the patient's uvula and arch of the soft palate when the patient says "ah." Note if the arch appears symmetrical (Fig. 8-6). If the uvula appears to be

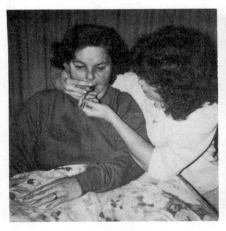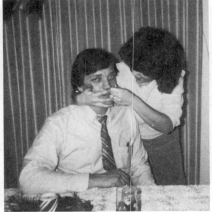

Figure 8-5. These two photographs show how a therapist can support a patient during feeding.

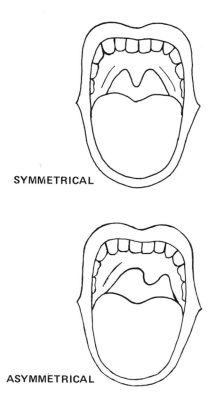

SYMMETRICAL

ASYMMETRICAL

Figure 8-6. A symmetrical soft palate and uvula and an asymmetrical soft palate and uvula (adapted from *Sensorimotor Evaluation and Treatment Procedures for Allied Health Personnel*, The Indiana University Foundation, Bloomington, IN, 1974).

weak on one side, the following helps to compensate for weakness: When the patient is swallowing, instruct the patient to position the head toward the weak side with slight cervical flexion and retraction. Alternatively, manually support the patient's chin with your hand. This is accomplished by standing beside the patient, with the therapist's arm behind the patient's neck and with the therapist's forefinger placed proximal to the patient's nose and upper lip. The therapist's remaining fingers are used to support the lower lip and mandible. This positioning allows the therapist to have complete control of the positions of the head, neck, mandible, and lips (see Figure 8-5).

The presence of a pharyngeal swallow is observed by palpating the rise of the larynx. If there is weakness, stimulate swallowing with a facial vibrator. Begin under the chin and vibrate down the laryngopharyngeal musculature in the direction of their fibers[22] (Fig. 8-7).

Look for the presence of saliva or drooling and the integrity of the mucosa. When thick or increased mucosa is present, avoid mucus-producing foods such as those that contain sugar, sweet citrus, or whole milk.

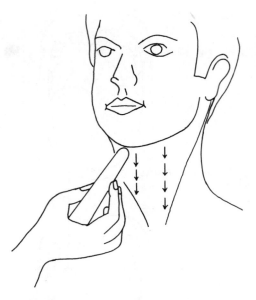

Figure 8-7. Vibration of the larynopharyngeal musculature (adapted from *Sensorimotor Evaluation and Treatment Procedures for Allied Health Personnel*, The Indiana University Foundation, Bloomington, IN, 1974).

Foods that are good for evaluation or swallowing are jello and frozen yogurt, if the patient does not have congestion or excess mucus.

Moderately textured foods should be used for feeding therapy because they form a controllable bolus. Cheese and hot dog chunks, canned fruits, and cooked vegetables are suggested. Be consistent with giving higher-textured foods because the same muscles that are activated for chewing are used for speech. Avoid hot foods. Spicy foods are acceptable because they increase sensory awareness. Avoid foods with varied textures—for example, jello with fruit, or vegetable soup—because those foods require higher functions of tongue coordination. If the patient is unable to chew, food can be prepared in a blender or a baby-food grinder. The ground food is preferred because it provides a more textured bolus.

Initially, liquids should be thickened to control the flow of the substance and to give increased sensory input. A "cut-out cup" is useful because it allows the patient to maintain the cervical spine in flexion while drinking (Fig. 8-8).

Self-feeding

If a patient is to feed oneself, the patient must be able to bring the hand to the mouth while holding a utensil or cup.

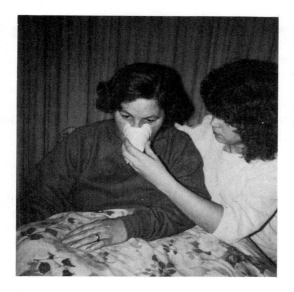

Figure 8-8. Patient drinking from a cut-out cup.

For patients with a weak grasp, a built-up spoon handle can help compensate for the weakness. Foam-rubber tubing, a foam curler, or a bicycle handlebar grip can be used to adapt a spoon for this purpose.

If a patient has difficulty using a spoon because of a weak wrist or improper forearm rotation, a swivel spoon may help prevent spillage. In addition, a therapist can place his or her hand on top of the patient's to facilitate smooth movement and to give tactile guidance as needed.

Foods such as cooked cereal or mashed potatoes are easier for the patient to handle because they do not slip off the spoon.

Suction cups or a rubber pad placed under a patient's bowl can be helpful in eliminating sliding dishes (bowls).

Positioning

When a patient has limited mobility, the therapist should work with the nursing staff to ensure that the patient is repositioned on a routine basis. Positions should include sidelying to the left and right, lying on stomach and back, sitting upright, and, if possible, brief standing.

Immobile stroke or diabetic patients with impaired circulation should be repositioned frequently to avoid decubitis ulcers.

Contracture of the joints and pelvic and scapular retraction in the hemiplegic patient are often attributed to infrequent or improper positioning techniques.

A waterbed is good for decreasing pressure areas and is useful in reducing spasticity. For the patient with Parkinsonism who has trunk rigidity, the waterbed helps normalize muscle tone. It is difficult, however, for a patient to assist in the performance of bedpan transfers, dressing, and coming to sit on a waterbed.

For the hemiplegic patient, place positioning illustrations above the head of the bed. Figures 8-9, 8-10, 8-11, and 8-12 are examples of techniques used for a left hemiplegic patient. The therapist instructs the nursing staff, the patient, and the family in these positioning techniques. A position needs to be changed at least every two hours. A schedule for changing positions can be posted with the positioning techniques.

While the patient is lying supine, and if he or she is flaccid or with flexor spacticity, a pillow is placed under the pelvis to prevent pelvic retraction and external rotation of the leg.[24] When the patient has extensor spacticity, the same technique is used in conjunction with a small pillow placed under the knee to facilitate flexion.

Also while the patient is lying supine, a pillow placed under the affected arm prevents shoulder retraction (See Figure 8-9).

Note that a lap tray is recommended for the patient sitting upright because it provides a weight-bearing surface for the upper extremity and prevents shoulder subluxation. Padded protection for the elbow and upper extremity range of motion exercises decrease ulnar nerve and skin pressure.

To reduce sacral pressure, a 2-inch foam cushion or a silicon pad may be used.

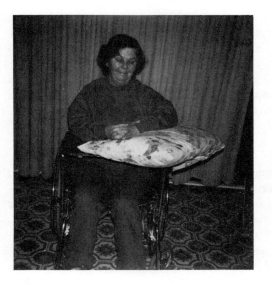
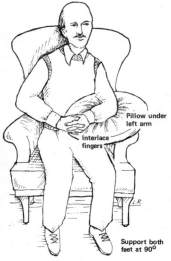

Figure 8-9. Positioning technique for a left hemiplegic patient sitting in a chair.

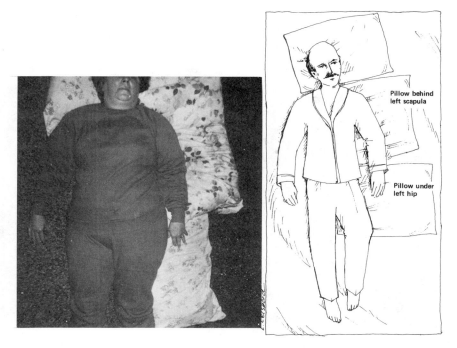

Figure 8-10. Positioning technique for a left hemiplegic patient lying supine.

Toileting

The most basic of all self-care skills which needs considerable attention is the independent care for bowel and bladder eliminations. When establishing a toileting routine, observe the patient's pattern of voiding and bowel movements. A schedule for placing the patient on the toilet can be arranged according to the patient's habits.

Encourage the use of the toilet for bowel movements. The act of transferring and changing to an upright position will help the patient be regular. The combination of movement and gravity are responsible for this being accomplished.

Therapeutic activities are given for toileting independence. While the patient is lying supine in the bed or on the mat with both hips and knees flexed, the patient is asked to raise the buttocks off the bed so that the bedpan can be placed under them.[24]

The therapist gives training for toilet transfers. When the patient is in the wheelchair, encourage him or her to move the chair from the bedside to the bathroom area. If the patient has regained enough strength and sensory awareness, encourage the patient to use all extremities for pushing the wheelchair. It is also feasible to use only the sound side to move the chair.

Therapists also observe how the patient enters the bathroom, the ability to reach and to open the door, to turn on the light, and to maneuver to the toilet.

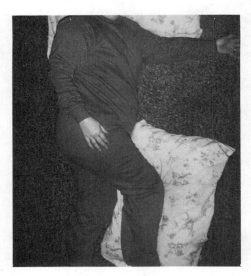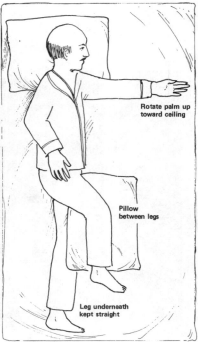

Rotate palm up
toward ceiling

Pillow
between legs

Leg underneath
kept straight

Figure 8-11. Positioning technique for a left hemiplegic patient lying on the left side.

The toileting area should be equipped with grab bars for patient safety and security. A raised toilet seat offers ease in moving to sit and to stand.

The patient should be instructed to lock the wheelchair prior to moving to stand. When the patient demonstrates inability to find the brake on the left side, he or she will need training to restore the ability to integrate and to use the perceptions from the left side of the body.[25] Have the patient practice locking the wheelchair and raising the foot rest before transferring. Be sure to use the same sequence of steps each treatment session.[25]

When the patient moves to the edge of the chair, the therapist should observe both sides of the pelvic girdle for symmetry. Often the affected side remains retracted. To bring the retracted side forward, the patient must shift weight to the sound side and, with the therapist's assistance, bring the retracted pelvis forward. The therapist helps by placing his or her hand under the buttock of the affected side and gently bringing the hip forward.

Before the patient stands, check the patient's foot placement and correct any malalignment, such as feet that are crossed or too close together. Proper foot placement helps the patient have a stable base of support.

It is advantageous to place the sound foot slightly forward. This technique will facilitate weight bearing on the affected side when the patient moves to stand.[24]

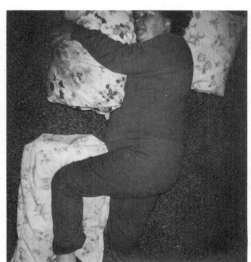
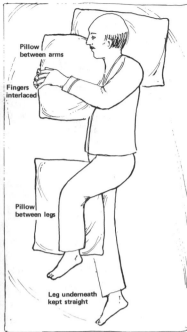

Figure 8-12. Positioning technique for a left hemiplegic patient lying on the right side.

Finally, the patient stands, turns, and moves to sit on the toilet. Never leave a patient unattended if he or she has poor sitting balance or impaired judgment.

The same sequence of steps that was described for transferring from the wheelchair to the toilet is used for getting off the toilet.

Dressing

When the patient begins self-dressing, it is beneficial for the patient to have the ability to move to a sitting position from a lying position, to have good sitting balance, and to have the ability to understand and to use concepts of left and right.

The therapist observes whether the patient has difficulty with the movement transition of moving to sit from lying supine. Preparation for learning to move to sit from lying can be given with activities such as segmental rolling combined with weight bearing on one upper extremity while lying on the side. The therapist gives tactile cues. The therapist's hand placement can be at the patient's head, shoulders, hips, or wherever the patient seems to need assistance with movement. When lying on the side, the patient's upper extremity is placed in a position of shoulder flexion and abduction and weight bearing on the elbow. The therapist assists the patient to bring the lower extremities over the edge of the bed. The patient is then ready to push up to a sitting position at the edge of the bed.

When the patient has difficulty sitting and is unable to sit without assistance, the therapist gives activities to improve the quality of sitting erect and equilibrium reactions. To improve sitting balance the patient may be placed on a program of rocking in a chair for a half hour each day. When the patient is sitting on a mat table, dynamic exercises, such as shifting weight from hip to hip, are given. The therapist places his or her hand under the patient's axilla of the weight-bearing side and brings the musculature into a position of elongation. For the patient who shows ability to maintain a position of sitting erect, the therapist uses a slight pressure to push the patient off the base of support, thus encouraging the patient to right himself or herself back to the neutral position.

Therapists are responsible for evaluating the patient's ability to discriminate and to use the concepts of left and right. The therapist asks the patient to point to the right eye, left shoulder, right knee, left hand, and so forth. When the patient has difficulty perceiving the concepts of right and left, the therapist recommends activities and compensatory devices. For instance, if the patient is hemiplegic on the left side, it is helpful to mark the left insides of dresses, shirts, pants, and so forth so that the patient will know which extremity to place in first. This also aids right-left discrimination.[25] Teaching the patient a routine for dressing and "finding a technique" that demands the least amount of turning of the garment facilitates independence with self-dressing.[25]

Bathing

When a patient is immobile, the patient will bathe himself or herself in bed until his or her strength improves. Place the basin, soap, and washcloth within the patient's reach. Give the patient a long-handled sponge when it is difficult for the patient to reach his or her back and lower extremities.

For safety in the bathtub and shower areas, devices such as rubber mats, safety grab bars, and bathtub or shower seats are recommended. While the patient is bathing, soap on a rope placed around the neck eliminates any bending over for soap that has been dropped. Soap on a rope can be made by drilling a hole through a bar of soap, putting nylon cord through the hole, and tying it together.

Integration of treatment for unilateral neglect can be given during bathing. If the patient is washing or drying the affected side, encourage the patient to look at it.[25] Following drying the affected extremity, have the patient rub it with hand lotion.

Emphasize the importance of thorough washing and drying between the fingers and in the palmar area of the hand in order to maintain good hygiene of the affected extremity. Suction cups attached to the bottom of a hand brush are useful for cleaning the fingernails.

CONCLUSION

When providing treatment to the elderly patient with neurologic dysfunction, it is important to be consistent and to develop a style that enables the patient to practice each skill until he or she has learned it.

It is important for the therapist to provide positive reinforcement when the patient can demonstrate safety and independence with regaining self-help skills.

The doctor, nursing staff, and the patient's family must also be made aware of the patient's progress so that they also can encourage the patient to be independent. Occasionally patients doubt their capabilities and need to be reminded that they are able to do more for themselves.

For the patient who is able to return home following a neurologic problem, the therapist will coordinate with the family or a social worker so that the appropriate self-help devices and equipment will be ordered. A home treatment program is instructed to the family or caretaker. Arrangements for home visiting therapy or outpatient office/clinic treatment may be discussed.

Encourage elderly patients to become active with leisure activities and social events. Through confidence built by regaining independence with self-care skills, readiness to return to the community is achieved.

REFERENCES

1. FROL'KIS, J AND BERZUKOV, V: *Aging of the central nervous system.* Hum Physiol 4(4):478, 1978.

2. GUTMAN, E: *Age Changes in the Neuromuscular System.* Bristol Ltd., Great Britain, 1972.

3. FINCH, C, BEHNLE, J, MOMENT, G: *The Biology of Aging.* Plenum Press, New York, 1978.

4. BRODY, H: Kliemer Lecture, Gerontological Society Meeting, November, 1979.

5. KATZMAN, R AND TERRY, R: *The Neurology of Aging.* FA Davis, Philadelphia, 1982.

6. DIAMOND, M: *The aging brain, some enlightening and optimistic results.* Am Sci 66(1):1, 1968.

7. MORTIMER, J AND PIROZZOLO, F: *The Aging Motor System.* Proeger Special Studies, New York, 1982.

8. GAITZ, C: *Aging and the Brain.* Plenum Press, New York, 1972.

9. ROSSMAN, J: *Clinical Geriatrics.* JB Lippincott, Philadelphia, 1979.

10. KETY, SS: *Aging in the nervous system.* J Chronic Dis 3:478, 1956.

11. WELFORD, A AND BIRREN, J: *Behavior, Aging and the Nervous System.* Charles C Thomas, Springfield, IL, 1965.

12. BIRREN, J: *The Process of Aging in the Nervous System.* Blackwell Scientific Publications, Oxford, 1954.

13. STEINBERG, F: *Cowdry's The Care of the Geriatric Patient.* CV Mosby, St Louis, 1976.

14. Murray, MP, et al: *Normal postural stability and steadiness: Quantitative assessment.* J Bone Joint Surg (Am) 57(A):510, June, 1975.

15. Brunnstrom, S: *Movement Therapy in Hemiplegics.* Harper & Rowe, New York, 1980.

16. Adams, G: *Essentials of Geriatric Medicine.* Oxford University Press, New York, 1977.

17. Bakerman, S: *Aging Life Processes.* Charles C Thomas, Springfield, IL, 1969.

18. Kunze, K and Desmedt, J: *Studies in Neuromuscular Disease.* S Karger, New York, 1975.

19. Naritomi, H: *Effects of advancing age on regional cerebral blood flow.* Arch Neurol 36(7):410, 1979.

20. Perry, B: *Falls Among the Elderly.* J Am Geriatr Soc 30(6), June, 1982.

21. Witte, N: *Why the Elderly Fall.* Am J Nurs, November, 1979.

22. Farber, SD and Huss, J: *Sensorimotor evaluation and treatment for the high risk neonate.* In *Sensorimotor Evaluation and Treatment Procedures for Allied Health Personnel.* The Indiana University Foundation, Bloomington, IN, 1974.

23. Buckley, JE, et al: *Feeding patients with dysphagia.* Nurs Forum 15:69, 1976.

24. Bobath, B: *Adult Hemiplegia: Evaluation and Treatment.* William Heineman, London, 1979.

25. Siev, E and Freishtat, B: *Perceptual Dysfunction in the Adult Stroke Patient.* Charles B. Slack, 1976.

BIBLIOGRAPHY

Aniansson, A, et al: *Muscle strength and endurance in elderly people with special reference to muscle morphology.* In Asmussen, E and Jørgensen, (eds): *Biomechanics VI-A.* University Park Press, Baltimore, p 100, 1977.

Asmussen, E, Fruensgaard, K, Norgaard, S: *A follow-up longitudinal study of selected physiological functions in former physical education students—after forty years.* J Am Geriatr Soc 23:442, 1975.

Astrand, I and Hedman, R: *Muscular strength and aerobic capacity in men 50–64 years old.* J Appl Physiol 19:425, 1963.

Astrand, P and Rodahl, K: *Textbook of Work Physiology.* McGraw-Hill, New York, p 386, 1977.

Birren, J: *Age changes in speed of behavior: Its central nature and physiological correlates.* In Welford, AT and Birren, JE (eds): *Behavior, Aging and the Nervous System.* Charles C Thomas, Springfield, IL, p 191, 1965.

Campbell, M, McComas, A, Petito, F: *Physiological changes in aging muscles.* J Neurol Neurosurg Psychiatry 36:174, 1973.

DeVries, H: *Physiology of exercise and age.* In Woodruff, D and Birren, J (eds): *Aging Scientific Perspective and Social Issues.* Van Nostrand, New York, p 257, 1975.

Gutmann, E, Hanzlikova, U, Jakoubek, B: *Changes in the neuromuscular system during old age.* Exp Gerontol 3:141, 1968.

LAUFER, A AND SCHWERTZ, B: *Neuromuscular response tests as predictors of sensory-motor performance in aging individuals.* Arch Phys Med Rehabil 47:250, 1968.

LIGHT, K: *Effects of mild cardiovascular and cerebrovascular disorders on serial reaction time performance.* Exp Aging Res 4:3, 1978.

MITOLO, M: *Electromyography in aging.* Gerontologie 14:54, 1968.

MUELLER, H: *Facilitating feeding and pre-speech.* In PEARSON, PH AND WILLIAMS, CE (EDS): *Physical Therapy Services in the Developmental Disabilities.* Charles C Thomas, Springfield, IL, 1972.

NORRIS, A, SHOCK, N, WAGMAN, I: *Age change in the maximum conduction velocity of motor fibers of human ulnar nerves.* J Appl Physiol 5:587, 1953.

ROBERTS, J, BASKIN, S, GOLDBERG, P: *Age changes in the neuromuscular system of rats.* Exp Aging Res 3:75, 1977.

RODSTEIN, M: *Accidents among the aged: Incidence, causes, and prevention.* J Chronic Dis 17:515, 1964.

SPIRDUSO, W: *Reaction and movement time as a function of age and physical activity level.* J Gerontol 30:435, 1975.

CHAPTER 9

IMPLICATIONS OF CARDIOVASCULAR AGING

ROBERT A. HABASEVICH, M.S., R.P.T.

BEHAVIORAL OBJECTIVES

Upon completion of this chapter, the reader will be able to
1. Recognize changes in the cardiovascular system occurring with age.
2. Identify the warning signs of cardiac failure.
3. Describe the effects of exercise on the cardiovascular system with age.
4. Explain the functional consequences of cardiovascular changes with age.
5. List the effects of decreased activity on the cardiovascular system.
6. Identify cardiovascular changes with age and to integrate modifications into treatment programs for the geriatric patient.

There comes a time in everyone's life when "how old" one is means nothing more than acknowledgment of the sum of birthdays endured. As we age, less significance is given to chronology, and functional ability becomes the standard to differentiate the young from the old. Cardiovascular disease (CVD) is the primary limiting factor in the elderly person's ability to maintain the same levels of activity experienced during youth.[1] Cardiovascular function in the elderly represents a compromise of physiologic functions resulting from both aging and cardiovascular disease. This chapter reviews the cardiovascular effects of aging with consideration of the pathologic changes common in elderly populations. Appreciation of these combined effects upon the elderly's functional capacity will offer the clinical guidelines with which therapists should approach treatment of elderly patients.

Clinical study estimates that over one half of the 25 million persons over the age of 65 in the US have heart disease,[2] an estimation supported by electrocardiographic evidence.[3] CVD prevalence in this population makes difficult the task of distinguishing between normal heart aging and pathologic change. Clinicians and researchers fail to agree upon a precise definition of the normal heart in the elderly. Thus, as a compromise, normal has become accepted to mean the least degree of cardiovascular abnormality for a specific age group.

The differentiation of change secondary to age or pathology is further complicated by the necessity to interpret cardiovascular function as it relates to the body's metabolic requirements. As one ages, he or she undergoes a decrease in lean body mass, beginning in the third decade and progressing throughout life, thus reducing the body's metabolic oxygen demand[4] as demonstrated at rest and varied levels of work.[5] The body's reduced demand for oxygen will stimulate both functional and morphologic adaptation of the cardiovascular system which must enter into the description of cardiac aging.

Many elderly persons decrease their activity levels, thinking that the "old" are supposed to slow down, a common misconception of society. Still others, limited by musculoskeletal problems, depression, or institutionalization, adapt to an imposed sedentary existence, thus giving rise to cardiovascular deconditioning and hypokinetic disorders. These activity-related changes frequently seen in the elderly represent a series of functional consequences upon which the therapist may have the greatest effect. This chapter addresses the role of prescribed exercise in maintaining optimal cardiovascular function in elderly individuals both with and without known CVD.

MORPHOLOGY OF THE AGING CARDIOVASCULAR SYSTEM

Heart

The appearance of the heart at autopsy provides unreliable evidence to determine accurately the individual's age.[6] Observation of the dissected myocardium demonstrates an accumulation of pathologic changes that have resulted over a lifetime. In the absence of pathology, an observer may have little evidence upon which to estimate age. Size of the heart is more likely reflective of pathology resulting in a thickening of ventricular myocardium than age-related changes.[6] Although study of European populations both with and without heart disease has shown that a general increase of heart weight occurs (males—1g per year, females—1.5g per year),[7] it is believed that this increase in gross weight of the myocardium represents an accumulation of myocardial fat, and true myocardial tissue weight is not affected by age.[8] Smith[9] further suggests that heart size is a function of body surface area and lean body mass rather than of age.

Aging, however, does produce a darkening of the myocardium caused by an accumulation of lipofuscin, a yellow-brown pigment within the nuclei of cardiac muscle cells. Lipofuscin is absent in children and is present in the elderly regardless of sex, race, heart size, or disease state.[10] As such, lipofuscin accumulations most likely represent true biologic aging. It is unclear whether lipofuscin provides any functional significance. However, its prevalence among patients dying of heart failure has given rise to suspicion of its negative implications.[11] Koobs and associates[12] have suggested its relation to mitochondrial damage, which causes reduced myocardial efficiency.

Basophilic degeneration produces a focus of insoluable substances in some myocardial cells universally present in elderly heart tissue.[13,14] These cellular changes suggest a strong aging association, although its quantity is also common to cardiomyopathy.[15]

Within the endocardium, the internal lining of the heart's walls, normal aging produces a proliferation of elastic fibers and collagen, creating a progressive thickening with advancing age.[16] Endocardial thickening most apparent in the atria results from the repeated mechanical events of myocardial tension generation and hemodynamic pressure changes.

The connective tissue and collagen that form the heart's fibrous skeleton and valve systems undergo very little change with normal aging. Pathologic changes of the valves characterized by fibrous proliferation, nodular thickening, lipid accumulation, calcification, and fragmentation is greatest where cusp movement is the greatest[17] and are more evident on the left side of the heart.[18]

Davies and Pomerance[19] and others[20,21] report a loss of muscle cells in the sinoatrial node with increased fibrous tissue occurring with increasing age. However, the correlation of fibrosis to conduction disturbances in the elderly remains low.[22,23] Similar changes in the atrioventricular node have not been identified. However, researchers have noted some loss of fibers in the main branches of the bundle of His and to a lesser degree in the terminal branches in aged populations.[24]

It is important to recognize that with the possible exception of the accumulation of lipofuscin, none of the age-related tissue, cellular, or structural changes present negative functional consequences; in fact, the morphologic changes described in human subjects fail to support the hypothesis that the aging process alone produces cardiac dysfunction. Therefore, in the absence of disease or pathologic process, the elderly heart appears similar to hearts of younger populations. It is the accumulated effects of injury or disease that will eventually present functional disturbances for the majority of the elderly.

Peripheral Circulation

Age-related reduced elasticity of the peripheral vasculature was described over a century ago.[25] Alteration of elastin fiber and its fibrotic replacement occurs in the major blood vessels, as in other body tissues.[26] The eventual collagen infiltration into the vessle walls reduces the vessel's ability to return to initial diastolic diameters during the cardiac cycle. With time and repeated cycles of distension, the process results in a chronic or residual increase in the vessel diameter; this structural change is most apparent in the aorta.[27]

Atherosclerotic disease further contributes to vessel wall rigidity and progresses with age. However, as plaque formation continues, vessel narrowing occurs and thus restricts blood flow. This increased resistance is met by an increased arterial pulse pressure, which is seen to increase both with age and disease.[28,29]

The venous circulation readily demonstrates varicosities in most elderly persons. Distension of the veins increases the volume of venous circulation.[30] Destruction of the venous valves seen with aging contributes to the increase of venous pressure, as the skeletal muscle pumping action ineffectively returns blood to the heart. In summary, age-related changes in the peripheral vascular system most likely present little or no functional consequence during rest or activity requiring submaximal efforts. However, as activity becomes more demanding and the heart attempts to increase the volume of blood pumped to working muscles, age and pathologic changes described above combine to alter the hemodynamic responses that will be described later in this chapter.

Consideration of true aging, therefore, presents little or no evidence that the elderly person's cardiovascular system differs significantly from the younger individual. Changes affecting the system's structure are results of the accumulation of time-induced effects of pathologies affecting equally both structure and function.

PHYSIOLOGY OF THE AGING CARDIOVASCULAR SYSTEM AND ITS FUNCTIONAL CONSIDERATIONS

Cardiac Energetics

The task of describing the physiologic changes which accompany aging is complicated by the problem of differentiation between normal and pathologic processes. Just as these changes contribute to alteration in structure, they also contribute to alteration of function. A review of the major physiologic changes with emphasis upon age versus pathologic processes is presented here.

The heart obtains the vast majority of the energy required to perform its work through aerobic metabolism, more specifically, oxidative phosphorylation.[31] Any disruption of the aerobic pathways, such as a reduced blood flow to the myocardium as seen with CVD, is poorly tolerated and presents a significant threat to life-sustaining cardiac function. In his review of the subject, Hansford[31] concludes that mitochondrial enzyme activity is reduced in the aging heart. However, these findings were obtained from study of the animal model and are not yet clearly applicable to humans. It is possible that as specific enzyme activity is decreased, the heart may undergo compensatory changes that alter its depen-

dence specific enzyme dependent fuel sources resulting in only minimal alteration of energy production. While these alterations are highly probable, they
have not been specifically identified in humans. In summary, it appears that age-
related changes in the aerobic energy pathways provide little limitation to elderly cardiac function.

Electrical Excitation

The true aging effect upon the heart's network of nervous tissues is unclear. As
previously mentioned, over half the population 65 years and older demonstrates
electrical abnormality upon electrocardiographic exam. In a review of the ani-
mal-based literature, Lakatta[32] concludes that interpretation of age-induced
electrocardiogram (ECG) changes is not definitive and emphasizes the need for
further study. Although the frequency of abnormal ECGs increases with age,
the cause is most likely due to pathologic change attributed to CVD rather than
to aging.

Cardiac Hemodynamics

The effect of age on resting heart rate is minimal, declining slightly with age.[33]
Researchers have eliminated autonomic influence by injecting cholinergic and
adrenergic blocking drugs into their subjects. They described the inherent
rhythmicity of the sinoatrial node as exhibiting an age-related decreased rate[34]
as well as prolonged recovery time.[35] Maximal heart rate decreases progressively
with age after the age of 25. Calculation of maximum heart rate has been expressed by the formula (220 − age in years). However, a recent study[36] suggests
these estimates are too low for the North American population and reports maximal heart rates of at least 170 beats per minute are attainable at 65 years of age.
Researchers have explained this decreased maximal heart rate as the effect of a
reduction of sympathetic activity.[37] It should also be noted that plasma norepinephrine has been shown to increase with age, and particularly during activity.[38] Another explanation is the decreased receptor sensitivity or reduction in
the number of receptor sites.[18] Finally, fibrosis of myocardium and resultant
stiffening may contribute a mechanical resistance to heart wall movement[37] and
thereby slow the pumping cycle. It is possible that reduced adrenergic and cholinergic sensitivity, mechanical stiffening, and decreased vagal stimulation all
contribute to the declining maximal heart rate seen with aging.

Ventricular stroke volume is the amount of blood ejected with each heartbeat. The effect of age upon stroke volume is minimal during submaximal effort.[39] However, as effort increases to maximum, the elderly heart demonstrates
a significant reduction in stroke volume.[39,40] At maximum work levels the stroke
volume of the elderly is 10 percent to 20 percent of young adults.[37]

The combined effects of heart rate and stroke volume determine how much
blood is pumped by the heart. Cardiac output is the product of heart rate and

stroke volume, and it is observed to decrease with age.[41,42] The average supine cardiac output of the elderly patient is 25 percent lower than younger adults. During exercise or activity, the increase in cardiac output in response to an increased workload is essentially the same for the young and the elderly. However, the average cardiac output at any given workload is reduced in the elderly.[43] Shephard[36] states that in the elderly peak cardiac output is attained at lower percentages of maximal oxygen consumption levels and is 20 percent to 30 percent lower than in young adults. The exact mechanism of reduced cardiac output is not well understood. At rest, heart rates of the elderly and of young adults present small differences which would implicate deficiencies in stroke volume. The volume of blood ejected with each ventricular contraction is influenced by the volume of blood entering the ventricle prior to ejection, myocardial contractility (or forcefulness of the ejection contraction), and the arterial pressure resisting the ejection of blood from the ventricle, all of which may contribute to decreasing the elderly persons's cardiac output.

Filling pressure of the left ventricle at rest is similar in the young and in the elderly. However, with increasing effort or exercise, filling pressure in the left heart increases, possibly owing to increased myocardial rigidity.[43]

The time from myocardial excitation of the left ventricle to the initiation of blood ejection into the systemic circulation is called the pre-ejection period. This measure provides a useful estimation of ventricular contractility.[44] In the elderly the pre-ejection period is increased, demonstrating a reduced capability for myocardial force generation.[45] The sluggish contraction may be due to mechanical slowing of the myocardial fibers secondary to decreased energy availability,[45] fibrotic infiltration,[43] or loss of coordinated contractile process.[46]

Systolic ventricular pressure and systolic atrial pressure have received the greatest effort of investigation. With age the aorta and adjacent vessels become more rigid and resist ventricular ejection with higher systemic pressures.[47] The effect is more marked with exercise.[41,42,48]

There is little doubt that the elderly heart is limited in its ability to respond to increased physical demands and that it is less efficient; however, these limitations remain slight in view of the major decrease in the total metabolic demand. In the absence of disease or pathology, the elderly heart demonstrates the ability to increase its output and maintain it sufficiently to meet its metabolic needs. Unless metabolic demand increases sufficiently to embarrass the pathologic heart, it may perform quite adequately without sign or symptom of underlying disease.

CARDIOVASCULAR ADAPTATION TO DECREASED ACTIVITY

The elderly become sedentary for many reasons—poor health, loss of a lifelong occupation, depression, institutionalization. In addition to aging and disease, a third variable of deconditioning must be identified for its contribution and effect on cardiovascular function in the elderly. The cardiovascular system exhibits a plasticity of complex adaptations to alter the physiologic and mechanical responses of that system to external work, a fact common to populations regardless of age. Simply stated, the function of the cardiovascular system is to maintain a state of total body homeostasis when presented with physical, emotional, or metabolic stress. If the total sum of metabolic requirement varies little or declines, the cardiovascular system will adapt by decreasing its functional output. If this state is prolonged, the system loses its ability to achieve previous levels of maximal performance. The most significant consequence of such change is a reduction in cardiovascular reserve, or the degree to which cardiac output will increase above resting levels. Unfortunately, many elderly persons reduce their levels of physical activity because of musculoskeletal problems, decline of nerve function, or depression. However, cultural variables have also generated a negative relationship between aging and activity. Old people are supposed to slow down. This perception is often perpetuated by inappropriate physician and family reinforcement.[49] Hence, voluntary inactivity may account for a significant portion of deconditioning of the elderly person, resulting in limited work capacity and self-sufficiency.[49] The accumulated effects of deconditioning upon the cardiovascular system may eventually impair function, giving rise to hypokinetic disease. The older patient is especially prone to cardiovascular effects of deconditioning. Confinement to bed for only brief periods of illness has a marked impact on cardiac reserve. Therefore, any illness that requires the elderly to be confined and inactive will also necessitate an intensive rehabilitative effort to restore the patient to pre-illness levels of cardiovascular function.[50]

Although the body of literature available on the subject of the physiology of aging continues to expand, specific information discussing true aging from the effects of disease and inactivity fails to account for the age-related functional losses.[50,51] This section will present discussion of the cardiovascular response to exercise stress in the elderly and impose upon the clinician the necessity of assessment of that response prior to employing exercise as a therapeutic modality to improve function.

Exercise is a physical stimulus that produces a metabolic increase above resting levels. In young healthy individuals the cardiovascular system responds quickly to such increases in metabolic rate by increasing heart rate, stroke volume, and peripheral blood flow to deliver oxygen to working muscles. The elderly commonly demonstrate variation of those responses and delayed response time for the cardiovascular system to restore homeostasis at the increased level of physical stress.[51,52]

As previously noted, elderly persons have a lower resting cardiac output than younger individuals. In the elderly, basal metabolic rate is reduced primarily owing to age-related loss of lean body mass[51] and inactivity.[53] As exercise progresses, the demand for oxygen by working muscles is met by a linear response in heart rate. And although the absolute level of cardiac output is lower for the elderly at any given level of submaximal effort, the oxygen uptake at that workload is the same for both young and old.[51] The elderly person's system supplies this increased oxygen demand (A-VO$_2$) with oxygen from the circulating blood.[43] As exercise reaches maximum levels, the age-related reduction in heart rate and stroke volume account for a reduced maximal oxygen uptake in elderly subjects. These limitations of oxygen transport capability will translate directly to reduction in the elderly person's physical work capacity.

The age-associated structural changes occurring in the connective tissue result in a progressive stiffness of the myocardium and blood vessels. For the exercising elderly person, this produces an altered hemodynamic response at rest and all levels of physical effort. A higher systolic blood pressure at any given level of cardiac output is observed in the elderly person, but diastolic pressures are similar in both the young and the elderly.[42] As effort and intensity of exercise increase, systolic blood pressure increases linearly for both the young and the elderly. Diastolic pressures in healthy young subjects change very slightly as effort increases, but elderly subjects show a tendency to increase in diastolic pressures to a greater extent.[54]

In summary, the primary difference between the responses of the young and the elderly to acute exercise in the absence of pathology is a reduction in the peripheral blood flow attributed to the elderly person's decreased cardiac output at any given workload. Increased oxygen extraction from circulating blood occurs to compensate for these blood flow reductions.[33,42,43] However, the prevalence of arteriosclerotic disease among the elderly and their sedentary existence may combine to create the situation in which abnormal responses to physical stress remain obscured by the limited functional demands. The physical therapist should accept the responsibility of assessing the elderly patient's cardiovascular response to acute exercise prior to embarking on any exercise program intended to benefit the patient.

Recognition of abnormal responses to physical stress is the basis of cardiovascular function testing. For the physical therapist this means anticipation and observation of abnormal responses each time an elderly patient with suspected heart disease is asked to perform exercise greater than resting metabolic limits.

It is good clinical practice to develop the habit of monitoring the elderly patient's heart rate before, during, and after exercise treatment. The resting pulse should be between 60 and 100 beats per minute. The rhythm should be regular and stable. Irregular or unstable rhythm is indication for electrocardiographic examination before exercising the patient. Whenever possible, resting blood pressure should be taken; systolic values above 150 mm Hg are indication to proceed cautiously when subjecting this patient to physical stress. Exercise should be limited whenever blood pressure exceeds 230 mm Hg.[54] Systolic pressure and heart rate will normally increase with intensity of physical effort. Sudden drop or increase in rate or pressure during exercise is indication of acute pump failure warranting immediate attention. Intensity of exercise should be reduced to minimal intensities to assist venous return via the muscle pump mechanisms.

Observe skin color and temperature. A cool clammy pallor is an indication of circulatory insufficiency and the need to reduce exercise intensity. Neuromuscular incoordination; dizziness; headache; and chest, arm, or jaw pain are reasons to terminate exercise.

Upon cessation of exercise, blood pressure and heart rate should return to resting levels within 5 to 10 minutes, depending upon the exercise intensity and duration. The elderly patient should be observed for the above signs of cardiovascular compromise during recovery from exercise.

Testing the elderly patient's cardiovascular response to acute exercise may be performed to diagnose inherent heart disease. Under such conditions it is necessary to monitor continuously the patient's electrocardiogram to detect early signs of myocardial ischemia. Exercise stress is quantitatively progressed, with physiologic responses recorded. When exercise stimulus creates a sufficient oxygen demand such that the cardiovascular capability to transport oxygen to the working muscles can no longer meet that demand, the maximal oxygen consumption (VO_2 max) level is reached. In individuals with ischemic heart disease, the supply of oxygen to the myocardium is limited by restrictions in coronary blood flow. Ischemic symptoms will appear if exercise is continued at this level. When this occurs the individual is said to have reached the symptom-limited exercise capacity, usually at a submaximal level of VO_2.

The reduced capability of the heart to perform its oxygen transport function is called a reduced cardiac reserve, or the degree to which the heart can perform beyond resting levels. For many elderly individuals with heart disease, reduced cardiac reserves can be significantly improved by chronic exercise, affording these elderly patients an increased physical work capacity with which they can endure and enjoy life. Exercise testing is required prior to treatment to identify appropriate limits of physical stress to stimulate the cardiovascular system safely and efficiently. Under these conditions exercise testing is performed to establish a target heart rate or intensity of effort for training.

CHRONIC EXERCISE AND ITS REHABILITATIVE IMPLICATIONS

Physical exercise and physical training should not be confused. Exercise may be performed at low levels of oxygen consumption. Physical training, however, implies activity performed at high levels of oxygen consumption that, when performed chronically, produces morphologic and physiologic changes that result in an increased physical work capacity. Although the benefits of physical training are desirable for all, individual appropriateness must be determined prior to attempting such training. All elderly persons require some form of exercise; however, there must be careful selection of those who would benefit from physical training if safe and effective enhancement of function is to result.

A primary goal of rehabilitation for the elderly patient with or without heart disease should include the preservation or improvement of physical functional capacity.[50] A program of regular exercise will contribute to the preservation of function; however, if improvement in function is to occur, therapists must employ the training principles of specificity, overload, individual differences, and transience. Above all, these principles must be applied with methodology to guarantee maximum safety of the participants. This section presents an overview of the principles and benefits of cardiovascular training as they apply to the elderly patient.

Physical training using repeated dynamic exercise has been studied most often in young and middle-aged adult populations. The findings of these studies provide the basis for understanding the cardiovascular adaptation to chronic exercise. More recent study of elderly populations demonstrates that physical training produces significant training effects enhancing cardiopulmonary function.[55-61] It is generally recognized that physical training will help maintain or improve physical work capacity in elderly subjects.[55,56] Physical training improves cardiopulmonary efficiency and oxygen transport.[57] And although even slight improvement in oxygen transport results in significantly increased work capacities for the elderly,[58] maximal oxygen consumption levels do not increase to the degree seen with physical training of younger subjects.[59]

The cardiovascular benefit of exercise training elderly subjects have been reviewed by Sidney.[60] He observed that although younger populations demonstrate a difference in resting heart rates between fit and unfit subjects, physical training does not significantly reduce resting heart rates in the elderly. Conversely, blood pressure is unaffected by training in younger subjects, but elderly subjects generally demonstrate reduced systolic and diastolic pressures at rest following training. In response to submaximal efforts, physical training reduces heart rate, diastolic blood pressure, and blood lactate levels in the elderly. The concentration of oxygen transported by the blood per heartbeat is known as the oxygen pulse. It is observed to increase in the elderly following training. This is seen to occur despite the failure of hemoglobin concentrations to increase with training. Training increases total blood volume and total hemoglobin content. An improved oxygen pulse is then explained by an improvement in ventricular contractility and stroke volume. Others[58] measured similar improvement in left ventricular function following 12 weeks of bicycle training, which supports Sidney's assessment that physical training in the elderly results in a set of physiologic adaptations to improve the efficiency of oxygen transport performed by the circulatory system. The therapeutic rationale of employing physical training to improve the elderly patient's functional performances dependent upon aerobic power is sound and is appropriate for many elderly.[60]

The application of physical training procedures for patients with heart disease is well documented.[62] The above benefits obtained by healthy elderly patients are attainable also by selected patients following acute myocardial infarction or coronary bypass surgery. For elderly patients with known or suspected heart disease, an exercise tolerance test is a necessity to determine appropriate and safe levels of training intensities. The intensity of training must be based upon the observed performance of the same metabolic intensity under controlled laboratory conditions. Although symptomatic heart disease presents an added concern to exercising the elderly patient, the risks involved can be minimized by appropriate supervision, monitoring closely physiologic responses, and strict adherence to the principles of exercise training methodologies. The fact that physical training of these patients may result in a reduced cardiac effort for any given level of submaximal external work is extremely important for preservation of optimal activity and performance levels.

Methodology for Training the Elderly

The prevalence of heart disease among the elderly would support the rationale that everyone over the age of 65 is at increased risk to a coronary event and should be cautiously approached with therapeutic exercise training. Patient selection should occur based upon certain criteria with regard to the presence or absence of ischemic cardiac symptoms.[63] Generally, the elderly can be classified into two categories:[64] (1) cardiac-prone patients and (2) cardiac patients. Cardiac-prone patients are individuals with diabetes, hypertension, hyperlipidemia, and family history of coronary heart disease. Cardiac patients are individuals with known heart disease.

The criteria for entry to cardiac training are that patients should be able to exercise, should have recent results of a laboratory-performed graded exercise test, should not be in congestive heart failure, should present a stable angina for over one month, and should be at least two months past acute myocardial infarction or at least two months past cardiac surgery.

Patients with poor control of minor coronary risk factors of smoking, physically sedentary lifestyle, obesity, and type A personalities are poor candidates for exercise training. Elderly patients with obstructive valve disease and marginal cardiac compensation should be excluded from the exercise training program.[64]

The objectives of exercise training for the elderly are to

1. reverse the physiologic effects of deconditioning
2. overcome depression or anxiety
3. improve cardiac function
4. eliminate ischemic symptoms (angina)
5. produce favorable metabolic changes
6. achieve secondary prevention of CVD.[63]

It should be established for each patient that he or she needs exercise and should demonstrate a high motivation to participate in exercise training.

Physical training should be presented to patients in an organized, professionally supervised program. Evaluation and training methods must be convenient, safe, inexpensive, and effective in producing desirable training results. Successful training has employed varied forms of exercise stimuli to achieve desirable effects, including walking,[56,57,61] jogging[56,61,64,65] calisthenics,[56,61,65,66] bicycling,[64,66] and sports.[56,65]

Regardless of the activity employed in training, each participant must have an individual exercise prescription based upon observed response to physical stress. The intensity of effort employed must be sufficiently high enough to produce a training effect and at the same time must afford maximum safety to the patient. It has become customary to refer to measurement of heart rate as indicative of exercise intensity response. By calculation of 60 percent to 80 percent of maximal attainable heart rate, a target heart rate is obtained by which exercise intensity is monitored and adjusted. When ischemic symptoms prevent attaining maximal effort, the target heart rate is established below the symptom-limited threshold. Establishing the target heart rate serves as a guideline for exercise intensity; however, good clinical judgment must prevail on the part of the therapist if abnormal cardiac responses should present during exercise sessions. It must be kept in mind that target heart rates apply only to individuals with normal cardiocirculatory response to exercise. Abnormal changes in exercise heart rate or blood pressure require prompt assessment by the therapist, followed by appropriate patient instruction.

The peripheral effects of training are confined primarily to the working muscles. Exercise employed should attempt to utilize muscle groups required to perform daily activities. Exercise employing both upper and lower extremities should be included in training programs for the elderly, with attention to avoiding isometric contractions and Valsalva maneuvers, both of which produce adverse rises in systolic arterial blood pressure at low levels of cardiac effort.[67]

At least 60 percent of the individual's maximum exercise intensity is required to increase maximal oxygen consumption and endurance.[63] Intensity of exercise influences the training effect to a greater extent than does duration of exercise. Exercise for long duration and at low intensity will have little or no cardiovascular training effect other than burning calories. Exercise intensity approaching 75 percent to 80 percent of maximal oxygen consumption levels when performed continuously for 30 minutes at least three times per week will result in significantly higher oxygen consumption levels after several months. It will also result in lowered submaximal effort heart rate responses and higher stroke volumes in elderly cardiac patients when compared with pretraining values.[63]

When elderly patients with ischemic symptoms of heart disease undergo similar training following the same principles, they are able to perform higher levels of external work before the onset of ischemic symptoms.[62,68] These same individuals demonstrate higher levels of myocardial work as indicated by increased values of the heart rate blood pressure product prior to ischemic threshold. The ability of the heart rate blood pressure product (HRXBP) to predict oxygen supply-demand disparity of the myocardium makes it the appropriate measure of exercise intensity for elderly patients with heart disease.[68] Exercise training at intensities that produce a HRXBP less than the ischemic threshold will avoid adverse ischemic responses and will minimize the risk of cardiac failure.

CONCLUSION

The effects of aging upon the cardiovascular system for all practical purposes must be considered along with the accumulative insults of heart disease and physiologic adaptations to habitual activity. Collectively, cardiovascular aging results in a progressive increase of arterial blood pressure and a reduction of functional cardiac output. The system's ability to respond to activity and physical stress becomes slowed and inefficient with age. Cardiac reserve is reduced, limiting the elderly person's maximal functional performance levels.

The physical therapist must consider these age-induced changes when planning exercise treatment for the elderly. With proper application and attention to the principles and methods of progressive exercise training, many age-related changes can be delayed or reversed in elderly men and women, affording preservation of higher levels of physical function during the aging process.

REFERENCES

1. TASK FORCE ON CARDIOVASCULAR REHABILITATION OF THE NATIONAL HEART AND LUNG INSTITUTE: *Needs and opportunities for rehabilitating the coronary heart disease patient.* DHEW Publication (NIH) No 75-750, December 15, 1974, p 3.

2. KENNEDY, RD, ANDREWS, GR, CAIRD, FI: *Ischemic heart disease in the elderly.* Br Heart J 39:1127, 1977.

3. KITCHIN, AH, LOWTHER, CD, MILNE, JS: *Prevalence of clinical and electrocardiographic evidence of ischemic heart disease in the older population.* Br Heart J 35:946, 1973.

4. SHOCK, NW: *The physiology of aging.* In POWERS, JH (ED): *Surgery of the Aged and Dehabilitated Patient.* WB Saunders, Philadelphia, 1968.

5. McGANDY, RB, ET AL: *Nutrient intakes and energy expenditure in men in different ages.* J Gerontol 21:581, 1966.

6. HUTCHINS, GM: *Structure of the aging heart.* In WEISFELDT, ML (ED): *The Aging Heart.* Raven Press, New York, 1980, p 7-21.

7. LINZBACH, AJ AND AKNOMOA-BOATENG, E: *Die Altersveranderungen des menchlichen Herzens.* I. Das Herzgewicht im Alter Klin Wochenschr 51:156, 1973.

8. REINER, L, ET AL: *The weight of the human heart.* I. *"Normal" cases.* Arch Pathol 65:58, 1959.

9. SMITH, HL: *The relation of the weight of the heart to the weight of the body and the weight of the heart to age.* Am Heart J 4:79, 1928.

10. STREHLER, BL, ET AL: *Rate and magnitude of age pigment accumulation in the human myocardium.* J Gerontol 14:430, 1959.

11. ROSE, GA AND WILSON, RR: *Unexplained heart failure in the aged.* Br Heart J 21:511, 1959.

12. KOOBS, DH, SCHULTZ, RL, JUTZY, RV: *The origin of lipofuscin and possible consequences to the myocardium.* Arch Pathol Lab Med 102:66, 1978.

13. Kosek, JC and Angell, W: *Fine structure of basophillic myocardial degeneration.* Arch Pathol 89:491, 1970.

14. ROSAI, J AND LASCANO, EF: *Basophilic (mucoid) degeneration of the myocardium.* Am J Pathol 61:99, 1970.

15. HAUST, MD, ET AL: *Histochemical studies on cardiac 'colloid.'* Am J Pathol 40:185, 1962.

16. McMILLAN, JB AND LEV, M: *The aging heart.* J Gerontol 14:268, 1959.

17. POMERANCE, A: *Pathology of the myocardium and valves.* In CAIRD, FJ, DALL, JLC, KENNEDY, RD (EDS): *Cardiology in Old Age.* Plenum Press, New York, 1976.

18. KENNEDY, RD AND CAIRD, FI: *Physiology of aging of the heart.* In NOBLE, RJ AND ROTHBAUM, DA (EDS): *Geriatric Cardiology.* FA Davis, Philadelphia, 1981.

19. DAVIES, MJ AND POMERANCE, A: *Quantitative study of aging changes in the human sinoatrial node and internodal traits.* Br Heart J 34:150, 1972.

20. LEU, M: *Aging changes in the human sinoatrial node.* J Gerontol 9:1, 1954.

21. RIDOLFI, RI, BULKLEY, BH, HUTCHINS, GM: *The conduction system in cardiac amyloidosis: Clinical and pathological features of 23 patients.* Am J Med 62: 677, 1977.

22. SIMS, BA: *Pathogenesis of atrial arrhythmias.* Br Heart J 34:336, 1972.

23. THERY, C, ET AL: *Pathology of sinoatrial node. Correlations with electrocardiographic findings in 111 patients.* Am Heart J 93:735, 1977.

24. DAVIES, MJ: *Pathologies of the conduction system.* In CAIRD, FI, DALL, JLG, KENNEDY, RD (EDS): *Cardiology in Old Age.* Plenum Press, New York, 1976, p 57.

25. ROY, CS: *The elastic properties of the arterial wall.* J Physiol (Lond) 3:125, 1880.

26. HASS, GE: *Elastic tissue III. Relation between the structure of the aging aorta and the properties of the isolated aortic elastic tissue.* Arch Path 35:29, 1943.

27. DOTTER, CT AND STEINBERG, I: *The angiocardiographic measurement of the great vessels.* Radiology 52:353, 1949.

28. MASTER, AM, DUBLIN, LI, MARKS, HH: *Normal blood pressure range and its clinical implications.* JAMA 143:1464, 1950.

29. LANDOWNE, M, BRANDFONBRENER, M, SHOCK, NW: *Relation to age to certain measures of performance of the heart and circulation.* Circulation 12:567, 1955.

30. CARLSTEN, A: *Influence of leg variocosities on physical work performance.* In CUMMING, GR, SNIDAL, D, TAYLOR, AW (EDS): *Environmental Effects on Work Performance.* Canadian Association of Sports Sciences, Ottawa, 1972, p 207.

31. HANSFORD, RG: *Metabolism and energy production.* In WEISFELDT, ML (ED): *The Aging Heart.* Raven Press, New York, 1980, p 25.

32. LAKATTA, E: *Excitation-contraction.* In WEISFELDT, ML (ED): *The Aging Heart.* Raven Press, New York, 1980, p 77.

33. BRANDFONBRENER, M, LANDOWNE, M, SHOCK, NW: *Changes in cardiac output with age.* Circulation 12:557, 1955.

34. JOSE, AD AND COLLISON, D: *The normal range and determinants of the intrinsic heart rate in man.* Cardiovasc Res 4:160, 1970.

35. BOLSON, R: *Pacing.* In HARMER, J (ED): *Recent Advances in Cardiology.* Churchill-Livingstone, Edinburgh, 1973.

36. SHEPHARD, RJ: *Human physiological work capacity.* IBP Human Adaptability Project, *Synthesis,* vol 4. Cambridge University Press, New York, 1978.

37. SHEPHARD, RJ: *Cardiovascular limitations in the aged.* In SMITH, EL AND SERFASS, RL (EDS): *Exercise and Aging,* Euslow Publishers, Hillside, NJ, 1980.

38. ZIEGLER, MG, LAKE, CR, KOBIN, LJ: *Plasma noradrenaline increases with age.* Nature 262:333, 1976.

39. BECKLAKE, MR, ET AL: *Influence of sex and age on exercise cardiac output.* J Appl Physiol 20:938, 1965.

40. NIINIMAA, V AND SHEPHARD, RJ: *Training and oxygen conductance in the elderly. I. The respiratory system. II. The cardiovascular system.* J Gerontol 33(3):354, 1978.

41. GRANNATH, A, JONSSON, B, STRANDELL, T: *Studies on the central circulation at rest and during exercise in the supine and sitting body positions in old men.* Acta Med Scand 176:425, 1964.

42. GRANATH, A, JONNSON, B, STRANDELL, T: *Circulation in healthy old men studied by right heart catheterization at rest and during exercise in supine and sitting position.* In BRUNNER, D AND JOKL, E (EDS): *Medicine and Sports: Physical Activity and Aging.* University Park Press, Baltimore, 1970, p 48.

43. STRANDELL, T: *Cardiac output in old age.* In CAIRD, FI, DALL, JLC, KENNEDY, RE (EDS): *Cardiology in Old Age.* Duncan Press, New York, 1976.

44. MONTOYE, HJ, ET AL: *Cardiac pre-ejection period: Age and sex comparisons.* J Gerontol 26:208, 1971.

45. ALBERT, NR, GALE, HH, TAYLOR, N: *The effect of age on contractile protein ATPase activity and the velocity of shortening.* In TANZ, RD, KAVALER, F, ROBERTS, J (EDS): *Factors Influencing Myocardial Contractility.* Academic Press, New York, 1967.

46. SILVER, HM AND LANDOWNE, M: *The relation of age to certain electrocardiographic responses of normal adults to a standardized exercise.* Circulation 8:510, 1953.

47. LANDOWNE, M, BRANDFONBRENER, M, SHOCK, NW: *Relation of age to certain measures of performance of heart and circulation.* Circulation 12:567, 1955.

48. KOENIG, K, REINDELL, H, ROSKAMM, H: *Heart volume and efficiency in 60–75 year old healthy men.* Arch Kreislanfforsch 39:143, 1962.

49. BASSEY, EJ: *Age, inactivity, and some physiological responses to exercise.* Gerontology 24:66, 1978.

50. WENGER, NK: *Rehabilitation of the elderly cardiac patient.* In NOBLE, RJ AND ROTHBAUM, DA (EDS): *Geriatric Cardiology.* FA Davis, Philadelphia, 1981.

51. RAGEN, DB AND MITCHELL, J: *The effects of aging on the cardiovascular response to dynamic and static exercise.* In WEISFELDT, ML: *The Aging Heart.* Raven Press, New York, 1980.

52. SHEPHARD, RJ AND SIDNEY, KH: *Exercise and Aging.* Exerc Sport Sci Rev 6:1, 1978.

53. FENTERN, DH, ET AL: *Changes in the body composition of elderly men following retirement from the steel industry.* J Physiol 258:29P, 1976.

54. AMUNDSEN, LR: *Assessing exercise tolerance: A review.* Phys Ther 59:534, 1979.

55. HODGSON, JL AND BUSHIRK, ER: *Physical fitness and age, with emphasis on cardiovascular function in the elderly.* J Am Geriatr Soc 25:385, 1977.

56. DEVRIES, HA: *Physiological effects of an exercise training regimen upon men aged 52 to 88.* J Gerontol 25:325, 1970.

57. SCHURER, J AND TIPTON, CM: *Cardiovascular adaptation to physical training.* Ann Rev Physiol 39:221, 1977.

58. ADAMS, GM AND DEVRIES, HA: *Physiological effects of an exercise training regimen upon women aged 59 to 74.* J Gerontol 28:50, 1973.

59. BENESTAD, AM: *Trainability of old men.* Acta Med Scand 178:321, 1965.

60. SIDNEY, KH: *Cardiovascular benefits of physical activity in the exercising aged.* In SMITH, EL AND SURFASS, RC (EDS): *Exercise and Aging: The Scientific Basis.* Euslow, Hillside, NJ, 1981.

61. SIDNEY, KH AND SHEPHARD, RJ: *Frequency and intensity of exercise training for elderly subjects.* Med Sci Sports 10:125, 1978.

62. HOSKINS, TA AND HABASEVICH, RA: *Cardiac rehabilitation: An overview.* Phys Ther 58:1183, 1978.

63. DOROSSIEV, DL: *Methodology of physical training: Principles of training and exercise prescription.* In KOENIG, K AND DENOLIN, H (EDS): *Advances in Cardiology: Cardiac Rehabilitation.* S Karger, Basel, 1978, p 67.

64. WILSON, PK: *Policies and Procedures of a Cardiac Rehabilitation Program.* Lea & Febiger, Philadelphia, 1978, p 9.

65. SOUMINEN, H, ET AL: *Effects of 8 weeks' endurance training on skeletal muscle metabolism in 56–70 year old sedentary men.* Eur J Applied Physiol 37:173, 1977.

66. BARRY, AJ, ET AL: *The effects of physical conditioning on older individuals. I. Work capacity, circulatory-respiratory function, and electrocardiogram.* J Gerontol 21:182, 1966.

67. LIND, A: *Cardiovascular responses to static exercise.* Circulation 41:173, 1970.

68. ROBINSON, BF: *Relation of heart rate and systolic blood pressure to the onset of pain of angina pectoris.* Circulation 35:1073, 1967.

PHYSICAL ASPECTS OF AGING

CHAPTER 10

PULMONARY REHABILITATION OF THE GERIATRIC PATIENT

CYNTHIA COFFIN ZADAI, M.S. R.P.T.

BEHAVIORAL OBJECTIVES

Upon completion of this chapter, the reader will be able to
1. Define and identify the pulmonary adaptations that accompany the aging process.
2. Specify the pathologic changes that accompany pulmonary disease.
3. Describe how pathologic changes that accompany pulmonary disease differ from the normal process.
4. Describe the response of the pulmonary system to exercise.
5. Examine and evaluate the pulmonary system of the geriatric patient.
6. Set goals and prescribe a treatment or training program for the geriatric patient with pulmonary complications.

Exercise for the geriatric patient requires consideration from many aspects as evidenced by both this text and the growing specialty field. Medical professionals in the past have considered rehabilitation or return to well-being for the sick and/or injured. But the larger question, "How can a burgeoning portion of our population, the geriatrics, be *kept* well?" has now presented a greater challenge.

Historically, the pulmonary system has not proved a limiting factor in the performance of exercise for the healthy adult or child; consequently, the respiratory response to exercise was simply observed and recorded but did not generally receive specific attention during evaluation or exercise program planning. Pulmonary patients, therefore, who are specifically limited by their respiratory system become difficult patients to treat because there is a paucity of information published regarding the specific physiology of the respiratory response in the individual with pulmonary disease. Only recently has the patient with pulmonary disease been considered a viable candidate for rehabilitation or exercise training.[1] Subjects who are short of breath sitting are not generally stimulated to get up and to walk for necessity, which seems to preclude the idea of exercise for recreation. This prevalent mode of thinking has carried over to the geriatric population, many of whom become exhausted with the simple activities of daily living. To understand the underlying mechanics of both the elderly and the pulmonary-impaired populations, it is helpful to examine the aging process of the pulmonary system. The first section of this chapter specifies the anatomic and physiologic changes consistent with aging, then discusses their similarity to or differences from familiar lung pathology. The next section covers the pulmonary response to exercise, illustrates specifics regarding thoracic physical exam of the geriatric patient, and discusses exercise testing and various training programs. The chapter concludes with a review of the current literature.

ANATOMIC AND PHYSIOLOGIC CHANGES OF THE PULMONARY SYSTEM WITH AGE

In view of the increased awareness regarding our environment over the last few years, it is not surprising that research has been directed to the effect of our atmosphere on the pulmonary system. However, researchers have found it difficult to separate the anatomic and physiologic changes of age from the pathologic response of the pulmonary system to both the passive environment and the created environment (for example, smoking). The lungs are in constant contact with all components of our atmosphere. They, more than any other organ, are exposed to the noxious effects of the air that we breathe. Hence, the changes of age also may be due to environment and the changes of disease, compounded by environment, and separation of the aging process from the environmental effect is difficult at best. Consequently, all changes cited here must be considered within their appropriate context.

Tissue Changes

The anatomic structure of the lung is very specific to its function. A vast surface area is divided into many segments to conduct gas appropriately warmed, filtered, and humidified into the arterial system. This conduction system is comprised of approximately 23 generations of lung tissue eventually leading to the terminal respiratory unit where diffusion and gas exchange occur through the thin-walled alveoli into the capillaries of the pulmonary arterial system.[2] Aging changes this system structurally through loss of elastic fibers from the alveolar walls and ducts, loss of alveolar walls and septra, and an increase in both size and number of the alveolar fenestra.[3,4] Additionally there is a thickening of the medial and intimal layers of the pulmonary arterial walls and an increased thickness of the mucosal bed.[5,6] These structural changes decrease the surface area available for gas exchange, decrease the efficiency of alveolar distension and recoil, and slow the diffusion of gas across thickened membranes. Clinically, these changes are observed and measured by pulmonary function tests. The older individual has an increased closing volume owing to the early collapse of floppier, or more compliant, airways during exhalation. Resting and exercise arterial oxygenation are lower owing to loss of surface area for gas diffusion and increased membrane thickness impeding gas transfer. The resultant mismatching of ventilation and purfusion increases the work of breathing for the elderly patient as well as reduces the patient's exercise capabilities.[7-9]

Functional Changes

Ventilation of the lungs is accomplished by the coordinated action of the diaphragm, ribcage, and underlying lung exerting forces that create the pressure changes necessary to inflate and to deflate the alveoli. The adult human accomplishes this through contraction of the diaphragm and expansion of the ribcage during inspiration. As the underlying lung inflates, the normal tendency of the lung to recoil increases during inspiration, much like a stretched elastic, creating increased elastic pressure and thereby assisting the act of expiration. Loss of elastic fiber with aging decreases the force of expiratory flow with age.[2,10] Specifically, aging produces a floppier lung internally, which will readily inflate but will collapse more slowly and retain a greater volume of air.

Opposing the increase in lung compliance is a decrease in chest wall compliance progressing from age 24 to age 48 years.[11] This stiffening is due to structural changes of the ribcage and its articulations. Because this change is relatively greater than the change in lung compliance, there is a resultant overall decrease in the thoracic system or total lung compliance by age 60.[11,12] Aging, therefore, produces a stiff thoracic cage and a lung with decreased recoil, resulting in an overinflated floppier lung inside a rigid support. In comparison, a 20-year-old person would use 40 percent of the total elastic work of breathing on the chest wall compared with the 70 percent expended in the older individual.[12] The clinical picture of these changes can be illustrated by an elderly individual with a stiffened ribcage held in a somewhat expanded lung state at end expiration. The stiff, partially inflated lung within the ribcage is harder to expand into inspiration and mechanically less efficient.

The efficiency of the musculoskeletal system and the energy expenditure available for breathing are also affected by the static and dynamic lung volumes.[2] Although the total lung capacity does not appear to change significantly with age, vital capacity (VC) is reduced while the functional residual capacity (FRC) and residual volume (RV) are increased (Fig. 10-1).

This may indicate that the increase in airway resistance caused by compression of lung parenchyma at low volumes leads to air trapping and a thereby greater RV. The consequence of an increased RV is a decrease in VC, assuming a constant total lung capacity (TLC). Tidal breathing (V_T) then occurs in a less efficient range on the length tension curve as the ventilatory muscles are shortened, which increases the work of breathing. To imagine this, the normal individual inhales a maximum breath to TLC then exhales half of the inspired breath. Tidal breathing continues on top of this retained air. It is difficult to imagine that this is the geriatric patient's "normal" work for resting ventilation.

If a decrease in V_T results from this excess work, there will be less ventilation of distal lung tissue and an increase in ventilation to perfusion mismatching. Breathing maneuvers involving a large portion of the VC may improve the uniformity of ventilation; however, this requires a greater muscle force and the ability to sustain a larger voluntary level of ventilation. This ability, or the muscle power required to sustain such an effort, decreases with age.[10,13,14] The results of these clinical changes are demonstrated well by the elderly population. The stress of exercise requires a relatively greater amount of work to achieve a smaller gain in function. Fatigue comes faster and at lower levels of stress.

GAS MIXING

Decrease in the partial pressure of arterial oxygen (PaO_2) is also reported with advancing of age.[15,16] The decline parallels the loss of elastic recoil. It is postulated that the loss of recoil and subsequent closure of dependent airways can lead to a shunting of pulmonary blood flow. The resultant ventilation to perfusion (V/Q) mismatch could be a primary reason for decreased PaO_2 in the elderly.[17] It is therefore important to establish the baseline PaO_2 both at rest and during exercise in geriatric patients.[18]

In summary, the geriatric patient has the anatomical disadvantage of an inefficient or energy-expensive lung-thorax pump mechanism and a debilitated gas delivery and exchange system. These handicaps lead to decreased functional ability and an understandable reluctance to participate in the hard work of physical activity.

PATHOLOGIC CHANGES OF THE PULMONARY SYSTEM

The anatomic and functional changes of aging already described are not dissimilar to the pathologic changes seen in patients with chronic lung disease. It is very

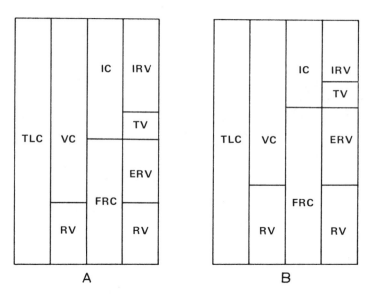

Figure 10-1. Comparison of standard adult lung volumes and capacities (A) with geriatric adult lung volumes and capacities (B) is shown schematically.

difficult, and, in fact, may be impossible, to separate the two entities in the earlier stages of chronic obstructive pulmonary disease (COPD) because both are characterized by insidious onset and similar symptoms. The proper identification of the severity of impairment is necessary, however, during evaluation and treatment of any elderly patient. The pathophysiologic changes of COPD may require the use of medications such as oxygen and bronchodilators as well as a modified exercise program. The risk of complications with exercise is also greater in a system compromised by COPD. The aged pulmonary system may require only a specific exercise program tailored to the patient's level of deconditioning. The compounding changes of COPD exacerbate the aging process and produce a more debilitated and compromised patient.

The symptoms of dyspnea and cough are commonplace among the elderly. People become routinely less active and therefore more short of breath (SOB) with activity as they age. The pathologic tissue changes seen with emphysema and chronic bronchitis are similar to the tissue changes of advancing age.[19] The necessary ability to recognize the additional compromise of COPD, then, is a matter of careful patient assessment and recognition of the disease process. Accurate pulmonary function tests, radiographic data, physical examination, and exercise testing data can contribute to an accurate diagnosis. Although emphysema and chronic bronchitis are pathologically separate, their clinical coexistence is far more familiar.

Emphysema and Chronic Bronchitis

"Emphysema is characterized by abnormal enlargement of the terminal air spaces. In part, the condition is an expression of normal senescence, a loss of elastic tissue from the lung leading to expiratory collapse of the larger air passages, difficulty in expiration and dilatation of the terminal airways."[20]

Chronic bronchitis has a clinical definition based on its symptoms. "If the subject has a chronic or recurrent productive cough on most days for a minimum of three months per year in not less than two successive years,"[21] the subject is considered to have chronic bronchitis.

The terms "chronic airways obstruction" (CAO) and "chronic obstructive pulmonary disease" (COPD) are used to describe the clinical phenomena resulting from the pathologic processes of both emphysema and chronic bronchitis. Both processes have an insidious onset and are frequently dismissed as the heralds of "old age." Functionally, they result in an increase in the work of breathing, whereby a large part of the maximum oxygen uptake (VO_2 max) is consumed by the respiratory musculature whenever exercise is undertaken.[22,23] Clinical symptoms of advanced disease include dramatic drop in PaO_2 with exercise; disproportionately high heart rate (HR) with exercise, coupled with less-than-anticipated increase in stroke volume; and extreme dyspnea.[24-26]

PULMONARY RESPONSE TO EXERCISE

The pulmonary system's response to exercise in the normal, healthy adult includes efficient function of three components: alveolar ventilation, lung and chest wall mechanics, and alveolar to arterial gas exchange. With the onset of exercise, each component steps up its contribution relative to the stress experienced. Initially, an increased tidal volume (V_T) provides more ventilation with light work. An increased respiratory frequency also can be provided by the musculosketal pump as the workload increases, allowing for improved alveolar ventilation. The increased volume of gas provided levels off and plateaus during "steady state" exercise. Alveolar to arterial gas exchange is produced by efficient internal and external respiration. Carbon dioxide produced at the tissues is transported via the blood, diffused across the large surface area of the lung, and eliminated by the lung-thorax pump.[27]

The above processes are slowed with age. The geriatric patient will have a higher ventilatory response for any given submaximal metabolic demand (VE/VO_2).[28] Similarly, the time to reach steady state and to return to resting levels after exercise are also delayed.[29] Once the person is exercising, the ability to sustain a high minute ventilation (V_E) is a factor of both the strength and endurance of the ventilatory muscles.[30] Strength and endurance decrease with age, thereby limiting both the amount and the duration of work a geriatric patient can perform.

The ventilatory muscles make a large contribution to the subject's ability to exercise. During quiet breathing the diaphragm appears to carry the major responsibility for flow of volume. As the stress of exercise is felt, contributions from the ribcage and adbdominals can reduce the diaphragmatic load. By active adbominal contractions in the normal individual, the contents of the abdomen are compressed, forcing the diaphragm into a more favorable position on the length tension curve and reducing its workload.[31]

Advancing age and CAO alter ribcage formation and function as previously described. The stiffened, overextended ribcage resists muscle action. Diaphragmatic movement is also less efficient. The lower, flatter diaphragm position caused by hyperinflation of the lung and expanded ribcage forces the muscle fibers into a shortened, less advantageous position.[32] Recent studies have demonstrated fatigue of the ventilatory muscles by electromyogram, resulting in discoordinated patterns of breathing with stress; however, further study is required to specify the exact mechanisms involved.[33]

Therapists planning exercise programs for elderly persons must therefore be cognizant of their slowed response to exercise, need for longer recovery period, and the specific segments of the ventilatory response which may require individual attention.

PATIENT EVALUATION

The key to success in treating the geriatric patient with or without pulmonary complications is an accurate and comprehensive evaluation. The examination includes observation, palpation, and auscultation.

Observation

Careful scrutiny of a patient's chart and/or family and patient interview can provide answers to many pertinent questions that will be extremely valuable for later program planning. An accurate medical history can specify whether this is a chronically ill patient with an acute exacerbation or an individual newly aware of the inability to exercise or to function on a daily basis. Answers to all pertinent questions (Fig. 10-2) will inform you not only of the patient's physical condition but of his or her mental attitude as well; for example, did the patient come here of his or her own volition or was the patient forced? Is the patient aware that there is a problem? Is the patient eager to participate in the program?

Searching out a social history can be enlightening regarding the patient's support system. The patient's financial circumstances will be useful for practical planning regarding the rehabilitation setting and potential equipment needs.

I. Patient interview
  A. Patient perception of problem/disease process
    1. specific didactic knowledge
    2. emotional reaction
      a. embarrassment
      b. anxiety
      c. preoccupation
      d. denial
  B. Family perception of problem/disease process
  C. Patient description of disease progress and physical performance ability
  D. Patient history of dyspnea/orthopnea

II. Chart review
  A. Medical history
    1. previous admissions and diagnosis
    2. present medical problems: active/inactive
      a. present medications
      b. admitting diagnosis/objectives/care plan
  B. Laboratory studies
    1. pulmonary function tests/ABGs
    2. metabolic studies/blood work
    3. recent ECG
    4. significant radiographic findings

III. Work/social history
  A. Present and past jobs/working environment
  B. Present and past living locations
  C. Social habits
    1. smoking
    2. alcohol
    3. physical activity

Figure 10-2. Answers to pertinent questions will inform the therapist not only of the patient's physical condition but also of the patient's mental attitude.

Once the background information has been solicited, a physical examination or observation of the patient follows (Fig. 10-3).

The patient should be draped appropriately so that thoracic skin surfaces can be adequately viewed (Fig. 10-4).

Examine head, neck, and thorax for signs of chronic musculoskeletal adaptations to pulmonary disease (Fig. 10-5) versus simple changes of age or other musculoskeletal processes.

Chronic pulmonary disease may also be accompanied by changes at the extremities, such as clubbing of the fingers (Fig. 10-6) or swelling of the feet and ankles (Fig. 10-7).

I. Observation
   A. Patient position
      1. use of upper extremities
      2. use of musculature
   B. Thoracic cage
      1. symmetry
      2. ratio of AP to Lat diameter
   C. Breathing
      1. rate and depth
      2. rhythm
      3. pattern

II. Palpation
   A. subcostal angle/AP to Lat diameter
   B. localized expansion/symmetry
   C. excursion/mobility
   D. locate painful areas

III. Auscultation
   A. Normal breath sounds
   B. Abnormal breath sounds
   C. Adventitious breath sounds

Figure 10-3. A physical examination is part of the patient evaluation.

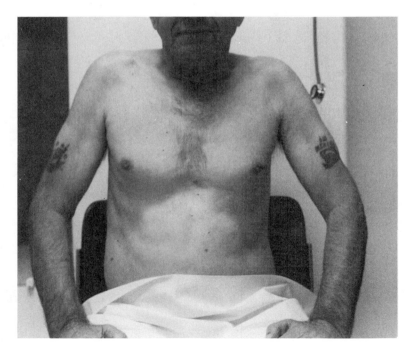

Figure 10-4. Shown here is a patient appropriately positioned and draped, thorax exposed.

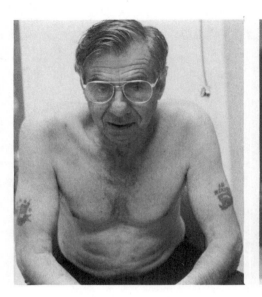
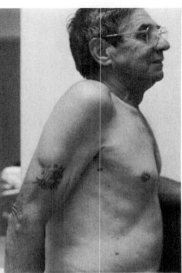
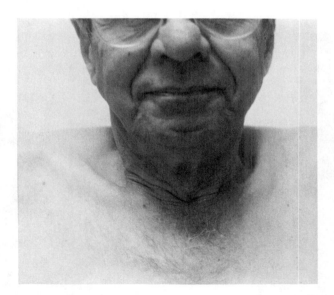

Figure 10-5. Signs of musculoskeletal adaptations to pulmonary disease are visible here: use of upper extremities to fix shoulder girdle, increased AP diameter, retraction above clavicles, and visible accessory musculature.

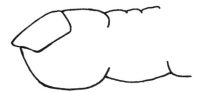

Figure 10-6. Clubbing, swelling of the distal phalanx is illustrated here. There is an increase of the base angle of the nail.

Palpation

Reduction in expansion and excursion can be evidence of decreased thoracic mobility and loss of compliance (Fig. 10-8). These symptoms are present with both CAO and advancing age.

An increase in the subcostal angle generally indicates a widening of the thorax in the anterior/posterior (AP) plane as the RV increases (Fig. 10-9).

These anatomic changes can be confirmed by palpation and comparison of AP/to lateral diameter. A 1-to-1 ratio is consistent with the term "barrel chest" (Fig. 10-10). These are changes that increase the work of breathing at rest, creating an extra workload during exercise.

The technique of palpation also can be used to assess the patient's level of relaxation, to locate areas of pain, or to test for voice sounds (Fig. 10-11). Fingertip pressure along the accessory muscles assesses the level of tension present in the muscle fibers. A rotating circular motion of the fingertips over thoracic surfaces assesses for areas of pain or musculoskeletal deformity. The use of the palmar surface or the ulnar border of the hand as the patient speaks will detect areas of voice transmission or "tactile fremitus." Increased transmission of voice

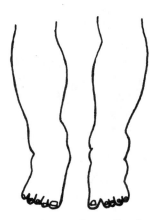

Figure 10-7. Illustrated here are chronically swollen feet and ankles.

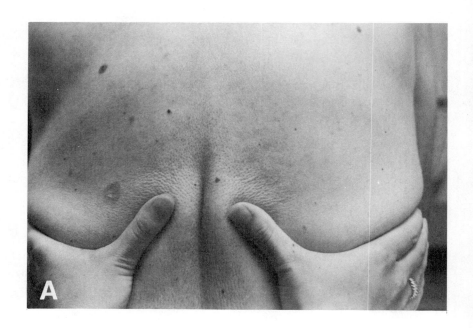

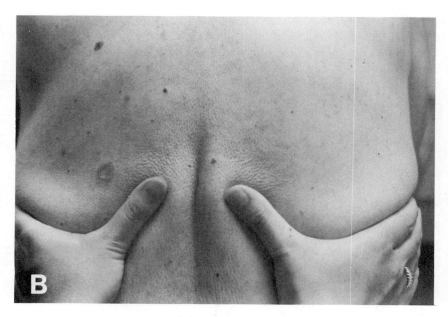

Figure 10-8. There is minimal motion observed before inspiration (A) and after inspiration (B).

PHYSICAL ASPECTS OF AGING

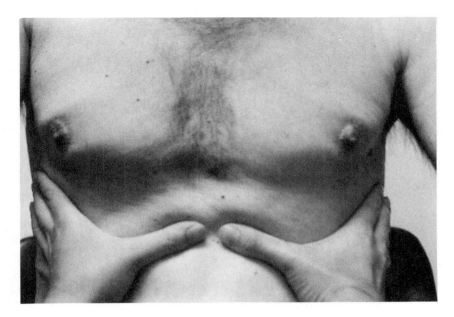

Figure 10-9. Measuring of the increased subcostal angle is shown here.

sounds indicates increased density of the underlying tissue, such as with an infiltrate, a consolidation, or possibly an effusion.

Auscultation

Auscultation is a useful technique to confirm the findings of both observation and palpation. Use of a stethoscope to auscultate breath sounds establishes a baseline level of normal or abnormal breath sounds. The presence of adventitious or additional breath sounds indicates acute or chronic pulmonary pathology. For example, the patient complaining of only morning cough can be assessed for presence or absence of secretions at the time of examination to establish chronicity. Many patients who cough chronically are so accustomed to their own cough that they don't notice it throughout the day.

Tidal breathing through the nose will provide vesicular breath sounds to the mid-lung fields in normal individuals. To auscultate the lungs accurately, the therapist must ask the patient to breathe softly and slowly through the mouth with an increased tidal volume. This increased ventilation creates vesicular breath sounds to the bases of the lungs in the normal individual. Both right and left lungs are ausculated to provide accurate baseline information (Fig. 10-12).

Elderly individuals or those with CAO many times present with decreased breath sounds at the lung bases owing to tissue loss and decreased air movement. Even when ventilation is increased to VC volumes, their breath sounds

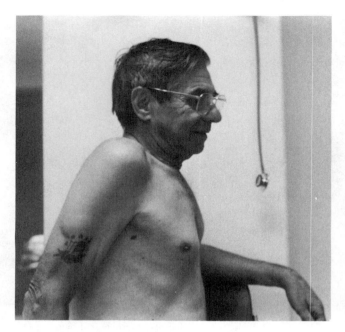

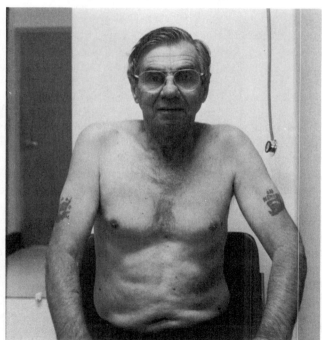

Figure 10-10. Comparison of AP with lateral diameter. Patient has 1-to-1 ratio, or a "barrel chest."

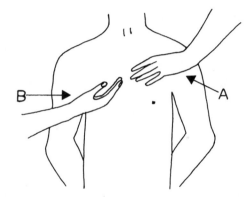

Figure 10-11. Palpation instructions: Use the palmar surface and fingers to locate deformities and areas of pain (A); use the ulnar border to palpate vocal fremitus: transmission of voice sounds through the chest wall (B).

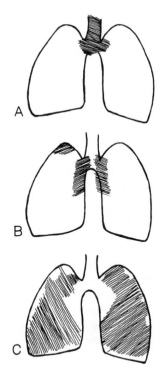

Figure 10-12. Auscultation: A, location of bronchial or tracheal breath sounds, B, location of bronchovesicular breath sounds, C, location of vesicular breath sounds.

remain distant or inaudible. Additionally, these patients may have rales caused by atelectasis or fluid overload and rhonchi resulting from excess or trapped secretions in the larger airways. These are adventitious breath sounds heard in addition to normal or abnormal breath sounds.

BRONCHOPULMONARY HYGIENE AND BREATHING EXERCISES

Although an increase in pulmonary secretions is not specifically linked to the aging patient, the other components of aging can lead to an inability to clear secretions. Decrease in muscle strength compromises the ability to cough; decrease in ventilation to the lung bases and patient immobility lead to atelectasis; and any degree of cardiac failure or fluid overload in the elderly patient can result in pulmonary congestion. Additionally, the geriatric population with concomitant lung disease requires evaluation and treatment for these problems. Presence of atelectasis and secretions can be determined by auscultation on physical examination and confirmed by chest x-ray examination. These patients require both a secretion drainage and a breathing exercise program.

Secretion Clearance

Postural drainage positions and manual techniques for the geriatric population are not different from those used with any other population. Location of secretions or atelectasis on physical examination followed by appropriate positioning to maximize secretion drainage and ventilation/perfusion relationships remains the procedure of choice. Attention is given to baseline values of blood pressure and heart rate considering the geriatric patient's ability or inability to respond to postural changes. If the Trendelenburg position is indicated but not tolerated, a compromise to the bed-flat, semiprone position can still provide improved gas mixing and some degree of drainage.

Manual techniques are chosen based on individual patient indications and contraindications. Percussion can be used to loosen excessive or inspissated secretions. Vibration and/or shaking is effective in augmenting the movement of secretions up the tracheobronchial tree.[34,35,36]

Careful evaluation of the patient, the patient's ability to tolerate manual techniques, and the patient's response to treatment are vital components of the program. Common orthopedic changes seen with aging that may affect a patient's tolerance include arthritis, bone degeneration, and loss of elastic/cartilaginous tissue. Elderly patients may experience pain or discomfort with manual techniques, which results in a decrease in both ventilation and cooperation with treatment. Initially, moderate intensity is better tolerated with careful attention to patient response. If the patient provides negative feedback, an alteration in the treatment program to emphasize breathing exercises and vibration may prove to be more tolerable and therefore more effective.

Breathing Exercises and Mobility

Breathing exercises are used either in conjunction with positioning and manual techniques or independently to increase strength of the respiratory musculature and mobility of the thorax. When they are used to aid in secretion clearance, the patient is positioned first for postural drainage. Breathing exercises with manual assistance are used to provide resistance to muscle contractions (both to the abdominals and lateral costal musculature) and to encourage maximum inspiration. Shaking throughout the expiratory phase followed by quick stretch (or rib springing) to initiate inspiration aids in increasing the volume of air moved as well as mobilization of the thorax (Fig. 10-13).

Breathing exercises used independently can provide a mechanism for relaxation and improved ventilation or as a strengthening technique. Manual stretch, resistance, and tactile stimulation to the abdominals increase a patient's awareness of diaphragmatic motion. This technique—used in conjunction with slow, deep nasal inspirations, a three-second hold at maximum inspiration, and relaxed exhalation—has been shown to improve gas mixing and oxygenation.[37]

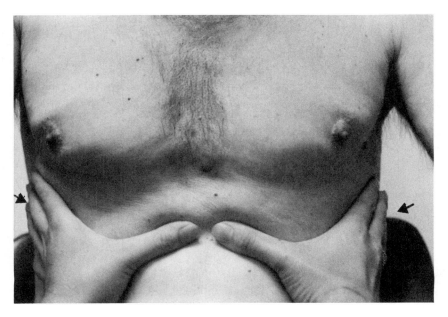

Figure 10-13. Arrows show palpation of abdomen (diaphragm) with participation of thumbs. Apply quick stretch with hands prior to inspiration.

Strengthening techniques using varied forms of inspiratory resistance also are proving useful to strengthen the muscles of respiration.[38]

Humidity and Bronchodilators

All techniques for secretion clearance and improvement of ventilatory function must be considered within the framework of the patient's overall medical condition. The bedridden geriatric patient frequently requires aggressive bronchopulmonary hygiene to maintain the patient's baseline pulmonary status and to prevent pneumonia. Elderly patients are frequently prone to neglecting routine personal and medical care including nutrition and chronic drug regimens.

Secretion clearance and ventilation are affected by the patient's overall hydration and level of bronchodilatation. Geriatric patients may require specific instructions regarding ingestion of both fluids and food. Recommended levels will depend on the chronic cardiac and renal conditions of the patient as well as the individual's baseline weight. Simple instructions, such as eating frequent, smaller amounts of food, can prevent shortness of breath and still keep up caloric intake. Fluid restriction or addition can be accomplished by premeasured amounts of fluid being kept in the refrigerator on a daily basis. Bronchodilators may be required prior to or during treatment for patients with reactive airways or CAO.

PHYSIOLOGIC PARAMETERS OF OLD AGE VS COPD

As previously described, it can be a perplexing clinical problem to separate the geriatric patient with uncomplicated aging of the pulmonary system from the more complicated patient with COPD. The evaluation and stress test process is actually an assessment to determine the degree of pulmonary impairment. Physical examination will aid this process by noting the degree of change in symptoms, that is, widening of the subcostal angle and decrease in breath sounds at the posterior bases. Table 10-1 lists guidelines for the normal changes seen with aging. Patients at their baseline who demonstrate progressively larger deviations from these parameters are frequently those with advancing COPD. The following sections describe stress testing and exercise prescription for geriatric patients in general terms. Examples are given at both ends of the spectrum to account for the geriatric patient with pulmonary impairment caused by aging and the geriatric patient with COPD.

STRESS TESTING

Indications for stress testing geriatric pulmonary patients are many and varied. The major goals are to assess functional impairment, disability, and dyspnea;

TABLE 10-1. Normal changes seen with aging

PARAMETER	CHANGE WITH INCREASED AGE	Standard Values
Vital Capacity (VC)	decreased*	
Functional Residual Capacity (FRC)	increased**	
Residual Volume (RV)	increased**	change dependent on size and sex
Forced Expiratory Volume ($FEV_{1.0}$L)	decreased*	
Forced Expiratory Flow ($FEF_{25-75\%}$ L/sec)	decreased*	
Partial Pressure of Arterial Oxygen (PaO_2)	decreased	80–100 mmHG
Partial Pressure of Arterial Carbon Dioxide ($PaCO_2$)	unchanged	35–45 mmHG
pH	unchanged	7.35–7.45

*Morris et al[13]: *Prediction nomogram: Spirometric values.* Amer Rev Resp Dis 103:57, 1971.
**Kenney, RA: *Physiology of Aging.* Yearbook Medical Publishers, Chicago, 1982.

however, the preliminary consideration in this patient population is safety. Many older patients have become so limited in their functional abilities or inaccurate at assessing their shortness of breath on activity that objective data are mandatory prior to beginning an exercise program or to making an exercise prescription. Establishing a baseline for documentation of progress; assessing oxygen requirements; and analyzing posture, gait, use of musculature, and balance are all integral indicators that comprise the assessment parameters of stress testing.

Protocol and Modality Selection

The appropriate protocol and method for stress testing the geriatric patient depend specifically on the patient's past medical history and present functional condition. Healthy, exercising geriatric patients will require a vigorous protocol such as the Bruce or Balke (Fig. 10-14) to elicit symptoms and to determine functional performance. Geriatric pulmonary patients with severe bronchoconstriction and obstruction will require modified protocols to demonstrate functional level and to record an accurate baseline (Table 10-2).

Consideration should be given to method of exercise as well as the best protocol for testing each patient. Bicycle ergometry and treadmill testing provide the simplest forms mechanically if they are available. Timed distance walking and step climbing can also be used if no equipment is available. Simple questions to the patient regarding their walking, bike riding or step climbing ability prior to protocol selection can aid your decision. Included are several test protocols and their advantages for any given portion of the geriatric population (See Figure 10-14).

Monitoring Parameters

Following protocol selection, monitoring needs are assessed to determine those measures of cardiopulmonary function that will indicate a patient's functional level most accurately and safely. Stable uncomplicated geriatric patients complaining of fatigue on exertion may require monitoring of HR, blood pressure (BP), electrocardiogram (ECG), and respiratory rate (RR) to demonstrate their functional level and ability to participate in an exercise program. The geriatric patient whose medical history includes frequent upper respiratory infections, two-pillow orthopnea, and dyspnea on exertion requires additional monitoring to include resting and exercise, pulmonary function tests (PFT's), minute ventilation, PaO_2, O_2sat, $PaCO_2$, and expired gas concentrations.

This monitoring can be accomplished with several types of equipment. Heart rate and ECG tracings are standard output for the oscilloscope and strip chart recorder. Arterial oxygen, arterial carbon dioxide, oxygen saturation, and pH are all obtained by drawing and analyzing arterial blood gases from an indwell-

200   PHYSICAL ASPECTS OF AGING

PROTOCOL

12-Minute Walk*	Level walking for 12 minutes, distance recorded.	No equipment necessary yet correlates well with study results of more complex tests; can be used for patients who cannot accomplish either treadmill walking or bike riding because of dyspnea.
Master's†	Stair climbing: up three and down two for a prespecified number of times in 1.5 min (number of times determined by weight, sex, and age).	Simple, requires little extra equipment, large volume of background data accumulated. Predictive value good. Geriatric patients may not be able to climb stairs because of orthopedic limitation.
Modified Naughton‡	Treadmill: speed constant at 2.0 mph; grade initially 0 percent increased by 3.5 percent every 2 min.	Slow speed allows patient with pulmonary impairment to be stressed without walking fast.
BIH Protocol	See Table 10-2.	Intermittent walk test for use with severely impaired patients. Allows flexibility of workload assignment and establishes an accurate baseline.
Balke Test‡	Treadmill: speed constant at 3.0 mph; grade initially 0 percent increased by 3.5 percent every 2 min.	Slight increase in speed for patient with less impairment allows pulmonary and cardiovascular stress to come before leg fatigue.
Bruce‡	Treadmill: speed initially 1.7 mph; grade initially 10 percent; both are increased every 3 min in a specified manner.	Can be used with relatively fit individuals to stress accurately all systems' response to exercise. Good to assess exercise-induced bronchospasm in fit individuals.
Bicycle Test§	Specific workload, i.e., watts or Kgm/min, patient rides for a preset time, next workload determined by patient response.	Intermittent subjective test based on patient response. Requires lower extremity strength and endurance to reach high metabolic response level.

*McGavin, CR, Cupta, SP, McHardy, GJR: *Twelve minute walking test for assessing disability in chronic bronchitis.* Br Med J 1:822, 1976.
†Master, AM: *Two-step test of myocardial function.* Am Heart J 10:495, 1934.
‡From *Physician's Handbook for Evaluation of Cardiovascular and Physical Fitness.* Tennessee Heart Association, 1972.
§Ellestad, NH: *Stress Testing: Principles and Practice.* FA Davis, Philadelphia, 1979.

Figure 10-14. Stress-testing protocols are summarized here.

TABLE 10-2. Exercise test protocol

Collect resting data: Supine and sitting	ECG, BP, PaO_2, $PaCO_2$, pH, A-aDO_2, A-$aDCO_2$, $\dot{V}O_2$, RQ, VE, RR, HR, VD, VD/V_T
Stage I:	Assessment of dyspnea/2 mph 0% grade Walk 6 min = 4 min stabilization + 2 min gas collection Rest: Patient returns to baseline HR, RR, and ABGs
Stage II:	Occupational assessment/treadmill set at speed and incline to equal functional work capacity Walk 6 min = 4 min stabilization + 2 min gas collection Rest: Patient returns to baseline HR, RR, and ABG's
Stage III:	Exercise tolerance/treadmill set to produce HR of 70–85% max Walk 6 min = 4 min stabilization + 2 min gas collection Rest: Patient returns to baseline HR, RR, and ABG's
Nitrogen washout:	Patient receives 100% O_2/draw ABG/calculate R-L shunt
Criteria to terminate test:	85% predicted HR_{max}, development of metabolic acidosis, fall in PaO_2 of 20 torr from resting, reaching a ventilatory maximum (35 × FEV_1), CO_2 retention of >10 torr from baseline, development of cardiac arrhythmias, or development of significant symptoms

*From Department of Pulmonary Medicine, Beth Israel Hospital, Boston, MA.

ing radial artery catheter.[18] Oxygen saturation can be monitored noninvasively with an ear oximeter. This accurately reflects saturation with a correlation coefficient of 0.99 between ear oximeter SaO_2 and arterial blood SaO_2.[39] Expired gases that are run through a spirometer can be collected to record both measurement of pulmonary function and analysis of gases. Several computerized metabolic monitoring systems can provide comprehensive gas analysis and other metabolic measures as needed. The severity of the patient's condition will dictate those monitoring parameters that will provide useful information and those that are necessary to assure a safe and clinically useful stress test (Table 10-3).

Patient Preparation

The entire process of the stress test, including the preparation, monitoring, effort necessary, and expected results is explained to the patient well ahead of time. Informed consent is required in the instances where invasive procedures are used. Step-by-step reminders throughout the process and supportive conversational encouragement can make a great difference in patient cooperation and achievement.

Beginning a Stress Test

Once a patient is set up with monitoring equipment, an explanation of the process is useful. If the patient has never walked on a treadmill, demonstration may

TABLE 10-3. Flowsheet for gas exchange and exercise

Patient: _____ DX: _____

Hospital #: _____ Date _____

	Supine	Resting	Ex. #1	Ex. #2	Ex. #3	100% O_2	Ex. on 100% O_2
Speed (MPH)							
Incline (%)							
PaO_2							
$PaCO_2$							
pH/$\dot{B}E$							
A-aDO_2							
A-aDCO_2 (calc/measured)							
$\dot{V}O_2$ (O_2 cons.)							
RQ							
$\dot{V}E$							
Respiratory Rate							
Heart Rate							
VD							
VD/V_T							
R-L Shunt (on 100% O_2)							

From Beth Israel Hospital, Department of Pulmonary Medicine, Boston, MA.

be necessary. Any hand signs or signals that will indicate patient stress should be reviewed, because patients may be using a mouthpiece and be unable to speak. When the first stage is begun and the patient is exercising, one team member is directly responsible for patient care. That person will monitor the patient's use of musculature and facial expression and will give the patient feedback and encouragement.

Stopping a Stress Test

Criteria for stopping an exercise test in the geriatric and pulmonary-impaired populations are more subjective or patient-oriented than for the young adult or strictly cardiac population.[40] As elderly or pulmonary-impaired individuals may not have exercised for many years, the simple activity of the test itself may elicit previously unrecognized symptoms. Knee or hip pain, shortness of breath, and muscle cramps are frequent complaints. A healthy, active geriatric patient may reach either the predicted maximum HR or 85 percent of predicted maximum according to protocol. A geriatric patient with pulmonary impairment frequently will be limited by dyspnea before reaching HR at or near maximum. This patient will also have a much higher HR at a much lower stress level than that of the normal individual.[41] If an individual patient states he or she is unable to continue, the test is terminated. The patient is recorded as having worked to "symptom-limited maximum," and the indication or reason for cessation of the test is recorded. Some examples of these symptoms include extreme dyspnea, wheezing, dizziness, or weakness or pain in the extremities. Once the patient's functional activity level has been determined, goals are set and a program is written.

SETTING GOALS

Analysis of the patient's performance during the stress test is essential prior to setting goals. The elderly individual who is significantly limited by shortness of breath must be evaluated within his or her performance context. For example, a geriatric patient whose shortness of breath specifically relates to inactivity and deconditioning may reach just a 3 MET (measurement of oxygen consumption; 1 MET = 3.54 ml/kg) level during the test and show no signs of desaturation or ECG change. A 3 to 4 MET functional level is needed to perform most activities of daily living (ADL). For patients with a maximum exercise capacity of 3 METS, short-term goals would be to improve baseline cardiopulmonary function for increased comfort with ADL. Once this goal is reached, long-term goals are set for training and/or maintenance of function based on that patient's particular needs and motivation level. A geriatric, pulmonary-impaired patient that exercised to 2 METS may have experienced both desaturation and ECG change. The goals in this program would be to treat the patient's cardiopulmonary pathology, to stabilize the medical condition, and then to provide an exercise program. A simple example for routine goal setting would be the elderly patient without pulmonary disease who is recently discharged from the hospital and lives alone in a second-floor walk-up apartment. Increased exercise tolerance and strengthening for this patient are necessary to maintain a functional level at home. Further goals to improve exercise tolerance are categorized as long term.

The geriatric patient whose shortness of breath relates to pulmonary disease as well as to advanced age is evaluated in a different context than the healthy geriatric patient. Short-term goals are related to stabilization of the medical condition and an understanding of the disease process. An educational component related to pulmonary disease is essential. Recognition of pulmonary processes as chronic and acceptance of the disease progression aids in setting appropriate goals. Long-term goals focus on an increase in exercise tolerance, improved feeling of well-being, and prevention of functional loss.

Other important factors to consider in setting goals relate to patient motivation, education, and compliance. If a patient does not feel safe in either the exercising environment or with the instructor, he or she will be reluctant to begin or to continue with the program. Patient education must be integrated into all phases of the program and delivered at the appropriate level. A basic comprehension of anatomy and physiology related to the aging process can provide both understanding and motivation. Consideration must be given to the patient's comprehension level and retention ability. Frequent review and reminders are beneficial. Goals must therefore be individual, realistic, and attainable. Patients who understand their own needs and capabilities will feel safer in the setting, enjoy the process, and be more likely to comply with the program and therefore succeed in attaining their goals.

TRAINING PROGRAM

Exercise prescription for the geriatric patient with pulmonary disease includes all the components utilized for programs that train young healthy individuals; yet the parameters, environment, and goals may be vastly different. Whether the patient is an elderly individual with the simple pulmonary changes of age or an elderly patient with long-standing COPD, the same elements are essential for consideration. The elements include appropriate settings, proper exercise modality, an exercise prescription, intensity, duration, frequency, and overall goals. Guidelines for each element of the program are determined by the patient's personal preference and performance during evaluation or stress test.

Setting

The most appropriate setting for patient training is determined by the geographic area of the country as well as by the facilities available. Warm, sunny, stable climates are conducive to outdoor walking, cycling, or swimming programs. Cold, wet, and unpredictable climates will require the frequent, continual use of an indoor facility. Pulmonary-impaired patients are educated to note response to temperature, humidity, and pollution index during exercise. As patient tolerance to both temperature and humidity is personal, there are no specific number guidelines recommended. Patients who note changes in HR or dyspnea owing to humidity should be encouraged to exercise indoors in controlled environments or in drier climates. Patients are also instructed to exercise in moderate temperatures rather than in extreme temperatures. Studies have shown that ozone levels of greater than 0.37 ppm create significant adverse health effects.[42] This level is usually broadcast as part of the Air Quality Index on local radio stations. Additionally, each patient should be assessed for group participation or individual work. Some elderly individuals respond well to a setting where others are "just as out of shape," using the group for support, but others will be intimidated and/or embarrassed in a group and cannot function unless they receive individual attention and consideration. Lastly, a particularly safe environment is a major consideration in the elderly population. Adequate supervision, quality medical personnel, and accessibility are three major factors to consider when beginning or recommending a program for referral.

Exercise Mode

Selecting the appropriate exercise modality also will be dependent upon personal preference and equipment or facility availability. Patients with a long-term love of cycling can be set up for indoor stationary-bike programs or outdoor cycling groups. Patients who love swimming and hate jogging are obvious candidates for swim programs, and the inner-city individual who prefers the apartment hallway and stairs to the great outdoors can participate in stair climbing. Patient familiarity and comfort with the type of activity can be useful motivation and an aid in compliance with any program.

Prescription

The three elements to be considered in exercise prescription include frequency, intensity, and duration. Based on the results of the stress test, an individual prescription is formulated incorporating all three. For a central cardiovascular training effect to occur, minimal criteria must be met in all three categories:[43] (intensity $\geq 60\%$ HR_{max}: duration ≥ 20 min: frequency $\geq 3 \times$/wk).[40]

Elderly patients without pulmonary impairment may be able to meet these criteria, exercise aerobically, and achieve this cardiovascular training effect. Because of their advanced age, geriatric patients can achieve this training effect at lower HRs than those of younger individuals, owing to the decline in HR_{max} with age ($HR_{max} = 220 - $ age).[19,40] Geriatric patients with pulmonary impairment, however, may be restricted from aerobic training by symptoms of dyspnea. At the present time, there remains the question whether patients with COPD ever reach anaerobic threshold even at the higher heart rates they demonstrate with exercise.[41] The improvements seen in COPD patients after rehabilitation are not consistent with the changes demonstrated by exercising normals (central cardiovascular training effect).[41] Their exercise training is presently directed toward an increase in functional capacity and an increase in performance with ADL.[44]

Intensity has been demonstrated the most significant factor in exercise prescription.[45] Elderly patients and those who are symptom limited by pulmonary disease receive exercise prescriptions with a training HR that allows them to exercise safely for at least 20 minutes. Heart rate can be related to oxygen saturation levels during stress testing and then used as a guideline for safety during exercise training. If desaturation occurs at a particular HR (intensity), the exercise prescription should acknowledge that level. Should desaturation (below 85 percent) occur that prevents exercise at a training level, the patient will require enough oxygen during exercise to maintain 85 percent saturation.[46] Patients with severe dyspnea or bronchospasm require modified programs. Modification occurs in the duration and frequency elements of exercise prescription. Geriatric and pulmonary-impaired patients who can walk for only 10 minutes without severe dyspnea at any prescribed HR are encouraged to increase their frequency of walking to twice a day, thereby cumulatively walking for a total of 20 minutes.[19] Exercise periods of less intensity and longer duration have also been demonstrated beneficial.[45] Elderly individuals with lower HR_{max} have shown increased function when exercising in lower HR ranges for longer periods.[19]

The goal in exercise prescription is to provide the individual with an exercise program that will include safe but beneficial intensity, duration, and frequency. This is true for both the deconditioned geriatric patient who may achieve a training effect and the pulmonary geriatric patient whose goal is an increase in functional performance.

The remaining components of a comprehensive exercise prescription include warm-up exercises (Fig. 10-15) and a cool-down period. These exercises should emphasize flexibility and thoracic mobility. Warm-up and cool-down periods should be longer for the geriatric patient because the system's response times are delayed with age.[28,29] Common programs include walking in place for 3 or 4 minutes, gradually lifting the knees higher; 3 or 4 minutes of rhythmic bend-and-stretch exercises, inhaling as one lifts the arms in flexion and exhaling on extension; and concluding with 3 or 4 minutes of trunk rotation, such as side bending and circling.

Considerations of present medical regime (use of drugs, such as bronchodilators), nutritional status, and mental attitude are also essential. If a bronchodilator is necessary for exercise, it should be administered prior to the rhythmic exercises, which mobilize the thorax, slow the breathing rate, and increase the inspired volume. Patients with reactive airways disease will require a baseline level of bronchodilatation to exercise safely. To maximize benefits of the drug,

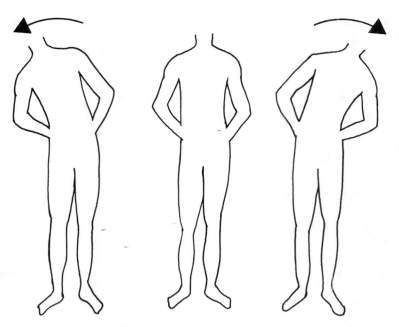

Figure 10-15. Rhythmic bend-and-stretch exercises are illustrated here. Patient can use either lateral flexion or anterior/posterior flexion and extension. Inspiration occurs through the nose while standing in the upright position. Exhalation occurs during flexion through pursed lips. Slow counting throughout the procedure helps maintain rhythm.

an inhalant used 20 minutes prior to exercise will enhance air movement, complement attempts to increase volumes of air moved, and so improve ventilation/distribution.

Initially, programs incorporating short activity periods followed by rest times may be used. The ideal exercise program begins slowly, increases in intensity, plateaus at a HR of 60 percent of maximum, continues for the designated time period (>20 min), works back down in intensity, and ends with a cool-down period.[19] This format practiced at least three times weekly allows both the geriatric and the geriatric pulmonary-impaired patients a physiologically safe and beneficial mode to improve exercise tolerance and to increase functional activities.

Once a patient has embarked on such a program, frequent assessment has proven beneficial.[19] Each patient should keep a log or diary of his or her own progress (Fig. 10-16). The log can include initial parameters such as HR, amount of work performed (for example, distance walked), and the patient's subjective response to the exercise program. As the patient progresses, other factors can be important, such as diet and weight; medications; and, most specifically, the patient's progress and achievements. Because this is the patient's own record, it should be a personal recording of the factors most significant to the individual. This written record keeps the patient honest about his or her program, allows the patient a degree of control with self-assessment, and visibly documents im-

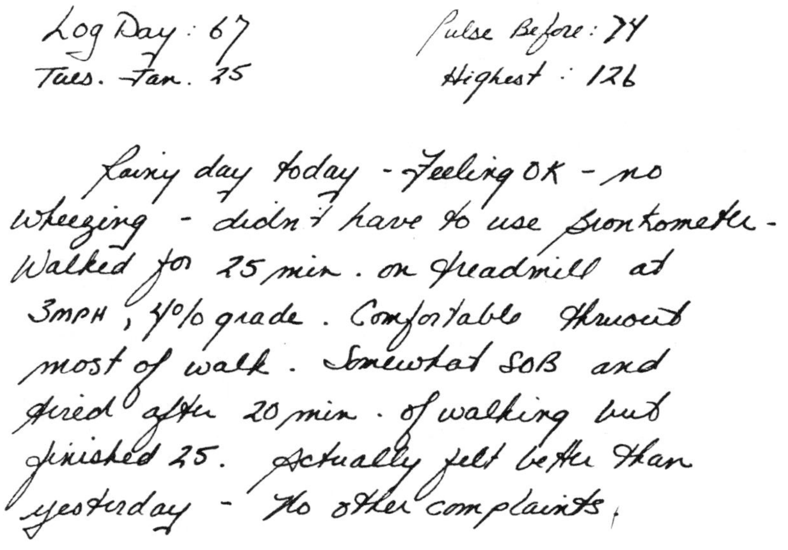

Log Day: 67
Tues. Jan. 25

Pulse Before: 74
Highest: 126

Rainy day today - Feeling OK - no wheezing - didn't have to use spirometer. Walked for 25 min. on treadmill at 3mph, 4% grade. Comfortable throuout most of walk. Somewhat SOB and tired after 20 min. of walking but finished 25. Actually felt better than yesterday - No other complaints.

Figure 10-16. Shown here is a sample of a patient log entry.

provements. This is especially important for the elderly and pulmonary-impaired patient, for whom increases in function may be small and take a longer time to occur.[19] The therapist also may find it helpful to have documentation of patient progress that allows accurate program changes.

Related Research

Study results regarding the efficacy of training programs for the pulmonary system of the elderly patient vary widely. In 1964, Hollmann reported that individuals over 60 years of age showed little improvement with training unless they had participated in conditioning at an earlier point in life.[47] Similarly, in 1965, Benestad found no gains in $M\dot{V}O_2$ maximum in a group of men 70 to 80 years old who participated in a six-week training program.[48] Conversely, several studies from the late 1960s to early 1970s reported large gains in maximum oxygen uptake of older individuals undergoing training after many years of inactivity.[49-51] Therefore, when assessing the current research, it is important to consider carefully the specific population studied, the training method used, and the variables measured.

Healthy, active geriatric patients who begin a specific training program are bound to show smaller gains than those completely sedentary prior to the program. Familiarity with the procedures is another factor. The older patient who has never walked on the treadmill before will have an increased HR and $\dot{V}O_2$ owing to anxiety prior to training on the equipment, thereby skewing the post-training test results.

In 1970, DeVries reported an increase of 5 percent in the VC of elderly subjects who had been in an endurance training program for six weeks.[50] The training continued and showed an overall 20 percent increase after 42 weeks. This study accounted for the learning effect and familiarity with equipment and procedures. They simultaneously followed a control group who demonstrated no change in VC, increasing the accuracy of this report. Other investigators[52] have reported no effect of training on the VC, but Niinimaa and Shephard concluded that their subjects initially fitted within normal chart standards for pulmonary function, which might account for the discrepancy.[53] An increase in VC most likely relates to increased strength of respiratory muscles and perhaps increased mobility of the thorax. Despite these positive changes with exercise, the capacity for change steadily decreases with age.

There is no evidence to date that training can alter lung function that is dependent on the specific anatomic aging process. Decrease in elastic fibers and lung recoil results in increased closing voumes regardless of training.[53,54] In addition, although there is a progressive loss of surface area for diffusion, some studies have shown a high resting pulmonary diffusing capacity in the well-trained individual.[54,55] Training of elderly subjects by Niinimaa and Shephard in 1978 demonstrated, however, a decrease in diffusing capacity at submaximal workloads which they predicted to be a result of the parallel decrease in cardiac output with training.[54]

The recognized benefits for elderly individuals are best described by patients themselves and specifically relate to increased ability to perform work, overall functional improvements with activities, and a greatly increased sense of well-being. Sidney and Shephard summarized their study of geriatric patients who were tested prior to and following a fourteen-week training program by noting that all patients scored improved grades on the Kenyon Attitude Tests. Overall improvement was seen in the specific category "Physical Activity as the Relief for Tension."[56] Patients also described changes of "improved body image, better routine health, better mood and decreased anxiety."[19]

In summary, it is reasonable therefore to suggest that there are many considerations to be made in each case. Aging is an inevitability with consistent, predictable physiologic changes. However, exercise can and does improve functional abilities and provides a healthy sense of well-being for those who are motivated and willing to work. Therefore, therapists and patients may find it a rewarding experience to evaluate the functional abilities of the elderly individual, to prescribe a treatment program adapted to the patient's needs, and to observe and to record the positive results.

GLOSSARY

1. **Adventitious breath sounds**. Those sounds heard in addition to the underlying normal or abnormal breath sounds.
2. **Compliance**. The volume change within the lung resulting from the application of pressure.

3. **Closing volume**. The lung volume at which airway closure starts to occur.
4. **Dyspnea**. Subjective difficulty with breathing.
5. **Fenestra**. An anatomical opening.
6. **Functional residual capacity**. The lung capacity comprised of the residual volume and expiratory reserve volume (FRC).
7. **Insidious**. A disease that progresses with few or no symptoms to indicate its progress.
8. **Inspissated**. Thickened by evaporation or absorption of fluid.
9. **MET**. Measure of oxygen consumption; resting level equals 3.54 ml per kg.
10. **Perfusion**. Flow of blood.
11. **Residual volume**. Air remaining in lungs that cannot be exhaled (RV).
12. **Respiration**. Exchange of gases across a membrane.
13. **Tactile fremitus**. Palpation of voice sounds transmitted through the chest wall.
14. **Tidal volume**. Air moved with a single breath (V_T).
15. **Total lung capacity**. Volume of air within the lungs at maximum inspiration (TLC).
16. **Ventilation**. Replacement of air or gas in a space by fresh air or fresh gas.
17. **Ventilation/perfusion**. Ratio of air moved to blood circulated.
18. **Vital capacity**. Volume of air expired from maximal inspiration to the level of FRC (VC).

REFERENCES

1. OFFICIAL ATS STATEMENT: *Pulmonary rehabilitation*. Am Rev Respir Dis 124:663, November, 1981.

2. MURRAY, JF: *The Normal Lung*. WB Saunders, Philadelphia, 1976.

3. JOHN, R AND THOMAS, J: *Chemical compositions of elastins isolated from aortas and pulmonary tissues of humans of different ages*. Biochem J 127:261, 1972.

4. PUMP, KK: *Fenestrae in the alveolar membrane of the human lung*. Chest 65:431, 1974.

5. SEMMENS, M: *The pulmonary artery in the normal aged lung*. Br J Dis Chest 64:65, 1970.

6. HERNANDEZ, JA, ET AL: *The bronchial glands in aging*. J Am Geriatr Soc 13:799, 1965.

7. ANTHONISEN, NR ET AL: *Airway closure as a function of age*. Respir Physiol 8:58, 1969.

8. MUIESAN, G, SORBINI, CA, GRASSI, V: *Respiratory function in the aged*. Bulletin de Physio-Pathologie Respiratoire 7:973, 1971.

9. HOLLAND, J, ET AL: *Regional distribution of pulmonary ventilation and perfusion in elderly subjects*. J Clin Invest 47:81, 1968.

10. REDDAN, WG: *Respiratory system and aging*. In SMITH, EL AND SERFASS, RC (EDS): *Exercise and Aging: The Scientific Basis*. Enslow, Hillside, NJ, 1981.

11. MITTMAN, C, ET AL: *Relationship between chest wall and pulmonary compliance and age*. J Appl Physiol 10:1211, 1965.

12. TURNER, JM, MEAD, J, WOHL, ME: *Elasticity of human lungs in relation to age*. J Appl Physiol 35:664, 1968.

13. MORRIS, JR, KOSKI, A, JOHNSON, LC: *Spirometric standards for healthy non-smoking adults.* Am Rev Respir Dis 103:57, 1971.

14. STORSTEIN, O AND VOLL, A: *New prediction formulas of ventilatory measurements: A study of normal individuals in the age group 20–59 years.* Scand J Clin Lab Invest 14:633, 1962.

15. SORBINI, CA: *Arterial oxygen tension in relation to age in healthy subjects.* Respiration 25:3, 1968.

16. NEUFELD, O, SMITH J, GOLDMAN, S: *Arterial oxygen tension in relation to age in hospital subjects.* J Am Geriatr Soc 21:4, 1973.

17. HARF, A AND HUGHES, JMB: *Topographical distribution of V/Q in elderly subjects using Krypton—81m.* Respir Physiol 34:319, 1978.

18. RIES, AL, FEDULLO, PF, CLAUSEN, JL: *Rapid changes in arterial blood gas levels after exercise in pulmonary patients.* Chest 3:454, 1983.

19. SHEPHARD, RJ: *Physical activity and aging.* Year Book Medical Publishers, Chicago, 1978.

20. CUMMING, G AND SEMPLE, SG: *Disorders of the Respiratory System.* Blackwell Scientific Publications, Oxford, 1973.

21. AMERICAN THORACIC SOCIETY: *Chronic bronchitis, asthma and pulmonary emphysema.* Am Rev Respir Dis 85:762, 1962.

22. FILLEY, GF: *Pulmonary ventilation and the oxygen cost of exercise in emphysema.* American Clinical Climatology Association J 70:193, 1958.

23. SHUEY, CB, PIERCE, AK, HOHNSON, RL: *An evaluation of exercise tests in chronic obstructive lung disease.* J Appl Physiol 27:256, 1969.

24. JONES, NL: *Pulmonary gas exchange during exercise in patients with chronic airway obstruction.* Clin Sci 31:39, 1966.

25. SPINO, SG, ET AL: *An analysis of the physiological strain of submaximal exercise in patients with chronic obstructive bronchitis.* Thorax 30:415, 1975.

26. BAKHJAVAN, FK, PALMER, WH, MCGREGOR, M: *Influence of respiration on venous return in pulmonary emphysema.* Circulation 33:8, 1966.

27. ASTRAND, PO AND RODAHL, K: *Textbook of Work Physiology.* McGraw-Hill, New York, 1970.

28. ASSMUSSEN E, FRUENSGAARD, K, NORGAARD, S: *A follow-up longitudinal study of selected physiologie functions in former physical education students after forty years.* J Am Geriatr Soc 23:442, 1975.

29. SHOCK, NW: *Physiological aspects of aging in man.* Annu Rev Physiol 23:97, 1961.

30. ROUSSOS, CS AND MACKLEM, PT: *Diaphragmatic fatigue in man.* J Appl Physiol 43:189, 1977.

31. GRIMBY, G: *Pulmonary mechanics: The load.* In DEMPSEY, JA AND REED, C (EDS): *Muscular Exercise and the Lung.* University of Wisconsin Press, Madison, 1976.

32. RIZZATO, G AND MARRAZINI, L: *Thoracoabdominal mechanics in elderly men.* J Appl Physiol 28:247, 1970.

33. ROUSSOS, CS AND MACKLEM, PT: *Response of the respiratory muscles to fatiguing loads.* Am Rev Respir Dis 113:200, 1976.

34. KIGIN, CM: Personal communication, Summer, 1980.

35. CHOPRA, SI, ET AL: *Effects of hydration and physical therapy on tracheal transport velocity.* Am Rev Respir Dis 115:1009, 1977.

36. BATEMAN, JRM, ET AL: *Regional lung clearance of excessive bronchial secretions during chest physiotherapy in patients with stable chronic airways obstruction.* Lancet 1:294, 1979.

37. KNELSON, JH, HOWATT, WF, DeMIRTH, GR: *Effect of respiratory pattern on gas exchange.* J Appl Physiol 29:328, 1970.

38. BELLMAN, MF AND MITTMAN, C: *Ventilatory muscle training improves exercise capacity in chronic obstructive pulmonary disease patients.* Am Rev Respir Dis 121:273, 1980.

39. SNEDECOR, GW AND COCHRAN, WG: *Statistical Methods: 6th Edition.* Iowa State University Press, Ames, Iowa, 1967.

40. ACSM: *Guidelines for Graded Exercise Testing and Exercise Prescription.* Lea & Febiger, Philadelphia, 1975.

41. BELMAN, MJ AND KENDREGAN, BA: *Exercise training fails to increase skeletal muscle enzymes in patients with chronic obstructive pulmonary disease.* Am Rev Respir Dis 123:256, 1981.

42. *Air Quality and Automobile Emission Control Vol. 2: Health Effects of Air Pollutants.* Coordinating Committee on Air Quality Studies, National Academy of Sciences, National Academy of Engineering, National Research Council, Washington, DC, US Government Printing Office, September, 1974.

43. POLLOCK, ML: *The quantification of endurance training programs.* In WILMORE, JH (ED): *Exercise and Sports Sciences Reviews,* Vol I. Academic Press, New York, 1973.

44. SAHN, SA, NETT, LM, PETTY, TL: *Ten year follow-up of a comprehensive rehabilitation program for severe COPD.* Chest 77:2 (Suppl), 311, 1980.

45. HELLERSTEIN, HK, ET AL: *Principles of exercise prescription for normals and cardiac subjects.* In NAUGHTON, J AND HELLERSTEIN, HH (EDS): *Exercise Testing and Exercise Training in Coronary Heart Disease.*

46. PULMONARY REHABILITATION MEDICAL MANUAL. University of Nebraska Medical Center, 1977.

47. HOLLMAN, W: *Diminution of cardiopulmonary capacity in the course of life and its prevention by participation in sports.* In Kato, K (ED): *Proceedings of International Congress of Sports Sciences, Tokyo, 1964.* Japanese Union of Sports Services, Tokyo, 1966.

48. BENESTAD, AM: *Trainability of old men.* Acta Med Scand 178:321, 1965.

49. BARRY, AJ, ET AL: *The effects of physical conditioning on older individuals. I. Work capacity, circulatory-respiratory function, and work electrocardiogram.* J Gerontol 21:182, 1966.

50. DeVRIES, HA: *Physiological effects of an exercise training regimen upon men aged 52–88.* J Gerontol 25:325, 1970.

51. STANFORD, BA: *Effects of chronic institutionalization on the physical working capacity and trainability of geriatric men.* J Gerontol 28:441, 1973.

52. SIDNEY, KH AND SHEPHARD, RJ: *Frequency and intensity of exercise training for elderly subjects.* Med Sci Sports Exerc 10:125, 1978.

53. NIINIMAA, V AND SHEPHARD, RJ: *Training and oxygen conductance in the elderly. I. The respiratory system.* J Gerontol 33:354, 1978.

54. ANTHONISEN, NR, ET AL: *Airway closure as a function of age.* Respir Physiol 8:58, 1969.

55. HOLMGREN A: *On the reproducibility of steady-state DL, CO measurements during exercise in man.* Scand J Clin Lab Invest 17:110, 1965.

56. SIDNEY, IH AND SHEPHARD, RJ: *Attitudes towards health and physical activity in the elderly: Effects of physical training programme.* Med Sci Sports Exerc 8:246, 1977.

CHAPTER **11**

IMPLICATIONS OF ONCOLOGY IN THE AGED

STEPHEN A. GUDAS, R.P.T., M.S.

BEHAVIORAL OBJECTIVES

Upon completion of this chapter, the reader will be able to
1. List the major types of cancer that commonly occur in the elderly population.
2. Explain why detection of cancer in the elderly is often delayed.
3. Modify rehabilitation treatment goals in the geriatric cancer patient in light of the physiologic changes that accompany aging.
4. Outline a palliative and supportive program for the terminal geriatric cancer patient.
5. List the various members of the cancer rehabilitation team and state their roles in the management of geriatric cancer, with emphasis on head and neck cancer.
6. Identify clinical symptomatology and physical rehabilitation interventions in the elderly patient with myeloma, colon cancer, skin cancer, breast cancer, lymphoma, head and neck cancer, complications caused by metastatic disease, and lung cancer.

For older age groups, cancer is a significant health problem.[1] Cancer incidence and death rates rise continuously with age and are highest among the elderly.[2] Although cancer occurs at any age, the disease most commonly affects middle-aged and older adults. In the latter age group, cancer ranks second only to heart disease as a cause of death in the United States.[3,4]

Each specific type of cancer tends to have a peak incidence regarding age, although there is wide variability. The carcinoma family of tumors, such as those of the lung, skin, gastrointestinal (GI) tract, breast, and prostate, occur almost exclusively in older individuals. In men 75 years of age and older, prostatic cancer accounts for 25 percent of all cancer, and GI cancer comprises an additional 25 percent. In women in this same age group, breast cancer is responsible for 20 percent of malignant tumor incidence, and GI cancer comprises an additional 25 percent.[2]

The probability that a given individual will develop a malignant tumor within a 5-year period rises from 1 in 700 at the age of 25 to 1 in 14 at the age of 65.[4] This fact alone demands that the elderly population be well educated in the warning signs and symptoms of cancer and that physicians and other health professionals become more knowledgeable in the manner of presentation of neoplastic disease, in screening for cancer in the elderly, and in the general principles of therapeutic management and treatment of malignant disease in the elderly. Unfortunately, cancer management in the elderly is a topic that has received relatively little attention in the past. This is surprising, considering that 50 percent of all cancers occur in patients over 65 years of age.[5]

CANCER IN THE ELDERLY

From the standpoint of therapeutic intervention, some authors recommend that cancer should be regarded similarly in all age groups.[6] Although this may well be an oversimplification of the cancer problem in the aged, no patient should be denied full comprehensive treatment on the grounds of age alone. Also, it should be remembered that malignant disease in the elderly may be only one of several life-threatening diseases present, and frailty and disability may coexist with the occurrence of malignancy, thus complicating the clinical picture.[4] For example, many elderly patients may not experience early detection of their disease, owing to the fact that warning symptoms are often unheeded or attributed to or masked by another disease process already present. This delay, caused by insufficient vigilance on the part of the patient or family, is believed to be a significant factor in cancer in the elderly population.[2] Statistics tend to imply that older patients must be particularly alert for symptoms of cancer at high-risk sites. Some tumors, such as melanoma and thyroid cancer, tend to have a more aggressive clinical course in older persons.[6]

The development in recent years of newer and more elaborate scanning devices, such as radionuclide imaging and computerized axial tomography (CAT), has enhanced the detection and recognition of cancer.[7] Conventional diagnostic procedures are still employed and have wide clinical usage; the importance of breast self-examination to detect early breast cancer and of periodic chest radiographs to detect lung cancer is fairly well established in the older person. Indeed, screening techniques may be more urgent and applicable in the geriatric population, in which patient delay in reporting symptoms is common, leading to late detection of cancer and less chance of cure. The inverse relationship of age to clinical stage in bronchogenic carcinoma, for example, suggests that appropriate screening by periodic chest radiographs and cytologic sputum examinations may be more appropriate for the high-risk elderly population than for a younger age group in whom these screening methods have yielded fewer positive results.[8]

Changes in the immune system may play a role in the development of cancer in the aged. A defect or decrease in T cell function and regulation with age has been reported, and there appears to be an association between immunodeficiency and increased cancer incidence.[9] Paradoxically, immune processes may also contribute to the geriatric cancer problem. A recent review suggested that T cell dysfunction in the aged may permit the simultaneous development of autoimmunity—in which the individual manufactures antibodies against one's own tissues—and neoplasia.[10] Although results are inconclusive, further research in immunology will undoubtedly shed new light in the area of cancer in the aged.

Multiple primary neoplasms, or the development of separate cancers in more than one organ system, are a common problem in old age; the longer a person lives, the more predisposed he or she is to become host to primary malignant neoplasms at various sites.[11] During a prolonged followup period, up to 36 percent of elderly patients treated for cancer will eventually develop a second or third primary tumor.[12] In a series of 676 patients, 34 showed more than one site of malignancy, and six of these demonstrated three primary sites.[11] Because the likelihood of additional separate cancer occurrence increases with each year, clinicians should be aware of the possibility of a second primary tumor when reviewing patients who have enjoyed long survival periods following the initial appearance of cancer.

Many of the treatment procedures used in cancer management carry significant and pronounced cosmetic and functional morbidity. In general, the rehabilitation of the geriatric patient and alleviation or palliation of dysfunction and disfigurement are of the utmost importance.[13] Each type of cancer, and, in essence, each individual, will present with specialized problems arising from the malignant process itself or iatrogenically from the effects of treatment. Cancer rehabilitation in the elderly necessitates the involvement of a multidisciplinary team, the members of which should have expertise in both gerontology and oncology.

Too often rehabilitative efforts are directed toward employment-oriented goals or major physical achievements.[14] In planning programs for geriatric cancer patients, the rehabilitative staff should modify goals according to the potential lifestyle and physical condition of the patient, keeping the physiologic changes of aging in mind. The geriatric cancer patient will gain from the rehabilitation procedure even if he or she does not meet the predetermined rehabilitative goal that had been set initially.[15] Rehabilitation that affords a degree of independence and increased function in daily living skills is of great importance; the value of coordinated rehabilitation services for the elderly person experiencing disabilities caused by cancer cannot be minimized. A comprehensive assessment of the patient, together with positive attitudes and frequent reevaluation, greatly enhances the likelihood of a successful treatment outcome.[15]

After it has been ascertained that additional radical medical or surgical treatment is unwarranted in the face of disease progression, the health care professional can design a palliative and supportive care program for the terminally ill geriatric patient. At this stage, the health professional can intervene to alleviate pain, and proper positioning and supportive devices can assist in keeping the patient comfortable.

When the dying process becomes inevitable, every health practitioner must seek the answer to the basic question of how to provide the highest quality care for the terminally ill older person. Although dying is a physical process, cognitive and behavioral clues are often evident in the terminal patient. In an older individual dying from cancer, at times an abrupt change in thought and/or behavior may signal the beginning of the terminal phase of the disease.[16] Also, with the withdrawal from the patient of the various health providers, which unfortunately is so common in terminal care, a shift by the patient toward anxiety or depression may receive less attention than in the younger age group. The elderly person, like all persons, will approach death from a distinctive and individualistic pathway and will respond and react in a manner commensurate with that individual's psychologic makeup. These patients' wishes and desires regarding care, disposition, and environment during the terminal phase of their disease should be respected within all possible and practical means.

Advances in detection and diagnosis and major breakthroughs in surgical, medical, and radiation oncology have afforded longer survival periods for many patients and, in some cases, complete cures, even in the face of systemic, metastatic disease. Admittedly, much success has been manifest in the pediatric tumor realm, but as research advances, more geriatric individuals with favorable cancers will experience longer survival periods during which the quality as well as the length of life are emphasized. This chapter will explore some of the more common tumors that occur in the aged population and offer guidelines concerning the clinical presentation, treatment, and rehabilitation of cancer in this population.

PRIMARY AND SECONDARY LUNG CANCER

The average age of onset of primary lung cancer is 60 years. This disease is responsible for 33 percent of male cancer deaths and 11 percent of female cancer deaths and has demonstrated a marked increase in incidence in the last 50 years. Approximately 100,000 new cases will occur in the United States each year, with an incidence of 4 to 10 times higher in cigarette smokers than in nonsmokers.[17] Cromartie and his associates[18] reported that only 6.8 percent of a series of 702 patients were nonsmokers, which strongly suggests that tobacco may be a contributory etiologic factor.

Lung cancer exhibits both hematogenous and lymphatic metastatic potential and often spreads widely before diagnosis.[19] Consequently, surgical resection may not be curable; this, combined with the low response rate of lung cancer to available chemotherapeutic modalities, makes treatment extremely difficult.

Symptoms of the disease include dyspnea (20 percent), cough (75 percent), weight loss (40 percent), and occasional hemotysis.[19] These clinical manifestations may mimic other pulmonary conditions, an additional rationale for the elaborate diagnostic and staging procedures that are employed.

Elderly patients, as others with primary lung cancer, undergo a sequential process of evaluation, which includes initial staging (liver, spleen, and bone scans, and CAT scan of the brain), and final staging (histologic verification of lymph node or distant organ metastases).[20] This complex process significantly improves the accuracy of determining the extent of disease in older patients who do not have obvious clinical evidence of metastases at the time of diagnosis.

Both preoperative and postoperative physical therapy treatment will be required in the majority of elderly patients undergoing a thoracotomy for primary lung cancer. A complete chest evaluation is performed preoperatively. The therapist notes the rate and depth of respiration, use of accessory muscles of respiration, and any asymmetry of chest wall movement during breathing. The physical therapist also assesses the preoperative shoulder range of motion, general posture, and frequency and effectiveness of the patient's cough. The latter is particularly important, because postoperative sputum retention is a significant cause of morbidity in the lung cancer patient. Palpation is systematically carried out to determine if structural abnormalities are present in the chest wall and thorax; vocal fremitus will be increased over the area of the tumor if the lesion is large and there is accompanying consolidation. Percussion over a tumor, used as an evaluative tool, often yields a dull, flat sound. Lastly, auscultation is performed by the therapist to determine the presence of abnormal or adventitious breath sounds. Normal breath sounds are frequently diminished over a large lung cancer. The postoperative program is explained to the patient, who is instructed in deep breathing, coughing, and splinting of the incision.[21]

Particularly in the geriatric patient, who might be frail, initially debilitated, and perhaps frightened of the surgical procedure, a preoperative visit by the physical therapist can allay some of the fears the patient may have, as well as familiarize him or her with the treatment procedures that will follow surgery. Post-thoracotomy complications are common enough to warrant both preoperative and postoperative programs designed to give attention to areas such as weak or ineffective cough, heavy secretion production, oversplinting of the chest incision, and drying of the respiratory mucosa.

The postoperative physical therapy approach to these patients is multidimensional. Postural drainage techniques may be employed to assist in removal of secretions and to insure adequate lung ventilation, but percussion and vibration are contraindicated directly over the tumor site if hemorrhage is present or if there is an ongoing course of radiation.[21] Modified drainage positions may be necessary; ultrasonic nebulization can be employed to liquify secretions. The therapist should realize the potential dangers of aggressive physical therapy procedures performed on cachectic, elderly lung cancer patients.[22] Hemoptysis, atalectasis, and exhaustion of the patient may occur if vigorous percussion and vibration are employed. If any complications ensue, the therapist should discontinue treatment and consult with the appropriate medical personnel. The postoperative program should include breathing exercises and instruction in coughing.

The incidence of post-thoracotomy pneumonitis in patients over the age of 65 is three times that of younger individuals. This suggests that the geriatric patient may need more attention in order to prevent this complication.[22] In the recumbent, semicomatose patient, positional rotation by the combined team is necessary both to prevent secretion accumulation and to avoid skin breakdown, the latter being of special concern in the older patient, who may have poor skin nutrition. Lung cancer patients who do not undergo surgical resection will need modified postural drainage, instruction in coughing, and breathing exercises to assure adequate lung expansion and secretion clearance and to prevent atelectasis and pneumonitis.

Following a lateral thoracotomy, range of motion to the ipsilateral upper extremity is indicated. Proprioceptive neuromuscular facilitation (PNF) diagonal patterns have been found beneficial in increasing functional shoulder range of motion. This ipsilateral shoulder may displace slightly downward, and the therapist should attempt to keep the shoulders level so that weight can be evenly distributed on the buttocks when the older person is in the seated position. A postural evaluation will assess the patient for shoulder displacement as well as postoperative scoliosis (rare), which can be treated with appropriate exercise.

In a recent article by Stanley,[23] which reviewed the cases of over 5000 patients with lung cancer, over 77 prognostic factors were considered. The three most important factors affecting survival were initial functional performance, defined as ability to carry out normal daily activities; extent of disease; and recent weight loss. The author substantiated the role of the rehabilitation team in assuring adequate functional ability prior to surgery or other treatment.

Early hematogenous, or blood-borne, dissemination is distinctly common in lung carcinoma, and blood-borne metastases may involve the brain, liver, skeleton, and opposite lung. In males, lung and prostate cancer are responsible for the majority of metastatic bone disease found clinically. Bone metastases may be osteolytic, or bone destroying, or osteoblastic, or bone producing. Osteolytic metastases may cause dissolution and resorption of extensive areas of bone and carry the threat of pathologic fracture, particularly in the long bones.

Lung carcinoma is the most common primary neoplasm to metastasize to the brain; the tumor cells embolize via the pulmonary veins and carotid artery, enjoying a fairly direct route to the central nervous system. In the elderly individual, any neurologic sign may be the presenting symptom of a silent lung tumor. In a recent review of 80 patients 65 years of age and older with a brain tumor, metastatic carcinoma was second in occurrence to glioblastoma.[24] Solitary metastatic tumors may be surgically extirpated, but brain irradiation is more commonly used in lung cancer metastatic to the central nervous system (CNS), because the tumor foci are usually multiple.[25] The older patient who presents with a hemiparesis or other neurologic syndrome caused by brain metastases should be treated by the therapist much the same way as a patient whose nervous system has been compromised by trauma, vascular accident, or infection. The neurophysiologic facilitative approaches should be used in an attempt to regain motion, to alleviate spasticity if present, and to provide more normal motor patterns for the patient. Brain metastases formulate a dynamic process; with treatment with steroids and irradiation, the clinical neurologic picture is frequently marked by remissions and exacerbations of neurologic deficit. For this reason, it is often difficult to assess the efficacy of rehabilitation intervention in affecting neurologic and functional improvement.

Metastatic lesions in the lung will eventually occur in 20 percent to 30 percent of patients dying with malignant disease.[17] Almost any primary tumor can be responsible, and the lungs provide the first resting ground via the pulmonary arteries after cancer emboli are released into the systemic circulation. Parenchymal metastases are notoriously asymptomatic for long periods of time until sufficient pulmonary tissue has been crowded out and the patient experiences progressive dyspnea. When severe shortness of breath ensues, deep breathing exercises and supplementary oxygen inhalation can be of considerable benefit to these patients.

In contrast to parenchymal lung metastases, lymphangitic metastases—usually from the breast, GI, or uterine cancer—cause an intense early pulmonary symptomatology consisting of severe dyspnea, tachypnea, and cough productive of large amounts of grayish sputum.[26] In these patients, the reason for the symptomatic pulmonary manifestations is that the cancer cells are dispersed throughout the perivascular and peribronchiolar lymphatic channels, interfering with the normal cleansing action of the lung. Elderly patients exhibiting this type of metastatic lung disease may be acutely ill, and chest physical therapy procedures, particularly postural drainage to mobilize secretions, can be significantly beneficial in relieving their distress.

Another complication of lung carcinoma is metastatic involvement of the vertebrae, which can result in epidural spinal cord compression, with resultant paraplegia or quadriplegia.[27] Metastatic spinal cord lesions, although not common, are not rare in the elderly patient suffering from cancer. The vast majority of these cases are caused by metastatic malignant disease, particularly of the lung.[28] Treatment is usually by surgical decompression and laminectomy, which may be combined with radiation therapy. The geriatric patient who presents with spinal cord symptomatology owing to metastatic epidural disease should be treated as any spinal cord injury; although the survival period is usually short, the patient can benefit both physically and psychologically from proper positioning, maintenance of range of motion, mobilization of extremities, and strengthening programs to enhance whatever functional abilities are present.

The paraneoplastic syndromes—such as polymyopathies, peripheral neuropathies, pulmonary hypertrophic osteoarthropathy, and hypercalcemia—occur more often in primary lung cancer than in any other type of cancer. Over 50 percent of elderly people who present with a polymyositis syndrome will be found to have an underlying carcinoma, usually in the lung, breast, large bowel, or prostate.[1] In polymyositis and its variants, the proximal muscles are swollen, tender, and weak. Patients with these syndromes may respond to a rehabilitation program of splinting, positioning, and judicious use of active assisted exercise.

It is clear that lung cancer, both primary and secondary, results in clinical problems that go far beyond the realm of pulmonary symptomatology. The elderly lung cancer patient may present with a wide variety of complications which will require the intervention of a coordinated, well-disciplined cancer rehabilitation team. Throughout the course of the disease, the patient's physical comfort and mobility are of prime concern; many therapeutic modalities can be utilized to achieve these goals. In the future, newer methods of diagnosis, staging, and treatment, including polychemotherapy, will result in longer survivals and a more hopeful outlook—further evidence for the place of rehabilitation efforts as a contribution to optimal patient management.

HEAD AND NECK CANCER

Cancer of the head and neck region constitutes 5 percent of all malignancies in men and 2 percent of all cancer in women, collectively comprising 70,000 new cases annually and resulting in 22,000 deaths.[29] Head and neck cancer is largely a geriatric problem, the majority of patients being over the age of 60 at diagnosis.[30] The most common location is in the larynx, and the vast majority of tumors are of the squamous cell variety.

The head and neck area, with its areas and organs of special senses, has a special significance in one's body image. Surgical mutilation which is frequently necessary to control or to eradicate neck and head cancer has a much greater psychologic impact than elsewhere in the body. In no other form of cancer is the team approach so greatly needed or appreciated. Cooperation of the entire team is mandatory in order for the full rehabilitation potential of the patient to be attained.

A summary of the major types of head and neck cancer is given in Table 11-1. Cancer of the oral cavity, anterior two thirds of the tongue, and lip is relatively common. Alcohol and tobacco are major etiologic agents, associated with age, sex, and ethnicity. The vast majority of tumors occurs in elderly men.[31] The increased cancer and precancer rates in older people may be due in part to age changes in the oral mucosa making it more vulnerable to the action of carcinogens.[30] Survival rates with localized disease, particularly in cases involving only the lip, are excellent.[32]

Disabilities resulting from surgery, such as problems in speech, swallowing, facial and masticatory muscle control, and sensation will necessitate the skills of various trained professionals. The speech pathologist evaluates and treats the

TABLE 11-1. Major types of head and neck cancer

LOCATION	PERCENTAGE HEAD AND NECK CANCER	5-YEAR SURVIVAL	COMMENT
Oral cavity	10%–15%	50%–80%	80% occur in males, mean age of 60
Paranasal sinuses	3%	30%–60%	90% occur in maxillary sinus
Nasopharynx	less than 1%	30%–40%	relative frequency of hematogenous spread is high
Oropharynx	10%–15%	20%–30%	in cancer of posterior 1/3 of tongue, 50%–70% will have positive cervical nodes
Larynx and hypopharynx	greater than 50%	Variable	good prognosis if lesion detected early

Adapted from Norante and Rubin,[29] p 163.

patient who has undergone a laryngectomy or resection of structures used in speech, such as the tongue, lips, hard and soft palates, and buccal surfaces. The dietician is needed both preoperatively and postoperatively to assess nutritional problems which are all too common when chewing and swallowing become painful or difficult following resection of head and neck structures. The occupational therapist may prescribe assistive devices which will aid the postoperative patient in achieving proper nutrition and motor control. Both physical and occupational therapists treat muscle dysfunction in the postsurgical head and neck patient and, by sensory stimulation and muscle reeducation and training, afford the patient optimal control and use of the muscles of expression and mastication.

Carcinoma of the paranasal sinuses is fortunately rare, comprising 3 percent or less of all head and neck cancer.[28] Over 90 percent of cases occur in the maxillary sinus but only 10 percent in the ethmoid sinus. Sphenoid and frontal sinus cancers are extremely rare. The relative frequency is higher in women than most other head and neck cancers. Symptoms include bloody nasal discharge, pain in the teeth or face, nasal obstruction, and a palpable swelling in the area involved. The treatment of these cancers demands complex methods of radiation and surgery.[33] The radical surgery required may include orbital exenteration with en bloc dissection of the tumor mass, producing considerable cosmetic and functional defects. Maxillofacial prostheses are used as an adjunct or as a replacement for reconstructive surgery, because the defect may be too large or the blood supply too poor to allow surgical reconstruction.[34] Too, the elderly person may not tolerate as well the multiple surgical procedures that may be required for adequate reconstruction. The use of maxillofacial prosthetic devices permits an early return of function for patients with severe deformities. Much research is needed in the area of muscle reeducation and training in the use of prostheses employed to treat the defects resulting from surgery for head and neck cancer. The logical place to begin would be for health professionals to perform a *detailed* assessment of motor ability and sensation in the operative area, so that the patient may make optimum use of remaining structures to provide acceptable use of the prosthetic device.

Tumors of the nasopharynx occur in a slightly younger age group, although cancers in this area may be seen in the elderly population. Nasopharyngeal cancer is particularly common in the Oriental races for reasons not completely understood.[34] The majority of patients seek the aid of a physician because of cervical adenopathy; the incidence of nodal spread from these lesions is 70 percent to 90 percent. Symptoms include cranial nerve impairment, hearing loss, pain, and nasal obstruction.[29] Surgical resection is difficult because of the anatomic location. Recent research has examined the occupation of patients with this tumor, and a somewhat higher incidence was reported in persons who worked with wood or leather.[35]

The oropharynx may be defined anatomically to include the soft palate, tonsil, and posterior one third of the tongue. Major symptoms of malignancy in these areas are sore throat, dysphagia, painful ulceration, or an exophytic growth that may be palpable by the patient.[29] A significant proportion (over 50 percent) of patients will have positive cervical nodes if the primary tumor is located at the base of the tongue, thus the survival rate remains low. When cancer in this area or in any head and neck location becomes unresponsive to treatment, the irreversibility of the disease becomes a challenging problem to the cancer rehabilitation team. The health care professional and the patient's family should respond with appropriate supportive measures in order to assist the patient in remaining independent and productive.[36,37] Engaging the patient's cooperation in rehabilitative efforts may be difficult in light of so distressing a lesion and a seemingly hopeless situation.

The vast majority of head and neck cancers occur in the larynx and hypopharynx, and the majority of cases occur in the sixth and seventh decades of life.[34] The major symptoms are hoarseness, dysphagia, and, in advanced lesions, dyspnea and stridor caused by respiratory obstruction. Any geriatric patient presenting with acute or gradual onset of hoarseness should be considered to have or at least should be highly suspected to have laryngeal cancer until proven otherwise. The 5-year survival is quite variable, but the prognosis is quite favorable if lesions are detected early.[29] The multidisciplinary approach to treatment is stressed, and protocols employing surgery, radiation, chemotherapy, and immunotherapy in various combinations are becoming increasingly more common.[38] In cases of early detection, conservative surgery, such as wide excision and subtotal laryngectomy, is used, thus sparing the patient the considerable morbidity and dysfunction of total laryngectomy and the creation of a permanent stoma. In all cases the judicious use of postoperative speech and physical and occupational therapies will afford the patient adequate communication techniques and acceptable physical function.

The majority of head and neck cancer patients require rehabilitation and treatment not for the effects of the primary tumor or its metastases but for the disabilities encountered after a radical neck dissection has been performed. This procedure usually requires the dissection of the cervical lymphatic chain, the internal and external jugular veins, the sternocleidomastoid muscle, and the spinal accessory nerve.[39] Because of the paralysis of the trapezius muscle, which is supplied by the spinal accessory nerve, there is a loss of ability to flex completely or to abduct the arm at the shoulder joint.[40] The degree of trapezius paralysis will depend on the amount of primary accessory innervation loss, because this muscle receives collateral innervation in some individuals from C-2, C-3, and C-4 spinal segments. The therapist employs active and active-assisted range of motion exercises and mobilization techniques to assure adequate capsular mobility. Inferior displacement of the ipsilateral shoulder joint may also occur, along with protraction of the scapula—the latter caused by a combination of the loss of trapezius as a scapular stabilizer and an uneven or unopposed anterior shoulder muscle pull. An already chronically protracted scapula and kyphosis, which are commonly found in the geriatric age group, will contribute significantly to the problem. Late scoliosis is possible.

Postural exercises emphasizing shoulder extension, external rotation, scapular retraction and adduction, and cervicothoracic extension are indicated. In one study of radical neck dissection patients, inferior shoulder displacement occurred in 50 percent, pain and discomfort in 42 percent, and reduction of active range of motion in the shoulder in 90 percent of the individuals studied.[39] Most often impaired are those complex acts involving the use of the arm over the head.

Recently a variation of the classical radical neck dissection has been proposed and tried with a small selection of patients.[41] In this variant, the jugular vein, accessory nerve, and sternocleidomastoid muscle are dissected out during surgery and preserved. The cosmetic advantage as well as the lessened physical dysfunction in these patients undergoing a "functional" radical neck dissection is significant. The smaller degree of surgery involved reduces the metabolic stress in the patient, and this procedure may find applicability in the geriatric patient who for medical reasons cannot tolerate extensive surgical procedures. The efficacy of this relatively new and innovative surgical technique remains to be established in future controlled trials.

For all patients undergoing a radical neck dissection, the therapist would perform posture evaluation, sensory testing, specific manual testing, and goniometric evaluation. The therapeutic rehabilitation approach would emphasize maintaining or increasing the shoulder range of motion, strengthening of the remaining musculature, and improving performance in activities of daily living (ADL). Strengthening of shoulder muscles is of great importance; no muscles can really substitute for the trapezius if the latter is completely paralyzed. The serratus anterior does help appreciably in stabilizing the scapula, and its strengthening should be emphasized. In light of the multiple problems that may occur, the geriatric patient may consider the cosmetic problems more significant than the functional ones. In these sedate patients, the shoulder disabilities may present seemingly little problem, and gentle ADL and functional activities may be all that is indicated. In all cases, goals should be mutually agreed upon by both therapist and patient.

Lastly, the importance of psychologic counseling should be entertained in the treatment approach to the geriatric head and neck cancer patient. There is need for consideration of emotional factors during all phases of diagnosis and treatment of head and neck cancer.[42] Attention should be given also to the psychologic needs of the staff and patient's family as well.

Head and neck cancer in the geriatric population will continue to be an engrossing clinical problem in the ensuing decades. The cosmetic, sociologic, psychologic, and physical ramifications are extensive, and older patients will present with complications requiring the services of various members of the cancer rehabilitation team. As with lung cancer, improved treatment regimes will afford longer survival periods; many patients with both localized and systemic diseases will require these rehabilitative efforts to continue for longer periods. In response to this need, newer rehabilitation strategies may have to be developed to treat the clinical disability and dysfunction that will be observed.

BREAST CANCER IN THE ELDERLY

Breast cancer is the most common type of cancer in women, one in eleven woman will develop a breast cancer at some time in their lives. These tumors account for 27 percent of female cancer deaths.[43] There is a wide geographic variation, with incidence being highest in the United States and Western Europe and lowest in Japan.[44] The disease occurs at a median age of 50; 60 percent of cases occur in those persons over 55 years of age,[45] and 13 percent occur in persons over 75 years of age. Another study reported that 36 percent of new breast cancer cases and 42 percent of deaths caused by breast carcinoma occurred in women 65 years of age and older.[46] The overall survival rate in breast cancer is approximately 50 percent, and despite advances in treatment, this figure has not changed appreciably in several decades. Herbsman and his associates[47] reported an absolute 5- and 10-year survival rate of 54 percent and 41 percent, respectively, in 138 female patients over 70 years of age.

The typical presentation of breast cancer is a lump or nodule in the breast which is isolated, movable, and usually painless in the early stages. In geriatric women with large, pendulous, or atrophic breasts, the early signs may not be appreciated as often; an early detection depends on self-examination and annual examination by the physician. Over 50 percent of tumors occur in the upper outer quadrant of the breast.[43] Frequent breast self-examination is as important in the geriatric woman as it is for her younger counterpart.

The treatment of primary breast cancer has become a complex process, combining the modalities of surgery, radiation therapy, hormonal manipulation, and chemotherapy. These combined approaches have offered significant prolongation of life in many patients, even those with disseminated disease. Survival periods of 5, 10, and even 15 years are becoming increasingly more common.

Kessler and Seton[48] stated that the management of operable breast carcinoma in women aged 70 years or more represents a unique problem. These patients often suffer from intercurrent diseases that reduce their life expectancy and increase their operative risk. They felt that treatment of breast cancer should be based partially on the life expectancy of the woman at each age. Some authors recently studied 94 patients over 65 years of age who were treated surgically.[49] They substantiated the contention that long-term survival was comparable with that in the general population with breast cancer, despite a high percentage of deaths from intercurrent disease. Elderly patients may present with advanced disease when first seen clinically, but this finding does not generalize to all geriatric breast cancer patients.

Other authors[50] have found no significant difference between older and younger patients regarding detection and patterns of spread in breast cancer. It appears, then, that breast carcinoma in the elderly woman is not a significantly different disease than breast carcinoma in younger populations.

The radical mastectomy, which removes the breast, pectoralis major and minor muscles, and ipsilateral axillary lymphatics, has been the mainstay in treatment for operable breast cancer for many decades. Extensive clinical trials have lent evidence to the observation that patients receiving a modified radical mastectomy, in which the pectoral muscles are left intact, affords equal survival rates in breast carcinoma and produces less morbidity.[43] In many centers the modified technique has replaced the standard Halsted radical mastectomy. Alternatives are lumpectomy, where the tumor alone is excised, and simple mastectomy alone. Many clinical trials are underway in which these less radical procedures are employed in conjunction with radiotherapy and/or chemotherapy. In one series, however, an elderly group treated with simple mastectomy did not fare as well (in terms of overall survival and disease-free interval) as a group composed of mixed ages who underwent a standard radical mastectomy. However, this may be a matter of patient selection; the older patients were treated by simple mastectomy. A study that compares various surgical procedures within a selected group of geriatric patients would assist in finding the most efficacious surgical operation for this age group.

The removal of the pectoralis major and minor muscles during a radical mastectomy results in a moderate degree of dysfunction for varying periods of time after the survery. It is the goal of the rehabilitation team, particularly the physical and occupational therapists, to initiate and to monitor exercises to ensure the return of range of motion and strength to the affected shoulder.

The usual disability encountered is an immediate postsurgical loss of abduction and forward flexion of the involved shoulder. This is mainly a result of the mastectomy incision extending up into the axilla; there is pulling on this incision when abduction and forward flexion are attempted. Edema in the operative area may also contribute to this loss of range of motion. The elderly patient may have a preexisting functional loss of range of motion in the operative shoulder, stressing the need for preoperative evaluation, if possible. Shoulder horizontal adduction, for which the pectoralis major is a prime mover, is seriously weakened. In time, the anterior deltoid and coracobrachialis muscle compensate for the loss of the pectoral muscles.

Exercises performed postsurgically assist in increasing range of motion and strength and also in reducing edema. The therapist should be attentive to the cardiovascular changes and decreased endurance in the elderly patient. An exercise program should be performed three times daily, starting on the second or third postoperative day. Exercises are performed *slowly* and to the limit of endurance. This is extremely important because overexercising causes fatigue and pain. This fatigue may cause the patient to splint during movement or to develop substitution patterns which might be detrimental to further function.

Shoulder internal rotation is frequently limited after a mastectomy and interferes with activities that involve the use of the hand on the upper back, such as bathing and hooking a bra. A manual muscle test is impractical during the first few weeks following a mastectomy; however, after this period the patient should be gently assessed for gross muscle weakness. Assessment of ADL and sensory testing are useful adjuncts to successful therapy.

Examples of exercises that are useful include ball squeeze with the elevated arm; pendulum exercises of the Codman's variety; wall climbing; which measures successive progress in shoulder range; exaggerated deep breathing to assist in chest expansion; bilateral external shoulder rotation; and pully exercises.[52] An individualized program for the geriatric patient is essential; not all patients will be able to perform all exercises. The patient should aim for smooth, rhythmical motions when exercising; performing movements in front of a mirror helps tremendously. The rehabilitation professional should foster a positive, assured attitude in the patient, which is a necessary component for good recovery of function. The sensitive therapist also will consider the psychologic and socioeconomic problems that may beset the breast cancer patient[58] and be prepared to refer the patient to appropriate team members who are trained to handle such problems.

Swelling of the ipsilateral arm occurs in one third to one half of mastectomy cases.[51,53] In 10 percent of cases, this edema may be severe, resulting in a grossly enlarged arm and loss of functional ability. The usual cause is surgical ablation of the lymphatic channels and nodes in the axillary region; but scarring, delayed wound healing, radiation fibrosis, venous obstruction, recurrent cancer, obesity, and infection may all be contributory. Elevation of the affected arm and frequent exercising will assist in lymphatic drainage and thereby reduce lymphedema. Intermittent compression with pneumatic devices and units is very effective in early or moderate lymphedema, but current research indicates that this treatment must be employed for several hours *daily* for any considerable or lasting benefit to be realized.[53] Treatment may need to be carried out for several weeks before improvement is noted. Meticulous hand and arm precautions—

such as avoiding injections, cuts, and infections, especially in the elderly—should be followed to prevent or to reduce lymphedema. Fortunately, the overall incidence and degree of lymphedema in the postmastectomy breast cancer patient is decreasing, perhaps owing to early detection, improved surgical technique, newer radiation therapy modalities, and comprehensive and early therapeutic management.

Breast cancer spreads both lymphatically and hematogenously; few cancers can result in as wide and varied a metastatic pattern as this tumor. Metastases are common in bone, lung, pleura, liver, brain, and soft tissue. Skeletal involvement occurs clinically in over one half of cases with disseminated breast carcinoma and can be found in up to 70 percent of cases coming to autopsy.[54] One theory states that older breast cancer patients tend to have a greater degree of soft tissue and bony metastases, as opposed to the visceral, liver, and lung metastases which are more common in the younger patient.[2]

Bone metastases may be of the osteolytic type, appearing as decorticated areas of decreased bone density, or osteoblastic, appearing as areas of scarring of increased bone density. In breast cancer, 70 percent of metastatic bone disease is osteolytic, 10 percent osteoblastic, and 20 percent mixed.[49] The axial skeleton is most frequently involved; metastases usually are found in the spine, pelvis, ribs, proximal femora, proximal humeri, and skull. Table 11-2 gives the frequency of metastases to specific bony sites in a sample of 25 patients with breast cancer

TABLE 11-2. Frequency of metastases to specific bony sites*

BONY SITE	NO. OF PATIENTS	PERCENTAGE OF PATIENTS HAVING BONY DISEASE, N = 25
Lumbar Vertebrae	15	60%
Thoracic Vertebrae	15	60%
Ribs	13	52%
Wing of Ilium	10	40%
Skull	9	36%
Ischium	8	32%
Femur—Head and Neck	8	32%
Femur—Intertrochanteric	7	28%
Acetabulum	6	24%
Pubic Bone	6	24%
Sacrum	4	16%
Shoulder girdle (clavicle, scapula, upper humerus)	4	16%
Femer—Subtrochanteric	2	8%
Cervical Vertebrae	2	8%
Sternum	1	4%

N = 25
*Detected by bone survey, bone scanning, or both.

metastatic to bone. These findings are comparable with larger series, in which metastases are most common in the vertebral column.[53]

In the elderly woman with disseminated bony disease, bone metastases may be asymptomatic. Pain usually heralds positive radiographs; it is usually deep and worsened by activity, particularly weight bearing. In geriatric patients, the clinician may dismiss bone pain as arthritis or muscle strain, and a careful clinical history of each patient is mandatory. Pathologic fractures occur in 50 percent of breast cancer patients with radiographic evidence of osteolytic metastases,[56] perhaps the greatest and most disabling complication in this disease. Fractures may rapidly incapacitate the elderly patient with decreased muscle mass and poor cardiac and pulmonary reserve. Femoral fractures are the most common and carry the greatest morbidity, chiefly because of the weight-bearing properties of this bone.

In the past, these patients rapidly became bedfast and had short survival periods. Little was done in the way of treatment for these patients because of the historically poor prognosis once a pathologic fracture occurred. However, the rationale for internal fixation of pathologic fractures of the long bones, followed by aggressive rehabilitative therapy, is now well established.[56-60] Surgery facilitates nursing, ambulation potential, radiotherapy, and transportation of the patient. The complications of the bedridden patient can be avoided.

Methyl methacrylate cement has recently been found to be useful adjunct in fixation of malignant neoplastic fractures.[58] Radiation therapy is usually employed in addition to surgical fixation and does not appear to alter fracture healing time.[57] The breast cancer patient with a hip nailing for metastatic fracture should be treated with the same rehabilitation efforts that would be used for any hip fracture patient. The therapist should employ early mobilization, early weight bearing (depending on the type of orthopedic device utilized), and graded exercises to restore strength and range of motion.

A fracture of a long bone is imminent if greater than 50 percent of the cortex of the bone is destroyed by the metastatic deposit. Metastatic bone tumors are best treated *before* the extent of malignant invasion permits a fracture to occur.[60] The concept of prophylactic internal fixation has gained wide favor.[59,60] Internal stabilization of an imminent fracture eliminates pain, displacement of fragments, and an emergency situation created by the fracture. Ryan and his associates[59] reported on 18 prophylactic nailings in 14 patients (11 of 14 patients had breast cancer); all but three ambulated postsurgery and continued to do so until 1 to 2 weeks prior to death. In most patients, immediate or early weight bearing is allowed, thereby greatly increasing their mobility and functional ability.

Metastatic disease can lead to additional complications, such as hypercalcemia and quadriplegia or paraplegia from epidural spinal cord compression, as in metastatic lung cancer. Lastly, it is important to note that metastatic bone disease can be caused by primary tumors in the lung, kidney, prostate, and thyroid, among others. The same complications outlined above for breast cancer can ensue and will require similar treatment and rehabilitation management.

In summary, the rehabilitation effort for the breast cancer patient is multifaceted and begins with initial diagnosis and continues throughout all phases of the disease. In the initial phase, the therapist will treat respiratory problems, shoulder dysfunction, and lymphedema. Later the management focuses on disabilities caused by metastatic deposits. In the later stages, the clinician will encounter neurologic deficit owing to brain metastases or generalized weakness owing to liver metastases, and these problems should respond to rehabilitation efforts. Lastly, supportive and palliative care for the terminally ill geriatric breast cancer patient cannot be underestimated, for it is integral for total cancer therapy and is most appreciated by the patients who seek it.

SARCOMAS COMMON TO THE GERIATRIC AGE GROUP

A wide variety of connective tissue tumors may affect the geriatric population. Although some of the primary soft tissue and bone tumors have peak incidences in childhood or early adulthood, many also have a high incidence in the elderly patient.

Adult pleomorphic rhabdomyosarcoma, a cancer of striated voluntary muscle orgin, occurs in the sixth and seventh decade, accounting for approximately 10 percent to 15 percent of malignant muscle tumors.[61] The tumors usually arise in the extremities; over half occur in the lower extremity.[62] The quadriceps, adductors, and biceps femoris are most commonly involved. The disease most often presents clinically as a hemorrhagic bruised area or soft tissue mass, which is characterized by nonencapsulation and local invasiveness. These tumors may metastasize both hematogenously and lymphatically; and even after wide surgical excision, they will recur in approximately 60 percent of cases.[63] At diagnosis, 30 percent of cases will already have pulmonary metastases, and metastases to regional lymph nodes will occur in 15 percent of patients.

In patients who undergo a wide surgical section, a considerable loss of muscle balk may be expected. In order to obtain a wide surgical margin, the surgeon may resect an entire muscle or muscle group. Muscle reeducation performed by the physical and occupational therapists will be important in restoring or increasing strength, mobility, and contour to the affected extremity. Ambulation training with appropriate assistive devices may be necessary, especially initially. Treatment should continue until the patient regains functional control of the limb or develops successful muscle substitution patterns to replace the function lost by muscle resection. The specific exercise approach will depend on the location and extent of surgery.

Because of their usual location in the extremities and their notorious ability to recur after local resection, these tumors may require amputation. The surgical procedure may include resection of regional lymphatics proximal to the stump.

The site and level of amputation will depend upon the location, extent, and invasiveness of the primary tumor. The principles of management of the elderly amputee who has an amputation because of cancer are the same principles that would apply to any geriatric amputee. An adequate program of stump wrapping and exercise is instituted immediately after surgery. Dietz[51] claims that preoperative training is of great value to the prospective amputee. During this period, the patient is not in any discomfort from a surgical wound, has not been immobilized, is not overmedicated for pain, and still has confidence in ambulation. Especially in geriatric cancer patients, the progress in rehabilitation can be facilitated by preoperative training in crutch or walker ambulation. This will be of great assistance in ambulation training in the postoperative recovery period. A diagnosis of malignancy should never in itself be a contraindication to prosthetic fitting. The overall 5-year survival rate for adult pleomorphic rhabdomyosarcoma is approximately 35 percent,[64] and many patients will live for significant periods of time, even with disseminated disease.

Either upper or lower extremity prostheses should be employed to assure maximal patient function and mobility. Fitting of the prosthesis can be done early or sometimes immediately in the postoperative period in selected cases; this relatively new approach affords early ambulation. In all cases, adequate upper extremity strength and balance are tantamount to a successful outcome. The therapist must instruct the patient in proper stump hygiene and correct stump wrapping, the latter to assure a conical shape for optimal prosthetic fit. The prosthetist becomes an important member of the cancer rehabilitation team, joining the oncology nurse, social worker, physical and occupational therapists, and physician in effecting good geriatric amputee care and rehabilitation.

Paget's disease is a disorder of unknown etiology, characterized by hyperactive destruction of bone and replacement of normal bone by expanded, soft, poorly mineralized osteoid tissue.[65] The disease rarely occurs under the age of 40 and usually involves the pelvis, skull, femur, spine, tibia, humerus, and scapula. One to 2 percent, and possibly as high as 7 percent, of cases will be complicated by the development of osteosarcoma. These tumors are most frequently located in the femur and humerus, occasionally in the pelvis and skull; occur at a mean age of 67.6 years; and carry a pathologic fracture rate of 33 percent.[65]

The prognosis in sarcomatous transformation of primary Paget's disease is unfavorable, with a mean survival of approximately 1 year following diagnosis. Nevertheless, the elderly patient with an orthopedic stabilization device for a fracture from osteosarcoma will respond well to therapy that is designed to increase functional range of motion, to maintain an increase in muscle strength, and to permit early ambulation. If an amputation is performed, the principles of geriatric amputee care and rehabilitation will apply. In an older patient, often prosthetic devices that are essentially more cosmetic than functional are prescribed, and this is acceptable from a rehabilitation standpoint if the patient's psychologic status and physical comfort are improved. In the terminally ill patient, positioning, frequent turning, pain relief, and other measures of palliative care are important.

Liposarcoma, the malignant tumor of fat cells, represents approximately 18 percent of all soft tissue sarcomas and occurs primarily after age 60.[64] Liposarcomas occur in the extremities—primarily the lower extremity—in over 60 percent of cases and in the retroperitoneum in an additional 15 percent of cases. Forty to 50 percent of tumors will metastasize to the lungs via the bloodstream.[66,67] Because the tumor frequently recurs after simple excision, radical soft part resection is frequently necessary, and large surgical and functional defects are common.[66] An individualized assessment of each patient and muscle reeducation in treatment are the mainstays in assuring as normal postoperative functioning as possible. Occasionally an amputation is performed to control an aggressive tumor. Research indicates that multimodality therapy employing radiation therapy, chemotherapy, and surgery may prolong life.[67] The overall 5-year survival rate is 35 percent to 40 percent.

Other soft tissue sarcomas, such as leiomyosarcoma, fibrosarcoma, angiosarcomas, and other rare tumors may be found in the geriatric population. Wide surgical excision or amputation are the primary treatment modalities for extremity tumors, and the resultant disabilities or amputations are managed similarly.

NON-HODGKIN'S LYMPHOMA AND CHRONIC LYMPHATIC LEUKEMIA

The maximum risk for the development of lymphoma (lymphosarcoma) is between 60 and 69 years, clearly making it a concern in the geriatric age group. It is somewhat more common than Hodgkin's disease, with an incidence of 9 per 100,000 and a greater male to female patient ratio of 1.7 to 1.[68] Older patients are more likely to present with advanced disease, and excessive symptomatology has been correlated with shorter survival.[69,70] The liver is involved in one third of cases, and 20 percent of patients will have systemic symptoms of fever, chills, and weight loss.

Multiple involvement of systemic nodes is common upon clinical presentation, and the involved nodes may lead to obstructive symptoms. The overall survival rate is approximately 20 percent to 30 percent at 5 years; aggressive treatment is recommended in many patients, especially those in poorer prognosis categories.[70] Radiation therapy and chemotherapy are used extensively, and there are several clinical trials currently under investigation.

Chronic lymphatic leukemia (CLL) is a complex disease, is the most commonly encountered leukemia (30 percent), and is clearly a disease of the aged.[71] Over 90 percent of the patients are over age 50 years of age, and 70 percent are over age 60 at diagnosis.[72] There is a 2.1 male to female patient predominance, and the median survival is between 3 and 5 years. Familial clustering, especially in siblings, has been demonstrated but has not been explained fully.

It is of interest that a large proportion of patients are asymptomatic when the disease is diagnosed. Symptoms do occur in most patients with time and include malaise and fatigue, weight loss, diaphoresis, enlarged lymph nodes, organomegaly, and general dysfunction.[72] In mild cases with few symptoms, patients may be quite functional, and medical treatment may be electively withheld. In active disease, cyclic and/or combination chemotherapy produces encouraging responses.[73,74] Interestingly, the 5-year survival rate appears to be better determined by response to initial therapy rather than by clinical staging at diagnosis.[73]

Both lymphoma and leukemia in the aged can produce a clinical picture in the patient of generalized weakness and reduced tolerance for stress, activity and exercise, and increased susceptibility to fatigue. The latter is also caused by the anemia that frequently accompanies these neoplastic processes. Cachexia, the syndrome of weight loss, anorexia, nitrogen and protein imbalance, and generalized wasting of body tissues—problems in any long-term disease—may ensue in these lymphproliferative disorders, causing further loss of strength and making mobilization difficult.

For the aged patient who has become dysfunctional from the general effects of leukemia, lymphoma, or any metastatic cancer, a program consisting of gentle active exercise, positioning and turning, functional ambulation, and pain control may be beneficial. Treatment is based on the patient's willingness and ability to participate. Keeping the seriously weakened patient mobilized and ambulatory for as long as possible has pronounced effects on his or her functional level, physical comfort, psychologic well-being, and overall condition. The patients then can become or remain active participants in the treatment of their disease.

Exercise programs and ambulation schedules are determined individually, inasmuch as no patient will present with the same patterns of weakness or level of dysfunction. The answer to the question of how long physical therapy or other rehabilitation effort should be continued in an obviously terminal patient is simple: as long as the patient desires it and as long as the treatment continues to be of benefit.

CANCER OF THE PROSTATE

The median age for clinically overt prostatic cancer is 70 years. It is the third most common cause of cancer death in men, with approximately 60,000 new cases per year and 20,000 deaths in the United States. Prostate cancer exists in two forms: common localized tumors without clinical significance and less frequent, overt disease with metastases.[74] Only those tumors showing progression, with increased cell size and loss of differentiation, appear to acquire clinically aggressive behavior. Initial symptoms include cystitis, pain, dysuria, and polyuria.

A reliable assessment of prognosis can be expected by combined evaluation of histologic findings and clinical staging.[75] One group[76] found that patients over 70 who have early prostatic carcinoma treated conservatively will have a normal life expectancy, but that patients under 70 live fewer years than expected.[76] Radical prostatectomy is widely employed; however, it fails to cure prostate cancer in many elderly patients because distant dissemination of the disease is often present at the time of diagnosis.[77]

Prostate cancer, like lung and breast carcinoma, spreads by both the circulatory system and the lymphatics. The regional lymphatics are involved in 60 percent of cases, and early hematogenous spread through the paravertebral venous plexuses leads to early bone disease; the osseous involvement is most commonly osteoblastic (osteosclerotic).

Fully 70 percent of men with prostate cancer will develop metastatic bone disease, occurring most commonly in the following, in order of decreasing frequency: pelvis, sacrum, lumbar spine, femurs, dorsal spine, and ribs. These osseous lesions carry considerable pain and morbidity, making management a challenging clinical problem.[78,79]

Although at the present time there is no curative treatment for patients with widespread bone or visceral metastases,[78] surgery, hormonal therapy, radiation therapy, and chemotherapy have all been used quite successfully in palliating this disease.[80] Prostate cancer, like breast cancer, is very commonly hormonally related, and for this reason orchiectomy and estrogens have been used in treatment. Preliminary reports indicate that chemotherapy can be palliative and give good symptomatic relief in many cases.[81] Most cell-mediated immunologic activity is depressed in many prostatic cancer patients.[82] Immunotherapy will undoubtedly play a yet undefined role in metastatic prostate cancer in the future.

Patients with widespread disease from prostate cancer are quite debilitated and will appear older than their stated age. The lungs, liver, pleura, and other organs may be involved via the bloodstream, but it is the bone metastases that cause the most pain and distress in these patients. Severe spinal involvement may lead to restricted motion and a bedfast condition; the patient may need considerable assistance and encouragement in turning and positioning. Light range of motion exercises are frequently indicated to keep the extremities mobile. Ambulation, with a walker if necessary, should be encouraged in all patients. Although the lesions are mostly osteoblastic, careful monitoring of radiographs is important so that weight bearing may be adjusted accordingly. Orthotic devices for the low back are not usually employed because they are generally not tolerated well and the weight and pressure of the brace may actually aggravate symptoms. Transcutaneous electrical nerve stimulation (TENS) is sometimes useful as an adjunct for pain control and may lessen the amount of narcotic analgesic required for effective pain relief.

MYELOMA, COLON CANCER, AND SKIN CANCER IN THE ELDERLY

Multiple myeloma is a malignant tumor of plasma cells in the bone marrow, usually occurring during the sixth to eighth decades of life; 90 percent of cases occur after the age of 40.[83] It is the most common primary malignant bone tumor, per se, and is extremely difficult to treat.[84] Localized and indolent forms of the disease may also occur.[85]

The osseous lesions in myeloma are multicentric and characteristic; moth-eaten-like, lytic, and well-demarcated punched-out areas appear radiographically.[83] The most common presenting symptom is back pain that becomes increasingly unresponsive to treatment. Systemic abnormalities are common, because 60 percent of patients will have hypercalcemia; renal impairment may be progressive; and repeated infections may occur owing to deficient antibody production. Unfortunately, pathologic fractures caused by extensive bony destruction are all too common to this disease. Although the skeletal disease initially responds well to radiation, chemotherapy is eventually utilized in management. The elderly patient with advanced disease will need assistance in mobility, transfers, and general functional activity. Orthotic devices are sometimes employed in painful areas to restrict motion and also to provide support where the diseased skeleton may be unable to maintain stability. Tolerance of these devices is variable. Because of the high incidence of pathologic fracture, the orthopedic surgeon should be in close attendance. Pain control is also of high importance, because the pain-free patient is more mobile and can participate more actively in rehabilitation activities.

Colon cancer is the second leading cause of death from cancer in the United States, with approximately 100,000 new cases per year resulting in 60,000 deaths. This represents 12 percent of male cancer deaths and 15 percent of female cancer deaths. The average age at diagnosis is between 60 and 70 years.[86] Although many factors may predispose an individual to the development of colon cancer, the majority of cases have an unknown etiology. It is of interest that colon cancer has replaced stomach cancer as the leading gastrointestinal cancer in the last 40 years.

One half of colon cancers occur in the rectum, but patients with lesions in the transverse colon tend to have the poorer survival of 28 percent after 5 years.[87] The most common surgery for colon cancer is resection of the distal colon and rectum and creation of a colostomy. A total colectomy and ileostomy construction may be performed for more extensive tumors. Chronologic age alone, in addition, should not be a deterrent to necessary surgical colectomy or colostomy. Although diminished or weakened organ function is common in the elderly, the majority of patients appear to tolerate the surgery well.[88] A hopeful attitude on the part of the patient, family, physician, and the cancer rehabilitation team is helpful in rehabilitation. Notwithstanding, more extensive surgical procedures, such as abdominoperitoneal resection, carry higher mortality and morbidity, especially in the elderly. Gingold[89] advocated electrocoagulation followed by radiation for small rectal adenocarcinomas in the aged.

Ileostomies and colostomies leave the patient without voluntary control of bowel elimination. Enterostomal therapy has become a specialized branch of nursing, and the diversification of collective devices, skin adhesives, and related appliances has been remarkable in the past decade, offering a wide range of therapeutic approaches to individual problems. The enterostomal therapist begins intervention preoperatively with patient instruction. The immediate postoperative care is highly specialized, and the patient gradually learns to irrigate and to care for the stoma. Regular elimination schedules, protection of the skin, and the elimination of odors are but a few of the many facets of ostomy rehabilitation.

Colon cancer frequently metastasizes to the liver via the portal vein, and the lungs and other organs may be secondarily involved. Metastases to the regional retroperitoneal lymph nodes are extremely common in the disease. The patient with widespread metastases from colon cancer may be cachectic and weak and should benefit from a therapeutic program stressing exercise, ambulation, and pain control.

Skin cancer is the most common type of cancer in human beings.[90] An enormous variety of carcinogens—physical, chemical, and environmental—have proven to be important in its etiology. Repeated exposure of the skin to solar ultraviolet radiation is responsible for most skin cancers, and these tumors become progressively more common in older people.[91] Skin damage occurs with each prolonged exposure to the sun, leading to changes characteristic of aged skin.[92] These changes are believed to form the foundation for later development of malignant lesions. The use of magnifiers and skin microscopes to detect early lesions in the elderly population is strongly recommended.[93]

The majority of skin cancers are squamous (epidermoid) and basal cell carcinomas. The former is more aggressive and may metastasize beneath tissue planes and via the lymphatics. Basal cell carcinomas rarely metastasize but are locally destructive. In a series of 1271 cutaneous carcinomas, 496 were recurrent basal cell carcinomas.[94] Older patients, then, tend to be at risk for persistent or recurrent basal cell carcinoma.

Patients who have undergone extensive facial surgery to eradicate skin cancer may need the services of the maxillofacial prosthedontist, speech pathologist, and physical therapist. In addition, because of the area involved and the considerable incidence of recurrence that may require additional surgery, psychologic support is of great benefit to the patient.

SUMMARY

The cancer problem in the geriatric age group is of multidimensional concern. Almost any cancer and its treatment will carry varying degrees of disability and dysfunction. Some tumors are more prevalent in the aged, and the local and systemic effects of cancer may be heightened in this age group. In general, the elderly respond well to medical therapy and rehabilitation, and most endure the taxing treatment regimes without undue strain or morbidity.

However, challenging problems—such as pulmonary dysfunction, loss of range of motion, lymphedema, pathologic fractures from metastatic bone disease, epidural spinal cord compression, and loss of joint function and generalized weakness—can occur and will need the services of professionals who are highly trained and skilled in providing appropriate cancer rehabilitation procedures. The tumors outlined in this chapter are only a representative example of the array of malignancies that can affect the aged individual. With continued progress, research, and specialization in cancer rehabilitation, the elderly with cancer-related dysfunction will be able to reach maximal functional potential.

REFERENCES

1. KURK, AE AND WARDLE, DF: *Management of malignant disease in old age.* In DENHAM, MJ (ED): *The Treatment of Medical Problems in the Elderly.* University Park Press, Baltimore, 1980.

2. RATNER, LH: *Management of cancer in the elderly.* Mt Sinai J Med 47:224, 1980.

3. RUBIN, P (ED): *Clinical Oncology for Medical Students and Physicians: A Multidisciplinary Approach,* ed. 5. American Cancer Society, 1978.

4. HODKINSON, HM: *Cancer in the aged.* In BROCKLEHURT, JC (ED): *Textbook of Geriatric Medicine and Gerontology,* ed. 2. Churchill Livingstone, New York, 1978.

5. BEGG, CB, COHEN, JL, ELLERTON, J: *Are the elderly predisposed to toxicity from cancer chemotherapy?* Cancer Clin Trials 3:369, 1980.

6. SERPICK, AA: *Cancer in the elderly.* In REICHEL, W (ED): *The Geriatric Patient.* HP Publishing, New York, 1978.

7. HORTON, J AND DAUT, M: *Detection and recognition of cancer.* In HORTON, J AND HILL, G (ED): *Clinical Oncology.* WB Saunders, Philadelphia, 1977.

8. HOLMES, FF AND HEARNE, E: *Cancer stage to age relationship: Implication for cancer screening in the elderly.* J Am Geriatr Soc 29(2):55, 1981.

9. GOOD, RA: *Cancer and aging.* Hosp Pract 15(11):10, 1980.

10. LIPSMEYER, EA: *Simultaneous development of autoimmune disease and malignancy in two elderly patients.* J Am Geriatr Soc 27:455, 1979.

11. RAO, DB, BATIMA, RR, RAY, M: *Multiple primary malignancy in the aged.* J Am Geriatr Soc 26:526, 1978.

12. HOWELL, TM: *Multiple primary neoplasms in the elderly.* J Am Geriatr Soc 28:65, 1980.

13. PAYTON, OD: *Geriatric rehabilitation.* In TEITELMAN, J AND YANCEY, K (ED): *Modular Gerontology Curriculum Series.* Health Sciences Consortium, High Point, NC. (In press)

14. HUNT, TE: *Practical considerations in the rehabilitation of the aged.* J Am Geriatr Soc 28:59, 1980.

15. HENRIKSEN, JD: *Problems in rehabilitation after age sixty-five.* J Am Geriatr Soc 26:510, 1980.

16. KASTENBAUM, R: *The physician and the terminally ill older person.* In ROSSMAN, I: *Clinical Geriatrics.* JB Lippincott, Philadelphia, 1979.

17. EMERSON, G, PHILIPS, C, RUBIN, P: *Lung cancer.* In RUBIN, P (ED): *Clinical Oncology for Medical Students and Physicians: A Multidisciplinary Approach,* ed. 5. American Cancer Society, 1978.

18. CROMARTIE, R, ET AL: *Carcinoma of the lung: A clinical review.* Ann Thorac Surg 30:30, 1980.

19. CONNORS, JP: INTRATHORACIC CANCERS. In HORTON, J AND HILL, G (EDS): *Clinical Oncology.* WB Saunders, Philadelphia, 1977.

20. MITZ, V, ET AL: *Sequential staging in bronchogenic carcinoma.* Chest 76:653, 1979.

21. HAMMON, L: *Oncology.* In FROWNFELLER, DL: *Chest Physical Therapy and Pulmonary Rehabilitation.* Year Book Medical Publishers, Chicago, 1978.

22. HAMMON, WE: *Total pulmonary hemorrhage associated with chest physical therapy.* Phys Ther 59:1247, 1979.

23. STANLEY, KE: *Prognostic factors for survival in patients with inoperable lung cancer.* Journal National Cancer Institute 65:25, 1980.

24. TOMITA, T AND RAIMONDI, AJ: *Brain tumors in the elderly.* JAMA 246:53, 1981.

25. SALEMO, TA, LITTLE, JR, MURO, DD: *Bronchogenic carcinoma with a brain metastasis: A continuing challenge.* Ann Thorac Surg 27:235, 1979.

26. JANOWER, ML AND STENNERHASSET, JB: *Lymphangitic spread of metastatic cancer to the lung.* Radiology 101:267, 1971.

27. GILBERT, RQ, KIM, JM, POSNER, JB: *Epidural spinal cord compression from metastatic tumor: Diagnosis and treatment.* Ann Neurol 3:40, 1978.

28. COX, ML, OGLE, SJ, HODKINSON, DM: *Paraplegia and quadriplegia in the elderly due to spinal cord lesions: Association with malignancy.* J Am Geriatr Soc 29:126, 1981.

29. NORANTE, JD AND RUBIN, P: *Head and neck tumors.* In RUBIN, P (ED): *Clinical Oncology for Medical Students and Physicians: A Multidisciplinary Approach,* ed 5. American Cancer Society, 1978.

30. PINDBORG, JJ: *Oral cancer and precancer as diseases of the aged.* Community Dent Oral Epidemiol 6:300, 1978.

31. SMITH, EM: *Epidemiology of oral and pharmyngeal cancers in the United States: Review of recent literature.* Journal of the National Cancer Institute 63:1189, 1979.

32. LOVE, JM, ET AL: *Surgical management and epidemiology of lip cancer.* Otolaryngol Clin North Am 12:81, 1979.

33. ROBIN, PE, POWELL, DJ, STARBIE, JM: *Carcinoma of the nasal cavity and paranasal sinuses: Incidence and presentation of different histological types.* Clin Otolaryngol 4:431, 1979.

34. SESSIONS, P, THAWLEY, SE, CIRALSKY, RM: *Head and neck.* In HORTON, J AND HILL, G (EDS): *Clinical Oncology.* WB Saunders, Philadelphia, 1977.

35. HUYGEN, PL: *Nasopharyngeal cancer: A clinical study with special reference to age and occupation.* Clin Otolaryngol 5:37, 1980.

36. PEARSON, PW: *The dying patient with oral malignant disease.* Otolaryngol Clin North Am 12:241, 1979.

37. KEITH, CF: *Wound management following head and neck surgery: The challenge of complex nursing intervention.* Nurs Clin North Am 14:761, 1979.

38. FERLITO, A, ET AL: *Therapeutic prospects in cancer of the larynx.* J Laryngol Otol 94:405, 1980.

39. EWING, M AND MAYES, M: *Disability following radical neck dissection. An assessment based on the postoperative evaluation of 100 patients.* Cancer 5:873, 1952.

40. AUDGEON, BJ, DeLISA, JA, MILLER, RM: *Head and neck cancer: A rehabilitation approach.* Am J Occup Ther 34:243, 1980.

41. ARIYAN, S: *Functional radical neck dissection.* Plast Reconstr Surg 65:16, 1980.

42. HERYON, FS AND BOSHIER, M: *Head and neck cancer—emotional management.* Head Neck Surg 2:112, 1979.

43. SAULOV, E: *Breast cancer.* In RUBIN, P (ED): *Clinical Oncology for Medical Students and Physicians—A Multidisciplinary Approach,* ed. 5. American Cancer Society, 1978.

44. MOULGAVKER, SH, ET AL: *Effect of age on incidence of breast cancer in females.* Journal National Cancer Institute 62:493, 1979.

45. ERDIECH, LJ, ASAL, NR, HOGE, AP: *Morphologic types of breast cancer: Age, bilaterality, and family history.* South Med J 73:28, 1980.

46. SCHOTTENFIELD, D AND ROBBINS, GF: *Breast cancer in elderly women.* Geriatrics 26:121, March, 1971.

47. HERBSMAN, H, ET AL: *Survival following breast cancer surgery in the elderly.* Cancer 47:235, 1981.

48. KESSLER, HJ AND SETON, JZ: *The treatment of operable breast cancer in the elderly female.* Am J Surg 135:664, 1978.

49. HUNT, EI, FRY, DE, BLAND, KI: *Breast carcinoma in the elderly patient: An assessment of operative risk, morbidity, and mortality.* Am J Surg 140:339, 1980.

50. CHU, SY AND CHOI, HY: *Causes of death and metastatic patterns in patients with mammary cancer. A ten year autopsy study.* Am J Clin Pathol 73:232, 1980.

51. DIETZ, JH: *Rehabilitation of the cancer patient.* Med Clin North Am 53:607, 1969.

52. HEALEY, J: *Role of rehabilitation medicine in the care of the patient with breast cancer.* Cancer 28:1666, 1971.

53. GRABOIS, M: *Rehabilitation of the postmastectomy patient with lymphedema.* CA 26(2):75, 1976.

54. VIADANA, M, BROSS, L, PICKREN, B: *An autopsy studdy of some routes of dissemination of cancer of the breast.* Br J Cancer 27:336, 1973.

55. GALASKI, CB: *Skeletal metastases and mammary cancer.* Ann R Coll Surg Engl 50:3, 1972.

56. SCHUMANN, DJ AND AMSTUTE, H: *Orthopedic management of patients with metastatic carcinoma of the breast.* Surg Gynecol Obstet 137:831, 1973.

57. HEISTERBERG, L AND JOHNSEN, TS: *Treatment of pathological fractures.* Acta Orthop Scand 50:6, II:787, 1979.

58. HARRINGTON, E, ET AL: *The use of methylmethacrylate as an adjunct in fixation of malignant neoplastic fractures.* Journal of Bone and Joint Surgery 54-A:1665, 1972.

59. RYAN, M, ET AL: *Prophylatic internal fixation of the femur for neoplastic lesions.* Journal of Bone and Joint Surgery 58-A:1071, 1976.

60. WIRTH, CR: *Metastatic bone cancer.* Curr Probl Cancer 3:1, 1979.

61. KEYHANI, A AND BOOKER, RJ: *Pleomorphic rhabdomyosarcoma.* Cancer 22:956, 1968.

62. LEE, ES: *Rhabdomyosarcoma in adults.* Proceedings of the Royal Society of Medium 59:414, 1966.

63. Bizel, LS: *Rhabdomyosarcoma.* Am J Surg 140:687, 1980.

64. Aust, JB: *Soft tissue sarcomas.* In Horton, J and Hill, GJ (eds): *Clinical Oncology.* WB Saunders, Philadelphia, 1977.

65. Brackenridge, CJ: *A statistical study of sarcoma complicating paget's disease of bone in three countries.* Br J Cancer 40:144, 1979.

66. Campbell, DA, et al: *Liposarcoma of the lower extremity.* Surgery 88:453, 1980.

67. Evans, HL: *Liposarcoma: A study of 55 cases with a reassessment of its classification.* Am J Surg Pathol 3:507, 1979.

68. Horton, J: *The lymphomas.* In Horton, J and Hill, G (eds): *Clinical Oncology.* WB Saunders, Philadelphia, 1977.

69. Elias, L: *Differences in age and sex distributions among patients with non-Hodgkins lymphoma.* Cancer 43:2540, 1979.

70. Ridders, RA, et al: *Nodular non-Hodgkin's lymphoma (NHL)—factors influencing prognosis, and indications for aggressive treatment.* Cancer 43:1643, 1979.

71. Paolino, W, Infelise, V, Rossi, M: *Chronic lymphoid leukemia: Clinical observation about its natural progression.* Acta Haematol 63:19, 1980.

72. Lictman, MA and Lemperer, MR: *The leukemias.* In Rubin, P (ed): *Clinical Oncology for Medical Students and Physicians: A Multidisciplinary Approach,* ed. 5. American Cancer Society, 1978.

73. Burghouts, J, Prust, E, Van Leir, H: *Response to therapy as a prognostic factor in chronic lymphocytic leukemia.* Acta Haematol (Basel) 63:217, 1980.

74. McNeal, JE: *The origin and evolution of prostatic carcinoma.* Cancer Detect Prev 2:565, 1979.

75. Kastendieck, H: *Prostatic carcinoma: Aspects of pathology, prognosis, and therapy.* J Cancer Res Clin Oncol 96:131, 1980.

76. Barnes, R, et al: *Conservative treatment of early carcinoma of the prostate. Comparison of patients less than 70 with those over 70 years of age.* Urology 14:359, 1979.

77. Walsh, PC: *Radical prostatectomy for the treatment of localized prostatic carcinoma.* Urol Clin North Am 7:583, 1980.

78. Distenma, DA and Bagshaw, MA: *Prostatic adenocarcinoma—considerations in management.* Postgrad Med 67:135, 1980.

79. Pollen, JJ and Schmidt, JD: *Bone pain in metastatic cancer of the prostate.* Urology 13(2):129, 1979.

80. Barnes, RW: *Endocrince therapy of prostatic carcinoma.* Cancer Detect Prev 2:761, 1979.

81. Luckland, AT, et al: *Sequential polychemotherapy for advanced prostatic carcinoma. A preliminary cooperative study on 30 patients.* Eur Urol 5:250, 1979.

82. Catalona, WJ: *Immunobiology of carcinoma of the prostate.* Invest Urol 17:353, 1980.

83. Klos, JR and Burtz, JW: *Multiple myeloma: An overview for the clinician.* Journal of American Osteopathic Association 79:113, 1979.

84. Osby, E, Codmark, B, Reizenstein, PL: *Staging of myeloma. A preliminary study of staging factors and treatment in different stages.* Recent Results Cancer Res 65:21, 1978.

85. ALEXANIAN, R: *Localized and indolent myeloma.* Blood 56:521, 1980.

86. BASSETT, ML, BENNETT, SA, GOVLSTON, KJ: *Colorectal cancer: A study of 230 patients.* Med J Aust 1:589, 1979.

87. DIHL, E, ET AL: *Carcinoma of the colon: Cancer specific long term survival: A series of 615 patients treated by one surgeon.* Ann Surg 49:432, 1979.

88. WEISS, MF AND LESNICK, GJ: *Surgery in the elderly: Attitudes and facts.* Mt Sinai J Med 47:208, 1980.

89. GINGOLD, BS: *Local treatment (electrocogulation) for carcinoma of the rectum in the elderly.* J Am Geriatr Soc 29:10, 1981.

90. BECHTEL, MA, CULLEN, JP, OWEN, LG: *Etiological agents in the development of skin cancer.* Clin Plast Surg 7:265, 1980.

91. FORBES, PD, DAVIES, RE, URBACK, F: *Aging, environmental influences, and photocarcinogenesis.* J Invest Dermatol 73:131, 1979.

92. WILLIS, I: *Sunlight, aging and skin cancer.* Geriatrics 33:33, 1978.

93. GOLDMAN, L: *Direct skin microscopy as an aid in the early diagnosis of precancer and cancer of the skin in the elderly.* J Am Geriatr Soc 28:337, 1980.

94. LEVINE, HL AND BAILIN, DL: *Basal cell carcinoma of the head and neck: Identification of the high risk patient.* Laryngoscope 90:955, 1980.

EXTERNAL VARIABLES:
THE CURRENT STATUS

CHAPTER 12

STRESS AND AGING

Z. ANNETTE IGLARSH, R.P.T., Ph.D.

BEHAVIORAL OBJECTIVES

Upon completion of this chapter, the reader will be able to
1. Define stress and stressors.
2. Discuss current stress theories.
3. Classify and define types of stressors specific to older persons.
4. Identify coping mechanisms of older persons.
5. Design a treatment protocol for the elderly patient.
6. Select appropriate relaxation techniques for elderly patients.

This chapter does not represent a distinct entity in this text. Actually, it serves to redefine many of the concepts presented in this text as stressors in the scheme of the mind-body connection. Stressors are the physiologic, psychologic, and social changes that occur as one ages and that force the individual to modify his or her behavior. These internal or external changes, stressors, trigger a stress response in the body. Stressors do not abruptly commence with graying hair or menopause but are part of the gradual progression of aging. These changes are complex and may not be as overt as the classic symptoms of disease. Many individuals fear aging and its diseases, but few see it as a phase of great stress. The patriarch of stress research, Dr. Hans Selye has redirected his studies into areas of stress and aging.

STRESS AND THE STRESS RESPONSE

Stress is not a new concept. Over 50 years ago Dr. Selye[1] first identified stress in hospitalized patients and described a mind-body connection. These patients manifested common physiologic and psychologic characteristics regardless of their diagnoses. These characteristics included decreasing appetite, dulling of psychologic affect, and increasing blood pressure. In a series of studies of laboratory rats, Dr. Selye[2] found similar physiologic changes in the rats when they were stressed. As a result, Dr. Selye[3] defined stress as "the non-specific response of the body to any demand placed upon it." Although researchers[4] disagree with Dr. Selye as to the nonspecific quality of the response, there is little dispute as to the physiologic changes caused by stressors.

The body's response to these demands has been labeled the General Adaptation Syndrome (GAS) by Dr. Selye[3] (Fig. 12-1). This syndrome consists of three stages: alarm, resistance and exhaustion. The initial response, the alarm reaction, is a response to the sudden exposure to a stressor. The first part of this initial stage, the shock phase, consists of the following physiologic changes: an increase in heart rate and decreases in muscle tone, temperature, and blood pressure. This is followed by the counter-shock phase, in which the body readies itself to meet the stressor by increasing corticoid hormone secretion. These hormones stimulate organs to increase blood pressure and to make stored energy more readily available. The stage of alarm is analogous to Cannon's fight-or-flight response.[5] In both the alarm stage and the fight-or-flight response the body prepares to either meet physical harm or to run from the threat. Early researchers thought that the response stopped as soon as the physical threat disappeared. This is not true in our modern society, where most of the stressors are psychologic as well as physical. These stressors (which will be described later in this chapter) remain in

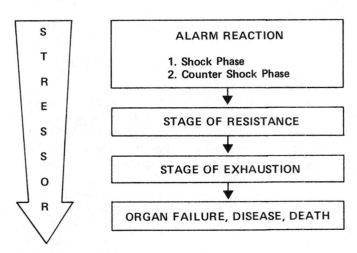

Figure 12-1. General Adaptation Syndrome is shown schematically.

the individual's mind, and therefore the stress response does not abruptly terminate. This sustained response leads to the remaining two stages of Selye's stress
response theory. The second stage, the stage of resistance, involves adaptation.
Here the body adjusts organ function to counteract the physiologic changes in
response to stress. These adjustments create a new homeostatic level of organ
function in the body. In this new state visable symptoms of stress may actually
disappear. However, if the stressor persists, the final stage, the stage of exhaustion, occurs. Here symptoms of physiologic adaptation to stress reappear and the
body's responses eventually fail with fatigue and disease. Organ failure and death
may result.

The body's physiologic response to stress is summarized and simplified in the
diagram of the neuroendocrine pathways (Fig. 12-2).[6] In this neuroendocrine
response the hypothalmus, a regulator of autonomic nervous system activity,
prepares the body to meet stressors via hormone release. These hormones affect
organ function and cause retrieval of needed materials from energy stores. These
hormones also alter cardiovascular function to redirect blood to organs essential
to the stress response and to survive blood loss from possible injury. Other major

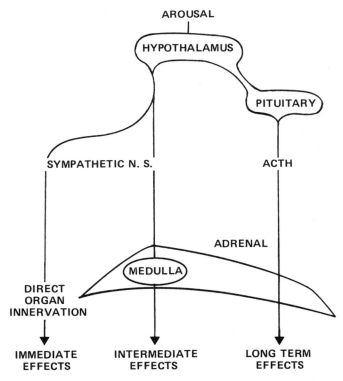

Figure 12-2. Basic neuroendocrine stress response pathways are illustrated here.
(From Allen and Hyde,[6] with permission.)

physiologic effects of stress are increased secretion of growth hormone, adreno-corticotrophic hormone (ACTH), prolactin, adrenalin, and cortisol; lowered sensitivity to insulin; lowered tolerance to carbohydrates; stimulation of lipolysis and neutralization of fatty acids; hypercholesteremia; and stimulation of thrombus formation.[7] It is ironic that these physiologic reactions, which are lifesaving at the time of the potential threat, can lead to disease if prolonged. The same lifesaving physiologic changes in the body that enable a pedestrian to dart out of the path of a speeding car can be sustained and consequently cause disease. The individual may sustain these physiologic changes each time he or she mentally relives the near accident as he or she crosses the street or reflects upon the traumatic event.

Physiologic responses are often thought to occur only with negative stressors. Surprisingly, this is not true. The body responds in equal magnitude to negative and positive stressors.[3] That is, a similar physiologic reaction will occur in the person threatened by a mugger as the fortunate person winning the state lottery. In addition, some level of stress is necessary for effective daily function; that is, simply to maintain a level of attention or cognitive focus.[6] Each person has his or her own point at which this functional stress level becomes destructive. This point will vary moment to moment as environmental conditions and the individual's physical status varies. Many people say that they work better under pressure, but they also speak of the "straw that breaks the camel's back." Disease, acute and chronic, will result from this prolonged or excessive stress state.

These diseases can actually be labeled as diseases of adaptation[8] and are results of faulty responses to stress. These faulty responses are both excessive or diminished physiologic changes in the stress response. The aging process presents a dual problem to these responses. As one ages, he or she is exposed to more incidents of stress as a mere function of time and experience. Each exposure leaves its mark and alters the degree of response system failure. Dr. Selye views these two aspects of aging as causing a gradual inability to remove the chemical scars of life and the stress response. In addition to the inability to remove these scars (for example, calcium deposits from blood vessels), the loss of irreplaceable tissue (for example, brain and heart tissue damage from micro infarcts or vascular failure) further limits adaptability with aging.

STRESSORS: THE SOURCE OF STRESS

Because aging is part of the life cycle and not a unique entity, many stressors are not unique to the elderly. Furthermore, experiences may occur as stressors only when they appear in conjunction with normal aging events or physiologic changes. Events that may have heralded independence or maturity in one's youth may become life-threatening stressors in later years. Striking out on one's own, moving, meeting new people, or changes in day-to-day routines are examples of this dichotomy. Stressors are simply life demands that are environmental, physical, achievement-based, and socially oriented.

Environmental stressors are those demands which originate outside the individual's body. These stressors can be as simple as a change in environment, for example, from familiar surroundings to a new home. This is often appraised as an exciting event in one's youth. However, it can be a trauma for the older individual, especially if the move is determined by need or circumstance, not by choice. A loss of personal and familiar surroundings, separation from supportive friends, and change in daily routine may result from a change in location. Increases in disease vulnerability or occurrence and mental disorientation may also result.[9] Health professionals are very familiar with the independently functional patient who cannot perform simple activities of daily life when hospitalized or admitted to a nursing home. The family who moves the aging parent into their home to care for the parent or the family that moves in with the older parent because neither can exist independently in difficult economic times may be creating more stressful or stress-potential situations than they realize. Crowding is another form of environmental stress that can lead to alienation and increased paranoia. This stressor is often encountered by people in urban areas and dwellers of high-rise apartment structures.[10] A change in environment and overcrowding expose the aging individual to a large number of new stimuli. Unfortunately, the elderly person must cope with this barrage of stressors by using the aging and decreasingly effective stress-control response. This is further exemplified by the older individual's response to physical stressors.

Stressors that originate within the body are classified as physical stressors. Fatigue, chronic illness, and failure of organ systems are common examples of these physical stressors. Because dulling or decreased sensory integration capabilities, as well as diminished reception ability of the five senses, alter perception of stressors, the older person is very prone to this category of stressors. The elderly individual may have distorted and often incorrect information, resulting in inaccurate assessment of the environment. Once again the normal consequences of aging compound the physiologic effects of stressors; in this case, they alter the stress response at its earliest phase, perception. The entire neuroendocrine response system actually functions less effectively with aging.[11] An example of this deficit is the disruption of the neuroendocrine feedback system, the hypothalamic-pituitary response to hormonal feedback, which creates an additional burden to the stress response system. Researchers[12,13] also showed that repeated exposure to physical stressors can actually hasten aging. Conversely, the lack or limited exposure to physical stressors[14] can contribute to greater longevity or a slowing of the aging process.[15]

In an industrialized society, achievement-based stressors are numerous and the most subtle types of stressors. These stressors tend to be characteristic of an individual's personality. The type A individual, common to this society, has been described by Rosenman and Friedman[16] as one who is

1. time urgent (time conscious, deadline oriented, impatient)
2. quantitative (describes things in terms of numbers)
3. polyphasic (does more than one activity at a time)

4. competitive
5. tense

These type A individuals do not change their ways but find themselves more frustrated. As physical and possibly cognitive abilities diminish, the goal-oriented type A individual will not be able to achieve the goals on which he or she bases his or her value and self-worth.[17] It is necessary for the older individual to reevaluate personal expectations. Youthful goals may go unaccomplished, never to be achieved. Sacrifices chosen for personal advancement in earlier years may be questioned as to their long-term value. Family, marriages, and relationships neglected to allow time and energy for personal professional growth may have suffered. They may not be viable social units when the individual finally has the time to assume these social responsibilities. Reinforcement that formerly came from the work environment must now be redesigned to maintain a sense of identity.

Often overlapping the achievement-based stressors are social stressors. As the husband finds time to direct attention to the family, he often finds his children moving away and his wife looking for her identity by returning to the work force. Our transient society has weakened social bonds, such as the ones between growing children and aging parents. These weakened relationships become social stressors as adult children may be forced to move in with parents when they become unemployed, divorced, or when they simply live beyond their earnings. These social stressors also occur in the reverse when aging parents move in with their adult children. This occurs when health impairs ability to function independently or when retirement financial plans are not sufficient to succeed in times of inflation. An opposite experience, the absence of social interaction, can be as stressful as excessive social relationships. Loneliness, a common social stressor, has also been correlated to a greater incidence of disease and high death rates.[18-20] Significant loss, especially of a loved one, has even caused sudden death, a severe stress response, as described in the giving-up syndrome.[21]

Retirement, often a long-awaited event, can be a harmful social stressor to many individuals.[8] Physical illness and premature organic brain syndrome can occur when an individual adjusts poorly to retirement. This occurs with such frequency that it has been labeled as "retirement disease." Retirement forces changes in an individual's relationship to his or her environment and the perception of his or her role in society. Consequently, the individual may face a change in personal income, potential for altered health as physical activity levels usually decrease, and lack of a daily schedule with a greater amount of free time.[22] Each of these major changes in the life of a retired person is a stressor. It is easy to see that the additive and interaction effects of these stressors can be overpowering and thus life threatening for the aging individual.

All of the aforementioned stressors can also be categorized as life events. Holmes, Rahe, and Masuda[23,24,25] compiled a list of life events (Fig. 12-3) which stresses an individual both positively and negatively. The numerical score attributed to the accumulation of the individual's life events over the preceding 24

LIFE EVENT SCALE

Sex: _____F_____   Age: _____68_____

(100)		Death of spouse
(77)		Divorce
(65)		Marital separation
(63)		Jail term
(63)		Death of close family member
(53)	x	Personal injury or illness
(50)		Marriage
(47)		Fired from work
(45)		Marital reconciliation
(45)		Retirement
(44)		Change in family member's health
(40)		Pregnancy
(39)		Sex difficulties
(39)		Addition to family
(39)		Business readjustment
(38)		Change in financial status
(37)		Death of close friend
(36)		Change to different line of work
(35)		Change in number of marital arguments
(31)		Mortgage or loan over $10,000
(30)		Foreclosure of mortgage or loan
(29)		Change in work responsibilities
(29)		Son or daughter leaving home
(29)		Trouble with in-laws
(28)		Outstanding personal achievement
(26)	x	Spouse begins or stops work
(26)		Starting or finishing school
(25)		Change in living conditions
(24)		Revision of personal habits
(23)		Trouble with boss
(20)		Change in work hours, conditions
(20)		Change in residence
(20)		Change in schools
(19)		Change in recreational habits
(19)		Change in church activities
(18)		Change in social activities
(17)		Mortgage or loan under $10,000
(16)		Change in sleeping habits
(15)		Change in number of family gatherings
(15)		Change in eating habits
(13)	x	Vacation
(12)		Christmas season
(11)		Minor violation of the law

Score: _____92_____   Stress Level: _____Mild_____

Figure 12-3.   Mild life event stressors are listed here.

months (some researchers and therapists use a 12-month period) will aid the therapist in identifying the person as prone to illness, acute or chronic (Figs. 12-4 and 12-5). Many of these identified sources of stress are common events of the life cycle: mortgage, marriage, death or loss of spouse, change in residence, and so forth. As a function of time the older individual will accumulate a large number of stressful events. Consequently, the older individual will compile a higher score on the Holmes and Rahe Life Event Scale and thus be more likely to suffer from stress-related illness (Fig. 12-6).

COPING MECHANISMS AND ADJUSTMENT TO THE STRESSORS OF AGING

Each person responds to stressful life events by utilizing different coping mechanisms. People often retreat to former or more immature coping mechanisms in the face of overpowering forces.[26] Common coping mechanisms are regression, conversion, denial, projection, and repression. Sigmund Freud listed examples of forces that may trigger utilization of these coping mechanisms as death of a loved one, separation, ill health, threatened body integrity (real or imagined), decreased cerebral and physiologic functioning, and environmental deprivation (owing to retirement or loss of money). Lowered sense of personal worth and loss of identity can lead to altered reality-testing ability, regression in behavior, and revival of infantile concerns. Health professionals are intimately aware of these changes in some elderly patients, especially those seen in nursing homes or retirement settings. As you read this paragraph, many of you may have nodded as you remembered your patient who clung to her deceased husband's pipe (transitional object) as she wheeled around your clinic or another patient who became noncompliant in a treatment session because you were unable to begin the treatment session at the precise time it was scheduled.

There is a great variability in the way one adapts to aging. Therefore, generalization among individuals or identification of an ideal lifestyle is not possible. However, by utilizing a common sense approach you can formulate some basic, positive suggestions for a maximal lifestyle for the aging individual. Maintenance of some level of activity is obviously important, although the level may be limited to some degree by the physical restrictions of aging. Development and presence of a positive, supportive social setting are also important. The individual should appropriately modify personal expectations and reflections of self. Design of a comfortable but structured schedule is needed. The schedule should be subject to change but instituted to promote continued activity. As at any stage in life, planning or creation of a secure financial status[27] will reduce life's stressors to some extent.

Researchers[28] recommend the adoption of a pet. Pets can serve as transitional objects.[29] Researchers have also found that a pet dog can cause a subject to respond with less anxiety in a stressful environment[30,31] and that touching a pet can act as an antianxiety agent.[28] Pets also further reduce stress by directing the

LIFE EVENT SCALE

Sex: ____M____   Age: ____60____

(100)	x	Death of spouse
(77)		Divorce
(65)		Marital separation
(63)		Jail term
(63)		Death of close family member
(53)	x	Personal injury or illness
(50)		Marriage
(47)		Fired from work
(45)		Marital reconciliation
(45)		Retirement
(44)		Change in family member's health
(40)		Pregnancy
(39)		Sex difficulties
(39)		Addition to family
(39)		Business readjustment
(38)		Change in financial status
(37)		Death of close friend
(36)		Change to different line of work
(35)		Change in number of marital arguments
(31)	x	Mortgage or loan over $10,000
(30)		Foreclosure of mortgage or loan
(29)		Change in work responsibilities
(29)	x	Son or daughter leaving home
(29)		Trouble with in-laws
(28)		Outstanding personal achievement
(26)		Spouse begins or stops work
(26)		Starting or finishing school
(25)		Change in living conditions
(24)	x	Revision of personal habits
(23)		Trouble with boss
(20)		Change in work hours, conditions
(20)		Change in residence
(20)		Change in schools
(19)		Change in recreational habits
(19)		Change in church activities
(18)	x	Change in social activities
(17)		Mortgage or loan under $10,000
(16)		Change in sleeping habits
(15)		Change in number of family gatherings
(15)		Change in eating habits
(13)		Vacation
(12)	x	Christmas season
(11)		Minor violation of the law

Score: ____267____   Stress Level: ____Moderate____

Figure 12-4. Moderate life event stressors are listed here.

Sex: _____ F _____   Age: _____ 70 _____

(100) _____	Death of spouse
(77) _____	Divorce
(65) __x__	Marital separation
(63) _____	Jail term
(63) _____	Death of close family member
(53) __x__	Personal injury or illness
(50) _____	Marriage
(47) _____	Fired from work
(45) _____	Marital reconciliation
(45) _____	Retirement
(44) _____	Change in family member's health
(40) _____	Pregnancy
(39) __x__	Sex difficulties
(39) _____	Addition to family
(39) _____	Business readjustment
(38) __x__	Change in financial status
(37) __x__	Death of close friend
(36) _____	Change to different line of work
(35) __x__	Change in number of marital arguments
(31) _____	Mortgage or loan over $10,000
(30) _____	Foreclosure of mortgage or loan
(29) _____	Change in work responsibilities
(29) _____	Son or daughter leaving home
(29) _____	Trouble with in-laws
(28) _____	Outstanding personal achievement
(26) _____	Spouse begins or stops work
(26) _____	Starting or finishing school
(25) __x__	Change in living conditions
(24) __x__	Revision of personal habits
(23) _____	Trouble with boss
(20) _____	Change in work hours, conditions
(20) __x__	Change in residence
(20) _____	Change in schools
(19) __x__	Change in recreational habits
(19) __x__	Change in church activities
(18) __x__	Change in social activities
(17) __x__	Mortgage or loan under $10,000
(16) _____	Change in sleeping habits
(15) __x__	Change in number of family gatherings
(15) __x__	Change in eating habits
(13) _____	Vacation
(12) __x__	Christmas season
(11) _____	Minor violation of the law

Score: _____ 451 _____   Stress Level: _____ Excessive _____

Figure 12-5. Excessive life event stressors are listed here.

Sex: ____M____   Age: ____80____

(100)		Death of spouse
(77)	x	Divorce
(65)		Marital separation
(63)		Jail term
(63)	x	Death of close family member
(53)	x	Personal injury or illness
(50)	x	Marriage
(47)		Fired from work
(45)		Marital reconciliation
(45)		Retirement
(44)		Change in family member's health
(40)		Pregnancy
(39)	x	Sex difficulties
(39)	x	Addition to family
(39)		Business readjustment
(38)	x	Change in financial status
(37)	x	Death of close friend
(36)		Change to different line of work
(35)	x	Change in number of marital arguments
(31)		Mortgage or loan over $10,000
(30)	x	Foreclosure of mortgage or loan
(29)		Change in work responsibilities
(29)	x	Son or daughter leaving home
(29)	x	Trouble with in-laws
(28)		Outstanding personal achievement
(26)	x	Spouse begins or stops work
(26)		Starting or finishing school
(25)	x	Change in living conditions
(24)	x	Revision of personal habits
(23)		Trouble with boss
(20)		Change in work hours, conditions
(20)	x	Change in residence
(20)		Change in schools
(19)	x	Change in recreational habits
(19)	x	Change in church activities
(18)	x	Change in social activities
(17)		Mortgage or loan under $10,000
(16)	x	Change in sleeping habits
(15)	x	Change in number of family gatherings
(15)	x	Change in eating habits
(13)	x	Vacation
(12)	x	Christmas season
(11)		Minor violation of the law

Score: ____741____   Stress Level: ____Excessive____

Figure 12-6. Excessive life event stressors are listed here.

individual's attention away from stressful thoughts and force the individual to maintain a daily routine, often lacking in the retired individual.

To analyze appropriately methods to positively modify the lifestyle of the aging individual, strategies to successfully adapt to retirement must also be considered. The individual should attempt to minimize the number and magnitude of changes that occur with retirement. Cultivating nonwork, leisure activities and early transition to the retirement income level are examples of this suggestion. The retirement process should be gradual, beginning with a reduction in the work week rather than a handshake and being "shown the door" on the last day. The retiring individual should attempt to participate in the retirement decisions rather than be the "victim of the deed." It would be helpful for the individual to decide the date of retirement and the retirement process. Individuals should plan their income and know their health (and how to maximize their physical abilities by such strategies as pacing physical activity and eating balanced diets). Involvement with other individuals who are retired and facing similar situations will help minimize loneliness, maintain identity, and solve some of the problems of experiences in this new lifestyle. Planning, positive attitudes toward the retirement, and successful experiences dealing with change and flexibility will also contribute to a successful, healthy, and low-stress retirement.[22]

STRESS MANAGEMENT IN THE CLINICAL SETTING

Establishing a Treatment Regimen

These suggestions for a maximal lifestyle and effective retirement will benefit the active, independent, aging individual. But how can you help the ill, dependent, aging individual being wheeled into your clinic for treatment? The aging patient experiencing stress will benefit from the following treatment sequence.

1. Identify major stressors; evaluate the stressors and determine whether the problems are within your capabilities or if it is more appropriate to refer the patient to another practitioner.
2. Identify and analyze the person's coping or adaptive mechanisms.
3. Instruct the patient in stress and stress-management theories.
4. Select and instruct the patient in the appropriate management theory.

IDENTIFICATION OF STRESSORS

Evaluation of stressors begins with a comprehensive intake interview with the patient and the patient's family members, if appropriate. Identify environmental (description of home setting and daily environment), physical (medical history and review of current symptoms and health status), achievement-based (personal expectations and accomplishments), and social (marital status and interfamily relationships) stressors. If they feel comfortable with their interviewer, patients will often clearly outline their stressors. Listen with an open mind. This will enable the therapist to hear the patient self-diagnose his or her stress problems. The use of standardized tests, such as the Holmes and Rahe Life Event Scale,[23] Minnesota Multiphasic Personality Inventory,[32] and the Cornell Medical Index,[33] can assist the health professional identify a patient's stressors if the patient is not communicating effectively. After analyzing the patient's intake and test data, the therapist can decide whether he or she can treat the patient effectively for stress management in conjunction with the therapy regimen or if a referral to a psychologist, psychiatrist, or social worker is more appropriate. For example, a person with severe personality disorders would be treated most successfully by a psychiatrist, and a person requiring a new residence modified for nonambulatory people would best be served by a social worker. Multiprofessional treatment approaches to stress management can be the most effective approach, giving the patient the strength of each discipline. Communication among the professionals and the patient becomes more complex but also more integral to treatment success.

IDENTIFICATION OF COPING MECHANISM

Once the stressors are identified, the next step is to identify the individual's current coping mechanism for each stressor or group of stressors. Has the individual chosen an effective or destructive coping mechanism? Is the patient aware of the stressor and the effects of the coping mechanism being used? Not all mechanisms selected are negative. Sometimes an infantile mechanism can shield an individual from a stressor until a time at which that person is better able to deal with it. Your patient may primp each day for a visit from her husband who died a few weeks ago; another patient may "bargain" to live until a grandson's wedding and apparently maintain his health status until that day but die soon after; and yet another patient refuses instruction in the use of assistive devices because he is "not going to need them" when he recovers from his flaccid paralysis after a massive cerebral vascular accident. Each stressor, despite the coping mechanism utilized, must be dealt with at some time because it may cause a subliminal stress response.

INSTRUCTION IN STRESS AND STRESS-MANAGEMENT THEORY

Identification of the stressor has limited value to the health professional unless the patient is aware of its existence. The patient will respond more effectively if he or she shares in the responsibility of recognizing and evaluating the coping mechanism being utilized and subsequently designing the treatment strategy. If the therapist identifies the patient's fear of financial uncertainty as a stressor but the patient repeatedly smiles and proudly states that her husband left her secure and free from want or concern, the therapist's treatment is rendered ineffective. It is obvious from this example that the patient is not aware of her stressor because of her denial. It is important to teach the patient responsibility for self, the existence of the mind-body connection, and the potential for modification of this mind-body connection in a positive manner to learn to relax at will or need. The practitioner can implement this goal by definition of stress terminology, graphic representations of the mind-body connection, and simplified relaxation experiences (for example, a slowed breathing pattern will allow the person to feel less tense and more in control of a physiologic parameter—respiration). If the patient is interested in additional information, refer the patient to selections from this chapter's bibliography or to less academic articles which often appear in weekly newsstand magazines. This patient involvement will extend beyond the clinical setting, beyond the length of the treatment program, and into the patient's day-to-day life experiences.

SELECTION AND INSTRUCTION IN RELAXATION TECHNIQUES

Once the stressor-coping mechanism is identified, the health professional and the patient can select the appropriate relaxation technique. There is an endless list of techniques and combinations of techniques from which to choose. Some of these are

1. meditation
2. progressive relaxation
3. selected awareness
   a. hypnosis
   b. autogenic training
   c. guided imagery
4. biofeedback
5. breath control
6. systematic desensitization
7. exercise or physical activity.

Meditation. Meditation is described as the focusing and maintaining of awareness on a repetitive or unchanging stimulus.[6] It is a combination of physiologic state, a psychologic feeling, a philosophy, a religious technique, and a state of mind. Meditation is not a technique that is successful for all people, but it does help all people to varying degrees. It has its origins in Eastern culture, and in this country it has been attributed to cults and free spirits of the 1960s and 1970s. Consequently this technique is often rejected by the older population. However, if the therapist selects a comfortable or familiar object of meditation, such as the internal object of one's own breath or the external object of a picture of their grandchild's smiling face or the sound of a number, the patient may be more accepting of this technique. Taking a moment to discuss which object of focus would allow the aging patient to feel most comfortable may help the patient accept this technique. The aging patient may also prefer a sitting or reclining posture in a quiet, secluded environment. Meditation is an effective relaxation technique because it induces a relaxation response,[34] which produces a physiologic state opposite to the physiologic changes of the stress response, and reduces somatic organ arousal.[6,35]

Progressive Relaxation. Progressive relaxation is a technique classically taught in most physical and occupational therapy programs. It was developed by E. Jacobson[36] and is intended to induce deep muscle relaxation. It is helpful for some people because it allows the subject to feel muscle tension. It is a good technique for type A people because they can compete with themselves in their ability to maintain relaxation while tensing another part of their body. It is also an effective technique for subjects with good body awareness, such as athletes and dancers, because they can easily recognize tension and fatigue in muscles. The technique is a combination of 5 seconds of tension and 45 seconds of gradual relaxation in a series of muscle groups. The therapist instructs the patients (one at a time or in small groups) to begin contracting the agonist muscles, followed by contracting the antagonist muscle groups (for example, contraction and relaxation of the biceps is followed by contraction and relaxation of the triceps). The entire sequence begins at the head and progresses downward or begins at the toes and progresses to the head and neck area. Once the technique is learned, the patient can recognize parts of the body that are tense and then the patient can progress to relaxation of these areas without tensing all the muscle groups of the body in sequence. This technique is often well accepted by the geriatric population because it clearly consists of a descriptive task followed by a physical action.

Selected Awareness. Selected awareness utilizes the biologic limitations of people to respond to a limited number of stimuli at one time.[6] Normally, the individual perceives and appraises the most threatening or interesting stimuli in the environment, which contains an endless number of stimuli. While reading this book you are concentrating on the words on the page and possibly the temperature of the room, but until the text mentions it, you are not aware of the street noise or your sensations of thirst or hunger. The therapist can direct the patient to perceive selected stimuli to induce a state of relaxation. Hypnosis, autogenic training, and guided imagery are all types of selected awareness techniques.

During hypnosis the therapist creates a relaxed atmosphere by giving the subject a mental task or a repetitive stimuli. Both activities will alter perception. The hypnotist restricts the subject's awareness and then focuses the awareness on a mental image. In addition, the hypnotist tells the subject what he or she will be feeling, overt physiologic changes of the relaxation response, to build credibility and trusting rapport. Once the patient has successfully experienced a hypnotic state, the patient can be instructed to reproduce the state without the presence of the hypnotist.[37]

Autogenic training is similar to hypnosis in its utilization of a therapist who directs attention. However, unlike hypnosis, the focus is on the patient's physiologic function. The patient concentrates on the sensations of the relaxation response. The patient is taught how the body is altered in the relaxation response and then tries to create those changes by imaging sensations such as warmth or heaviness.[38] This technique increases the effectiveness of progressive neuromuscular relaxation and biofeedback.

In another selected awareness technique, guided imagery, the focus is on the subject's imagination. The therapist asks the patient to concentrate and to visualize a place, real or imaginary, that helps the patient feel relaxed. The place can be an exotic foreign hamlet or a quiet, private room at home. The feeling of relaxation attained and the image can be reproduced by the patient as needed. This technique is often very difficult for the type A patient and may be rejected as a time waster. To overcome this problem the therapist can establish a "contract" with the patient. Two possible strategies are (1) asking the patient to perform the technique for a very short period of time—5 minutes—which can be extended as patient comfort increases with successful relaxation experiences, and (2) by acknowledging to the patient that the therapist is aware of the patient's potential difficulty relaxing and asking for the patient's cooperation in spite of this difficulty.

Biofeedback. Biofeedback is a much more overt form of relaxation therapy than those discussed as examples of selected awareness. In biofeedback the individual receives information on the dynamic state of several possible physiologic functions to help gain control over that function.[39] These functions range from muscle tension to heart rate and blood pressure. Allied health professionals use electromyography (EMG) (muscle tension) biofeedback to reeducate muscle function impaired by disease or trauma. Electromyogram biofeedback can also be used to induce general muscle tension, reducing the muscle tension secondary to the stress response. In all types of biofeedback a device is used as transducer, converting a physical state into a monitorable mode via oscilloscope, audio signal, or digital readout. Once the physical state is perceived by the patient, the patient can then alter it into the desired physiologic response. In many settings mechanical devices are not available, but biofeedback need not be ignored. By holding a patient's hand you can monitor changes in hand temperature. By palpating a patient's upper trapezius or other areas of muscle spasm, the therapist can perceive the changing levels of muscle tension which can be verbally relayed to the patient.

These preceding techniques can be conducted by the therapist or by a recorded tape. Researchers[40] have found that the therapist's live voice is a more effective tool, but a tape is appropriate for homework sessions and for use in sessions once the patient is familiar with the technique being taught. The elderly patient may be intimidated by the operation of the tape recorder, and detailed instruction may be necessary. The patient should be able to choose from a variety of voices (both male and female) because some may be more conducive to relaxation for the individual than others. The therapist should try to listen to the content, as well as to experience each tape. Some tapes will contain phrases and approaches to relaxation that will be more appealing than others. Asking an elderly patient to let the abdominal muscles "sag and feel flabby" or to try "to be mellow" may be inappropriate.

Breath Control.   A simple, non-device-oriented technique is breath control. This is an essential feature of yoga instruction and can be simple or complex. An individual can be trained to breathe in different levels of the lungs, to modify the timing or rhythm of the breath, or to alternate the nostril utilized.[41] A simple modification of the breathing pattern, elongation of the expiration phase of the breath, will promote relaxation. Prolongation of the momentary pause between the inhalation and exhalation will allow the patient to feel in control of the breath and thus more in control of the self. Often the patient can be taught to think of something positive, relaxing, or encouraging during the pause. This simple technique allows the patient to quickly gain control of a physiologic parameter respiratory rate, which will induce a greater feeling of relaxation. Modification of breathing patterns can also be used with other relaxation techniques, such as progressive neuromuscular relaxation or biofeedback.

Systematic Densensitization.   Systematic desensitization is actually a problem-solving strategy.[42] In this technique the patient is asked to write down a list of personal problems, fears, or stressors (Fig. 12-7). The list is then to be rewritten in order of subjective magnitude of difficulty, beginning with the least stressful item. Once the list is formulated, the patient is to solve those stressors with feasible solutions. Those stressors remaining are dealt with by utilizing any of the previously described relaxation techniques, beginning with the least-threatening unsolved item. Once this item can be thought of without producing a stress response, the individual can move on to the next, more difficult item. By utilizing this technique the patient has productively dealt with some of his or her problems and can think about the nonsolvable problems without inducing a stress response. The patient usually feels great sense of accomplishment and control over the self. These are often infrequent achievements of elderly individuals who often feel a loss of independence and self-determination.

Exercise or Physical Activity.   The final relaxation technique is an activity that researchers only recently have identified as a stress-reducing event.[43] Exercise has always been recommended as an activity to improve and to maintain general body function, with special emphasis on the cardiopulmonary system.[44] Physical exercise removes the metabolic by-products of stress, minimizes response to new stressors, and gives the individual a sense of well-being.[43] However, these positive effects will occur only if the physical activity is noncompetitive, because competitive activity itself can be a stressor. This relaxation technique should not be ignored when treating elderly patients. Many individuals who have been active throughout their lives continue this lifestyle as they age. This is exemplified

A. *Problem List*
   money
   loneliness
   sad, depressed
   general aches and pains
   scared to go out alone
   fear of falling
   fear of dying
   can't handle my bank statement
   don't like to eat alone
   can't sleep well

B. *Organized Problem List*
   1. don't like to eat alone
   2. can't handle my bank statement
   3. can't sleep well
   4. scared to go out alone
   5. fear of falling
   6. fear of dying
   7. general aches and pains
   8. sad, depressed
   9. money
   10. loneliness

C. *Possible Solutions*
   1. don't like to eat alone: Join an organized eat-together program or simply arrange to eat with friends on a frequent basis.
   2. can't handle bank statement: Ask a friend or your bank's manager for assistance.
   *3. can't sleep well: Maintain some activity level during the day, limit daytime naps, and practice relaxation just before going to sleep.
   *4. scared to go out alone: Arrange walks and shopping trips with friends, join organized community activities, and follow police suggestions to maximize safety.
   *5. fear of falling: Use adaptive devices (glasses or care) as needed; limit travel in inclement weather; when walking, concentrate on foot placement and potential obstacles.
   *6. fear of dying: Join discussions with friends, community groups, and religious counseling sessions.
   *7. general aches and pains: Schedule a complete physical with a physician and maintain an activity level but do not overdo it.
   *8. sad, depressed: Participate in counseling sessions, keep busy.
   *9. money limitations: Watch for sales, participate in community and government support programs as needed, and get investment counseling.
   *10. loneliness: Participate in community activities and get a pet.

*The starred items have solutions to some degree, but the individual must use relaxation strategies to minimize the residual stressor effects to safer (non-disease-prone) physiologic levels.

Figure 12-7. Outlined here is a clinical example of systematic desensitization.

by the number of retirees who complete the Boston Marathon each year. Obviously the majority of the patients are not silver-haired marathon runners, but what about walkers, bikers, and dancers? A clinician[44] has found that rhythmic movements performed by wheelchair patients stimulates cardiovascular function and induces a pleasant relaxation state. Physical activity performed in small groups can accomplish relaxation as well as socialization. As with any event of therapist-patient interaction, the therapist's enthusiasm for the activity is essential and will encourage greater patient involvement.

A common-sense approach should be utilized when establishing the criteria for selection of the appropriate relaxation techniques. The therapist's comfort with the techniques, the patient's personality, the patient's specific stress problem, and the environment in which the technique will occur should all be considered.

The following outline may assist the therapist and the patient in this decision-making process.

1. Meditation
   a. general relaxation technique
   b. easier to learn in quiet environments
   c. when teaching older patients, consider minimizing the training techniques so that patients do not feel out of place doing "hippy things"
   d. example of effective application: the patient is anxious about living with her children but is unable to live alone and must learn to relax in her stressful environment
2. Progressive relaxation
   a. can be general or specific technique
   b. good to replace maladaptive behavior, for example, overeating
   c. good for patients with good body awareness
   d. good for type A person—relaxation becomes goal
   e. example of effective application: the patient is recently retired and finds himself feeling tense in non-goal-oriented routine
3. Selected awareness
   a. can be general or specific technique
   b. select approach based on therapist's or patient's comfort
   c. may need to convince the patient of the value of such a cognitive technique
   d. example of effective application: the patient has rheumatoid arthritis and would benefit from directing thoughts away from her painful joint condition
4. Biofeedback
   a. type selected depends on patient problem and equipment available
   b. can be general or specific
   c. train patient to the equipment and then wean the patient so that the patient can relax without the monitoring device
   d. often the devices, gadgets, motivate the patients

e. patient must be capable of monitoring the physiologic event and capable of altering the physiologic state (neurologic cognitive abilities)

f. example of effective application: the patient suffers from muscle tension headaches and has intact cognitive ability

5. Breath control
   a. can be used with other techniques
   b. can be used as an immediate stress-intervention technique without anyone else being aware of its being used
   c. allows the patient to regain control over a physiologic function when the patient may feel he or she is losing control of self
   d. example of effective application: the patient is overwhelmed by the concept of learning how to relax and needs to feel quick reduction of tension and control of self

6. Systematic desensitization
   a. should be used formally or informally with all patients
   b. promotes use of more productive coping mechanisms
   c. example of effective application: see Figure 12-7

7. Exercise
   a. extent of utilization will depend on patient status, but creative thought will allow the therapist to apply it to all patients in varying degrees
   b. group teaching and musical accompaniment promote more effective patient involvement
   c. group activities may reduce social stressors
   d. an example of effective application: a group of physically capable but physically uninvolved women would benefit from an early morning brisk walking activity

The therapist will be able to select an appropriate relaxation treatment for any patient from the previous list of stress-management techniques. However, the therapist should not apply these techniques without the same prudent judgment that would be used when applying a more traditional clinical modality. The therapist should analyze the effect of relaxation therapy on the patient's physiologic status, which is altered by normal aging and disease states. What will be the effect of altered blood pressure, heart rate, respiratory rate and depth, oxygen consumption, and blood content (glucose and hormone levels)[6] on the patient's physical condition? Patients with diagnoses such as hypertension, hypotension, diabetes,[45] hypoglycemia, and epilepsy should be evaluated by their physician before relaxation therapy begins and then monitored periodically by their physician as relaxation therapy continues. In addition, the therapist should have the patient describe any changes in physiologic status during, after, and between treatment sessions. Including these descriptions with the objective data from EMG biofeedback, thermometer, or blood pressure devices in the patient's records is essential for treatment documentation.

Instruction in relaxation techniques for outpatients follows a simple progression. Each series should begin with the patient's being instructed in stress, the mind-body connection, and the relaxation technique. The therapist should familiarize the patient with the technique, the environment, and any devices that will be used. The sessions begin with close patient-therapist interaction. Homework or patient assignments should be given after each session and reviewed at the beginning of each new session. These assignments range from keeping a stress diary to practicing the techniques using tapes supplied by the therapist. Accordingly, these assignments will reinforce the training sessions and encourage the patient to use the techniques in daily activities. Training sessions continue until the patient approaches a level of relaxation below which he or she can no longer reduce tension, their relaxation potential. At that time the therapist begins to spend less time with the patient during the training session and allows the patient to perform the techniques independently. As the series comes to a close after 5 to 7 weeks, the patient and therapist should discuss training termination and future patient responsibilities. Patients appear to be more compliant with the relaxation program if periodic return visits are conducted to evaluate patients' ongoing competence at controlling stress. This training sequence can be carried out in conjunction with standard therapy treatment and can be integrated into treatment regimens.

You may even be more effective using relaxation therapy with your inpatients. Fortunately, unnecessary stressors in the inpatient setting can be reduced, and the inpatient may have greater opportunity for relaxation therapy practice in this structured setting. All the patient's caregivers should be involved in stress identification and reduction of stressors with the patient. As health professionals may be stressors or "stress inducers" as well as "stress reducers," helping the patient recognize his or her stressors may inadvertently reveal to the caregiver that person's role as stressor. The caregivers can encourage the patient to practice the relaxation techniques and positively reinforce the patient's control of stress throughout the day if they are knowledgeable about stress theory. Small group in-service presentations on relaxation principles will help the health professional assist the patient to manage stress as well as give the caretaker insight into his or her stress status.

An additional benefit of relaxation exists for the therapist. In order to teach relaxation to others, the therapist also must relax prior to the instructional session and will feel more relaxed as the relaxation session progresses. This positive aspect of relaxation therapy can make these sessions the highlight of the working day and also can reduce professional burnout.[46]

This chapter has given the therapist an added responsibility in the course of clinical practice. Stress and stress-management theories are appropriate concerns of therapists treating the older patient for physical dysfunction and the associated psychophysiologic problems or complications. It challenges the therapist to look beyond the patient's loss of motion or disruption of cognitive function to identify the patient's stressors. Once the stressors are identified, the therapist can refer to other appropriate members of the health care team for solution or treatment of these stressors. Concurrently, the therapist educates the patient about his or her stress status and teaches the patient stress-control techniques. These new treatment modalities should not be thought of as added techniques but as complementary techniques which treat the "whole" patient. This will dramatically add to the therapist's treatment effectiveness and thus improve the elderly patient's prognosis. In addition, the therapist may discover a new dimension to the aging patient: a patient experiencing the stressors of a lifetime.

To cope with these stressors of a lifetime, Dr. Selye[8] has formulated a "code of behavior . . . to minimize distress and maximize eustress" (functional stress).

1. Find your natural stress level.
2. "Altruistic egoism . . . love of our neighbor is the most efficient way to give vent to our pent-up energy and create enjoyable, beautiful or useful things."
3. "Earn they neighbor's love."
4. "Fight for your highest attainable aim, but do not put up resistance in vain."

These final concepts should cultivate further your thoughts regarding stress and your aging patients. They are concepts related to patient care but can also be generalized to life—to the quality of your life and of your patient's life.

REFERENCES

1. SELYE, H: *A syndrome produced by diverse nocuous agents.* Nature 138:32, 1936.

2. SELYE, H: *Stress and aging.* Geriatr Soc 18:9, September, 1970.

3. SELYE, H: *The Stress of Life.* McGraw-Hill, New York, 1959.

4. LAZARAS, RS: *Psychological Stress and the Coping Process.* McGraw-Hill, New York, 1966.

5. CANNON, W: *Traumatic Shock: Surgical Monographs.* D. Appleton, New York, 1923.

6. ALLEN, R AND HYDE, D: *Investigation in Stress Control.* Burgess Publishing, Minnesota, 1982.

7. DILMAN, VM: *Transformation of development: Program in the mechanism of aging pathology.* Practitioner 4:465, 1979.

8. SELYE, H: *Stress, aging and retirement.* Journal of Mind and Behavior. 1:93, Spring 1980.

9. RIEGLE, GD AND HESS, GD: *Chronic and acute suppression of stress in young and old rats.* Neuroendocrinology 9:175, 1972.

10. MILGRAM, S: *The experience of living in cities.* Science 167:1461, 1970.

11. RANGELL, L: *Discussion of buffalo creek disaster: Course of psychic trauma.* Am J Psychiatry 133:313, 1976.

12. CURTIS, HJ: *Biological mechanisms underlying the aging process.* Science 141:686, 1963.

13. Timeras, P: *Aging*. In Cox, H (ed): *The Physiology of Aging*. Dushkin, Guilford, CN, 1980.

14. Davis, R: *Stress homeostatic mechanisms*. In Eliot, RS (ed): *Stress and the heart: Contemporary problems in cardiology*. Futura, Mount Kisco, New York, 1974, p 97.

15. Trujillo, TT: *A study of radiation induced aging*. Radiat Res 16:144, 1962.

16. Rosenman, R and Friedman, M: *Overt behavior pattern in coronary disease: Detection of overt behavior pattern A in patients with coronary disease by new psychophysiological procedure*. JAMA 173:1320, 1960.

17. Howard, J, et al: *Adapting to retirement*. J Am Geriatr Soc 30:488, 1982.

18. Maddison, D and Viola, A: *The health of widows in the year following bereavement*. J Psychosom Res 12:239, 1968.

19. Clayton, PJ: *Mortality and morbidity in the first year of widowhood*. Arch Gen Psychiatry 30:747, 1974.

20. Lynch, J and Convey, W: *Loneliness, disease, and death: Alternative approaches*. Psychosomatics 20:702, October, 1979.

21. Engel, G: *A life setting conducive to illness: The giving up—given up complex*. Ann Inter Med 69:293, 1968.

22. Howard, J, Marshall, J, Rechnitzer, P: *Adapting to retirement*. J Am Geriatr Soc 30:488, August, 1982.

23. Holmes, T, Rahe, R: *The social readjustment rating scale*. J Psychosom Res 11:213, 1967.

24. Rahe, R: *Life events and mental illness: An overview*. J Human Stress 5:2, September, 1979.

25. Holmes, T and Masuda, M: *Life changes and illness susceptibility*. In Dohrenwend, BS and Dohrenwend, BF (eds): *Stressful Life Events: The Nature and Effects*. W. Ley, New York, 1974.

26. McGrae, R: *Age differences in the use of coping mechanisms*. J Gerontol 37:454, 1982.

27. Barfield, R and Morgan, J. *Trends in satisfaction with retirement*. Gerontologist 18:19, 1978.

28. Katcher, A and Friedmann, E: *Potentiali health value of pet ownership*. Compendium on Continuing Education 11:2, February, 1980.

29. Winnicot, DW: *Transitional objectives and transitional phenomena*. Int J Psychoanal 34:89, 1953.

30. Sebkova, J: *Anxiety levels as affected by the presence of a dog*. Unpublished thesis, Lancaster, PA, 1977.

31. Friedmann, E: *Pet ownership and coronary heart disease*. Circulation 168(Suppl 2):57, 1978.

32. Dahlstrom, W, Welsh, G, and Dahlstrom, L: *An MMPI Handbook, Vol 1, Clinical Interpretation (rev ed), Vol 2, Research Applications*. University of Minnesota Press, Minneapolis, 1974.

33. Brodman, K, Erdmann, A, Wolff, H: *Cornell Medical Index Health Questionnaire*. Cornell University Medical College, New York, 1949.

34. Benson, H, Beary, J, Carol, M: *The relaxation response*. Psychiatry 37:37, February, 1974.

35. GIRDANO, D AND EVERLY, G: *Controlling Stress and Tension: A Holistic Approach.* Prentice-Hall, Englewood Cliffs, NJ, 1979.

36. JACOBSON, E: *Progressive Relaxation.* University of Chicago Press, Chicago, 1938.

37. BARBER, T: *Physiological Effects of Hypnosis.* Psychol Bull 58:360, 1961.

38. LUTHE, W (ED): *Autogenic Therapy: Volume 5.* Grune & Stratton, New York, 1969.

39. GAARDNER, I AND MONTGOMERY, P: *Clinical Biofeedback: A Procedural Manual for Behavioral Medicine.* Williams & Wilkins, Baltimore, 1981.

40. PAUL, G AND TRIMBLE, R: *Recorded vs. live relaxation training and hypnotic suggestion: Comparative effectiveness for reducing physiological arousal and inhibiting stress response.* Behavioral Therapy 1:285, 1970.

41. RAMA, S, BALLENTINE, R, HYMES, A: *The Science of Breath.* Himalayan International Institute, Honesdale, PA, 1979.

42. GOLDFRIEND, M: *Systematic desensitization as training in self-control.* J Consult Clin Psychol 37:228, 1971.

43. DUSEK-GIRDANO, D: *Stress reduction through physical activity.* In GIRDANO, D AND EVERLY, G (EDS): *Controlling Stress and Tension: A Holistic Approach.* Prentice-Hall, Englewood Cliffs, NJ, 1979.

44. SWITKES, B. *Senior-Cize: Exercises and Dances in a Chair.* Betty Switkes, Washington, DC, 1982.

45. FOWLER, J, BUDZYNSKI, T, VANDENBERGH, R: *Effects of an EMG biofeedback relaxation program on the control of diabetics.* Biofeedback Self Regul 1:105, 1976.

46. WOLFE, G: *Burnout of therapists inevitable or preventable?.* Phys Ther 61:1046, July, 1981.

CHAPTER 13

DRUGS AND THE ELDERLY

NANCY M. O'HARA, M.A.
DIANE WHITE, P.D.

BEHAVIORAL OBJECTIVES

Upon completion of this chapter, the reader will be able to
1. Explain why the elderly are a high-risk population with regard to drug use.
2. Describe the normal physiologic changes that occur with aging and how these changes affect drug functioning.
3. Recognize how drugs function (for example, drug interactions).
4. Delineate between generic and nongeneric drugs, as well as over-the-counter and prescription drugs, commonly used by the elderly.
5. List complications of drugs commonly taken by older patients.
6. Outline how caregivers can help minimize the potential for adverse drug reactions in older persons.

One axiom of aging is that growing older means changes in physical and psychologic functioning. Gradual physiologic changes occur throughout adulthood with a slow decline in function of all body systems. The rate of change is individual, and different systems within one person will age at different rates. Generally, though, the body's ability to ward off disease is lessened. Consequently, approximately 80 percent to 86 percent of persons over age 65 suffer from one or more chronic health conditions.[1] Cardiovascular disease, cancer, and cerebrovascular accidents, or strokes, have their greatest impact among older persons. Because of the multiplicity of their disease processes, the elderly are likely to be taking a variety of drugs. Persons over 65 years of age comprise only 11 percent of our population, yet they consume more than 25 percent of all medicines prescribed. It is estimated that the elderly use a similar proportion of over-the-counter (OTC) drugs. An average elderly person spends more than $100 for prescribed and OTC drugs annually and has more than 13 prescriptions filled per year.[2]

There are many reviews, portions of books, and journal articles on the topic of drugs and the elderly; this chapter on drugs and the elderly will highlight some general areas of concern. Particular emphasis will be placed on the elderly person's increased sensitivity to drugs of all kinds. This chapter will discuss several aspects of drug therapy in the elderly population and will provide references for further study of this subject.

OVERVIEW OF DRUG CONCEPTS

Drugs are obtained either over the counter or by prescription. Over-the-counter (OTC) medications are those medications which can be purchased without the written or oral consent of a physician.[3] These include such products as aspirin, Tylenol, Sominex, and Contac. They are sold in pharmacies, chain drugstores, grocery stores, airports, and even in some restaurants. The purchase of these products may result from the recommendation of a friend, a physician, a pharmacist, or from an advertisement seen on television or in a magazine. Prescription drugs (Lanoxin, Percodan) are those drugs which are dispensed to the patient only via written or oral consent of a physician. There are legal limitations on who may sell medications. Doctors and dentists may dispense from their offices, but, in general, drug sales are limited to pharmacies under the supervision of a registered pharmacist.

Drugs come in many different forms. Listed below are brief descriptions of each.

1. Aerosol sprays or powders. These products depend on the power of a liquified or compressed gas to expel the contents from the container. An example is Tinactin powder (an antifungal agent).
2. Tablets. These are drugs in solid pill form and are usually intended to be taken orally. Lanoxin (a cardiac medication) is an example of this form. There are many different types of tablets, including enteric-coated tables (Ecotrin), prolonged action tablets (Polaramine, an antihistamine), sugar-coated tablets, and tablets for solution (potassium permanganate tablets).
3. Sublingual and buccal tablets. These are small, flat, oral tablets. Tablets intended for buccal administration are inserted into the buccal pouch and dissolve or erode slowly. Progesterone tablets may be ad-

ministered in this manner. Sublingual tablets, such as nitrostat (a vasodilator used to treat angina), are placed under the tongue. These tablets dissolve rapidly and are absorbed locally.

4. Capsules. These are solid dosage forms in which the drug is enclosed in either a hard or soft solution container or shell of a suitable form of gelatin. Indocin (an anti-inflammatory agent) and Sinequan (an antidepressant) fall into this category.

5. Ointments. Ointments are highly viscous or semisolid substances used topically. Nitropaste (used to treat angina) is an example of an ointment.

6. Solution. A solution is a homogeneous mixture that is prepared by dissolving the active ingredient in an aqueous or nonaqueous solvent. An example is Dimetapp elixir (a cough and cold remedy). Ear, nose, and eye drops are also included in this category.

7. Emulsions. An emulsion is a dosage form in which the medicine is incorporated into one of the two phases of an oil-and-water mixture. A lotion is an example of an emulsion.

8. Suspensions. The drug is suspended in an appropriate medium or solvent. Many of the antibiotics used in the treatment of infections are suspensions.

9. Creams. Creams are solid emulsions containing suspensions or solutions of medicines for external application. Many of the antiinflammatory compounds that are prepared as ointments are also prepared as creams. Patients may prefer the cream because it is less greasy.

10. Suppositories. Suppositories are solid dosage forms for insertion into the rectum, vaginal cavity, or the urethral tract. Preparation H and Anusol are examples.

11. Injections. These are drug preparations intended to be given by a parenteral route or administration. Parenteral means injected directly into a vein, intramuscularly, or into the subcutaneous tissue. Insulin is an example of a drug administered subcutaneously.

All drugs have a brand name and a generic name, also called the official name. Generic names are usually contractions of a complex chemical name; brand names are generally short, easy to remember, and often devised to suggest the pharmacologic action of the drug.[4] The brand name is used to advertise a drug to the medical profession, although the generic name must appear in the advertising and labeling also. Aspirin, for example, is the generic name for acetylsalicyclic acid; Bayer and St. Joseph's are brand names for different manufacturers' aspirins. Generic products contain the same active ingredients as brand name products. Generally, the only difference between the two products is cost and manufacturer. Whether you buy a discount drugstore's brand of aspirin or a nationally advertised brand, there will generally be no difference in the pain-killing quality of the products. Any drug that is labeled aspirin must meet specific Food and Drug Administration (FDA) standards.

AGING PROCESSES AND DRUG THERAPY

The aged have a sensitivity to drugs that is related to a combination of factors.[5] Older persons are more susceptible for several reasons:[6]

1. They are more likely to have multiple diseases that can alter the way the body handles drugs.[7] For example, a patient with congestive heart failure does not perfuse his or her liver normally; accordingly, metabolism of some drugs, such as Coumadin (an anticoagulant), is slowed, and higher blood levels of the drug result.[8]
2. They are more likely to take a large number of different drugs, which increases both the risk of adverse drug effects and the risk of drug interactions.
3. Increased numbers of medications also increase the probability that mistakes in taking the medication will occur. Furthermore, patients taking many medications tend to be less compliant, that is, they may take their medications less frequently than prescribed. Indocin can cause problems if older patients do not tell their doctors about any OTC drugs they may be taking, including aspirin. The taking of aspirin and Indocin at the same time can be dangerous to the patient; this combination can cause extreme stomach upset and gastric bleeding.[9,10]
4. With age, there are changes in physiology that lead to changes in the ways drugs affect the body. Aging produces several physiologic changes that can affect pharmacokinetics. Pharmacokinetics refers to the rate of drug absorption, distribution, biotransformation, and excretion.[11] In general, aging changes the effect drugs have on elderly persons. For example, because of a gradual decline in the efficiency of the liver and the kidneys, drugs are not metabolized or eliminated by older persons as quickly as they were in earlier years. By age 70, kidney function may be reduced by as much as 40 percent. Harmful accumulations of drugs in the bloodstream may result from a reduced rate of elimination. The physiologic changes of aging do not occur at the same rate for everyone, thus, it is impossible to determine how drugs will affect every older person. Therefore, adverse drug reactions are unpredictable and become more likely with advancing age.

Absorption

Absorption is the passage of drugs from the intestine to the bloodstream.[12] The route of administration, either enteral (oral) or parenteral (intramuscular, subcutaneous, or intraveneous), determines the site of the drug's absorption. With age, the lining of the digestive system becomes less cellular and the secretion of gastric juice decreases.[11] These changes alter the solubility and ionization of drugs which in turn affect the degree and rate of absorption.

Distribution

In the normal distribution process, a drug first enters the portal circulation and passes through the liver, where it may be changed by enzymes. The drug then enters the systemic circulation, where it may bind to proteins in the blood or in cells, be dispersed in body water, or accumulate in certain organs. Two processes of aging alter this response:[11] (1) Drugs are absorbed more slowly in older persons, and (2) after absorption, some drugs are stored in increased body fat. In the elderly, functional tissue is replaced by fat cells, which have a greater attraction for some drugs than do other cells. This may cause drug accumulation and may extend the duration of effect of the drug.

Biotransformation

Biotransformation (metabolism is often used synonymously with biotransformation) is a process that converts substances in the blood into a form that can be excreted more readily.[11] Biotransformation usually occurs in the liver microsomal enzyme systems but may also occur in the intestinal wall during absorption, in the muscles, and in the blood. With age, the process of drug metabolism can be slower because of a decrease in metabolic capacity of and a decrease in perfusion of the liver or other metabolizing tissues.

Excretion

Small amounts of a drug may be excreted through saliva, lungs, and perspiration, but the main excretory routes are through the kidneys and gastrointestinal (GI) tract. Kidney filtration decreases with age because nephrons in the kidneys gradually shrivel and become replaced with scar tissue.[11] Therefore, drugs cannot always be excreted as rapidly and may accumulate to toxic levels.

Drug Therapy for Common Medical Problems

The most common medical problems that occur among the elderly as part of this aging process are listed as follows:[13]

1. arthritis
2. hearing loss
3. heart conditions
4. high blood pressure
5. visual impairment
6. psychiatric disorders
7. digestive disorders

8. chronic sinusitis
9. nervous disorders
10. genitourinary problems
11. circulatory problems.

This section will discuss some of the most common drugs used to treat the above conditions. Each health care provider can build on the basics presented here as deemed necessary for individual practice.

DRUG THERAPY FOR CARDIOVASCULAR DISEASE

Cardiovascular disease continues to be the number one cause of death in the United States despite the decline in the rate of death from coronary artery disease. Atherosclerosis and hypertension account for nearly one million deaths annually. A large proportion of the 30 million Americans estimated to have diseases of the heart and blood vessels are elderly.

The term cardiovascular disease includes several diseases. One is coronary heart disease, which is characterized by the narrowing of the blood vessels that nourish the heart muscle, causing angina, myocardial infarction (heart attack), rhythm disturbances, or even cardiac failure. Hypertension, which is simply high blood pressure, is one of the most common serious health problems in the United States. Despite the fact that it usually does not have symptoms, high blood pressure does contribute to many degenerative changes that increase the risk of heart attack, stroke, or kidney disease.

Arrhythmia is an irregularity in the rhythm of the heartbeat. It can manifest itself as either bradycardia (abnormally slow heart rate) or various forms of tachycardia (abnormally fast heart rate). Quinidine, procainamide, disopyramide, and bidocaine are the most widely prescribed of the antiarrhythmic medications. They act to prevent or to alleviate the cardiac arrhythmia. Dilantia is primarily an anticonvulsant but is also used as an antiarrhythmic agent. Proprandol is used as an antiarrhythmic agent, although it is more commonly used for hypertension and angina.

Despite the fact that these drugs have different mechanisms of actions, many of their side effects are similar.[9] Hypotension, light-headedness, nausea, and vomiting are potential side effects, although hypotension is less common with procainamide. Fatigue, weakness, mental depression, and emotional instability are also seen. Unfortunately, many of these side effects can also be caused by other medications the patient may be taking or by other diseases.[4] Procainamide therapy presents two additional concerns. First, a total agranulocytosis has been reported. Second, the drug can cause systematic lupus erythematosis. If a patient complains of any soreness of the mouth, throat, or gums, unexplained fever or arthritis, he or she should be referred to his or her physician immediately. Drugs from digitalis (for example, Lanoxin) slow the rate of the heart but increase the force of contraction. They may be used to regulate erratic heart rhythm and to increase the output of the heart in heart failure. Digoxin (Lanoxin) and digitorin (Crystodigin) are two commonly used cardiac glycosides. They have similar side effects, most commonly anorexia, nausea, vomiting, and diarrhea.[14] These symptoms may also be caused by the underlying heart disease, so each patient must be assessed carefully when such symptoms are present. Other adverse reactions are headache, weakness, apathy, and visual disturbances.

The antilipidemics are drugs used to treat abnormally high blood levels of cholesterol and triglycerides. Antromid-S, Choloxin, and Questran fall into this category.[14] The most common side effect of Atromid-S is nausea. Other side effects are flulike symptoms, anemia, and biliary system disorders. Questran may cause constipation, hemorrhoids, decreased fat-soluble vitamin absorption, and possibly bleeding tendencies. Most of the side effects of Choloxin are related to the increased metabolic rate seen with the drug (for example, Choloxin's actions stimulate the body's metabolic rate). Cardiac changes, insomnia, nervousness, and palpitations are just a few examples.

Vasodilators are used in the treatment of angina pectoris. Angina is a condition in which the heart muscle receives an insufficient supply of blood, causing pain in the chest and often in the left arm and shoulder. Nitroglycerin and Isordil are the drugs of choice here. Headache, palpitations, and cutaneous vasodilation with flushing are the most common side effects. Another medication used in the treatment of angina is nadolol (Corgard). Its potential side effects are those seen with other beta-adrenergic blocking agents (bradycardia, hypotension, congestive heart failure, and bronchospasm).[14]

Hypertension is common in the elderly population of the United States. Several population studies indicate that the prevalence of hypertension in the elderly ranges from 35 percent to 69 percent. Although there is no cure for hypertension, the disease can now be controlled in most patients. Sometimes all that is necessary is for the patient to be on a dietary and exercise regimen. In other patients, drug therapy is necessary. The treatment of high blood pressure is lifelong. Even though hypertension itself is asymptomatic, its effects do damage the heart, arteries, and kidneys. Therapy is designed to prevent this damage. Once therapy is stopped, however, the blood pressure returns to pretreatment levels or higher.

A number of drugs and combinations of drugs are commonly used to lower blood pressure. The major categories include the diuretics, beta-adrenergic blockers, centrally acting drugs, vasodilators, alpha-adrenergic blockers, and combination agents.[15] The availability of such a wide variety of drugs permits the physician to choose one that has the desired effects in a patient without too many untoward effects.

The diuretic drugs—such as Aldactazide, Aldactone, Diuril, Dyazide, Esidrix, Hydrodiuril, Lasix, and Hygroton—lower blood pressure by acting on the kidneys to reduce the body's sodium chloride (salt) and water volume.

Thiazide diuretics are the most commonly used antihypertensive diuretics and are usually the first drugs tried in the patient. This group includes Esidrix, Diuril, and Hydrodiuril.[15] The main adverse effects of long-term thiazide diuretic use are potassium depletion, increased risk of gout, and impaired glucose metabolism. Potassium balance can sometimes be maintained by reducing the salt intake. Eating potassium-rich foods (oranges, bananas, tomatoes) or taking a potassium supplement may be recommended. There are also potassium-sparing diuretics, such as spironolactone (Aldactone), which cause potassium retention by the kidney.

Other drugs act much like thiazide diuretics. One of them is Hygroton. It lasts longer than Diuril and also seems to be effective if taken only once every other day. This may be an important factor for patients who are not compliant with their medications. It side effects are similar to those of the thiazides.

The so-called loop diuretics have a different mechanism of action than that of the thiazides, although they also reduce blood pressure by promoting the excretion of sodium chloride from the body.[15] Edecrin and Lasix fall into this category. Lasix is a very potent blood-pressure-lowering drug and is therefore used sometimes in hypertensive crisis. It has also been used in patients with impaired renal function. The side effects attributed to this drug are very similar to those of other diuretics except that potassium depletion may be more severe. Edecrin, in addition, can be ototoxic with possible loss of hearing.

The beta-adrenergic blocking agents are among the newest drugs to treat hypertension.[4] The three beta-blocking drugs used in the United States are propanolol (Inderal), metroprolol (Lopressor), and nadolol (Corgard). They are frequently prescribed in conjunction with a diuretic when a diuretic alone does not sufficiently lower blood pressure. They can, however, be prescribed alone for patients who cannot tolerate diuretics. Because beta-blocking agents also are effective in treating angina and arrhythmias, these medications are prescribed for hypertensive patients with coronary artery disease as well.

Tenormin and Blocadren are the newest beta-blocking agents developed for this reason. Tenormin appears to be more beta selective as well as longer acting than the other drugs. This means that the drug acts primarily on the heart and less on the lungs than do other agents. Therefore, patients with bronchospasm (asthma patients) can be treated with this agent more safely. In addition, because the drug is longer acting, it can be administered as a once-daily dose.

Centrally acting antihypertensive drugs—clonidine (Catapres), reserpine (Serpasil), and methyldopa (Aldomet)—lower blood pressure by working through the sympathetic nervous system. They usually are given in conjunction with a thiazide diuretic. All these medications tend to decrease the heart rate and output of blood from the heart. Side effects of any of these drugs can include sedation and orthostatic hypotension. Reserpine, in addition, can cause depression. It should be remembered that elderly persons tend to be more sensitive to such side effects as the central nervous system depressant effects.

The vasodilators act by dilating or expanding the blood vessels. This enables the blood to flow through the vessels with less resistance. Drugs in this category include minoxidil (Loniten), hydralazine (Apresoline), and nitroprusside (Nipride). These agents are often used in combination therapy with other antihypertensive agents.

Prazosin (Minipress) is an alpha-adrenergic blocking agent.[15] The blood pressure is lowered by blocking constriction of the vessels. Nausea, palpitations, dizziness, headaches, and drowsiness are frequent side effects of this medication.

Antihypertensive agents are sometimes combined into one tablet or capsule. This may promote compliance with the medication—something which is sometimes hard to accomplish with hypertensive patients.[16]

THERAPY FOR GASTROINTESTINAL DISORDERS

With few exceptions, there are no specific diseases of the gastrointestinal tract that can be attributed directly to the aging process. The most common gastrointestinal disorders will be considered here: constipation, ulcers, heartburn, indigestion, and hemorrhoids. Constipation is a common gastrointestinal complaint in the elderly; 30 percent to 50 percent of patients 60 years old and older are said to complain of constipation and to use laxatives at least intermittently. Most laxatives are sold as OTC medications. There are stimulant, lubricant, saline, bulk-forming, and stool-softening laxatives. Generally, it is recommended that dietary measures be tried first in alleviating a constipation problem. However, if occasional laxative use is necessary, the bulk-forming laxatives or stool softeners are safest and most effective. Fluids should be taken with either one.

Ulcers are primarily treated by neutralizing the gastric acid and/or reducing its secretion. Regular use of antacids, as well as frequent small meals of foods unlikely to cause further irritation, usually will accomplish this goal. Tagament is the most commonly used antacid.

Hemorrhoids are the single most common disorder affecting the lower gastrointestinal tract of Americans. Recent studies indicate that more than half of all Americans over the age of 40 have hemorrhoids. There are many preparations available to treat hemorrhoids. Most cases can be controlled by hygenic measures with the use of drugs (HC, Anusol, Proctoform HC) to relieve uncomplicated symptoms. Sometimes surgery is indicated.

THERAPY FOR RESPIRATORY DISEASES

Lung disease in the elderly population occurs as a result of several factors related to the aging process. They are

1. age-related changes in lung function
2. increased susceptibility to infection
3. end effects of smoking
4. presence of other diseases that affect lung function.[1]

These changes alter the therapeutic and toxic drug responses as well as drug dose requirements of the elderly. Furthermore, some medications that are taken by the elderly can affect lung function, causing bronchospasm (for example, Inderal, Corgard).

Some common lung diseases are asthma, a condition marked by recurrent episodes of wheezing owing to spasmodic contraction of the bronchi, and chronic bronchitis and emphysema, which are generally caused by long-term cigarette smoking. Patients with chronic bronchitis have a chronic cough and are predisposed to infectious bronchitis and pneumonia.

Medications used to treat asthma and chronic bronchitis are similar. Adrenergic bronchodilators (sympathomimetic agents) are agents that reverse bronchospasm by relaxing bronchiolar smooth muscle.[4] Many drugs in this category contain ephedrine and epinephrine. Other drugs in this class include isoproterenol, metaproterenol, terbutaline, and isoetharine. These agents are found in tablet, capsule, or liquid form. When taken properly, then can reduce the frequency and intensity of asthmatic attacks. Quicker-acting aerosols containing these agents are used to stop an attack or to limit its severity. Subcutaneous or intraveneous epinephrine sometimes has to be administered in emergency rooms to reverse a severe case of asthma.

Many of these adrenergic agents stimulate the central nervous system as well as the cardiovascular system. The elderly may be more sensitive to these effects. Possible adverse effects are excitability, nervousness, tremors, palpitations, and loss of appetite. These symptoms are dose related and may appear in mild form when these agents are administered within prescribed doses.

Another class of drugs used to treat bronchospasm are the xanthine compounds (Bronkodyl, Slophyllin, Elixophyllin).[4] Theophylline relaxes bronchiolar smooth muscle and also stimulates the cardiovascular and central nervous systems. Its clearance rate from the body is decreased in patients over 55 years of age (especially men), and therefore smaller doses are usually required. Because the drug's absorption, activity, and secretion varies from person to person, each patient must have an individualized dose. Nausea, vomiting, diarrhea, abdominal pain, and headaches may represent drug toxicity.

Corticosteroids are anti-inflammatory medications that are used to treat a variety of diseases.[4] They are the most potent drugs available to treat asthma. They are, however, used primarily for short-term therapy for moderate to severe asthma because of their potentially severe adverse effects. The inhalant form (beclomethasone is one example–brand names are Vanceril and Beclovent Inhaler) is usually prescribed instead of the tablet or liquid forms. These inhalant medications deliver the drug directly to the bronchioles and thereby minimize systemic side effects.

Some medications used to treat asthma are combinations of agents, usually a combination of bronchodilators with an expectorant and/or decongestant. Antianxiety agents or barbiturates also may be added. Some of these drugs are nonprescription. In all cases, especially with the elderly, a physician should be consulted before a medication is used. Some examples of combination antiasthma medications are Bronkolixir, Tedral, DuoMedihaler, and Quibron Plus.

There are a number of allergic disorders that can occur among the elderly. Some of these allergic reactions are secondary to drugs, such as penicillin; other etiologies are food, certain types of clothings, bee stings, and pollen from the air.

The severity of the allergic reaction can range from a red rash to life-threatening bronchospasm.

Two modes of treatment are available to the allergic patient besides avoidance of the known allergen. One is desensitization with the known allergen, and the other is symptomatic treatment aimed at suppressing the allergic response.

The primary ingredient in almost all allergy medications is some type of antihistamine. These agents (such as Benadryl, Dimentane, and Periactin) act by blocking the effects of histamine. It is the release of histamine and not actually the antigen itself that causes the inflammatory process seen in the allergic reaction. Thus by blocking histamine effects the inflammatory response can be subdued.

Common antihistamines found in both nonprescription and prescription products include diphenhydramine, brompheniramine, tripelennamine, and chlorpheniramine.[4] The major drawbacks to these medications are that they all tend to produce drowsiness as a side effect and they become less effective when taken orally over long periods of time. Most people experience anticholinergic effects, especially the elderly (dry mouth, blurred vision.)[9] Dizziness, sedation, and hypotension also occur more frequently in patients over 60 years of age.

The most common respiratory ailment in the elderly is the common cold or flu. We have emphasized the point that the elderly patient often is taking several medications on a chronic basis. It is important to remind the elderly patient as well as the health care provider that the physician or pharmacist should be consulted before a treatment for a cold is begun. This ensures safety against drug interactions as well as adverse effects. Acetaminophen (Tylenol) or aspirin are used to relieve the aches and pains or to reduce the fever. Antihistamines act to dry up the postnasal drip and runny nose. Decongestants clear up the stuffiness. There is a wide variety of expectorants and cough syrups. Most products on the market today consist of one or more of these ingredients. The multi-ingredient quality of these drugs increases the risk of possible side effects. When taken in conjunction with other medications, the potential for drug interactions is also increased.

ANALGESICS/ANTI-INFLAMMATORY AGENTS

In 1978, more than 31 million Americans suffered arthritis, and another 6 million individuals had related disorders requiring the use of analgesic and anti-inflammatory drugs. A large population of geriatric patients require drug treatment for arthritis.

Aspirin is usually the first drug of choice for most types of arthritis. This drug is an anti-inflammatory and is also a mild analgesic that exerts its effects by central and peripheral mechanisms. In addition to pain and inflammation relief, the aspirin also acts to inhibit prostaglandins, to inhibit platelet aggregation, and to reduce fever.

The most common side effects of aspirin are gastrointestinal problems, such as heartburn, nausea, cramps, and intestinal bleeding abnormalities.[4] When taken in high doses, the drug may cause ringing in the ears (tinnitus), dizziness, and headache. These adverse effects can always be eliminated by lowering the dose or stopping the drug. Because of the possibility of hemorrhage, aspirin is generally not used for patients with ulcers or for patients on anticoagulant therapy.

Ibuprofen, fenoprofen, and naproxen are classified as nonsteroidal anti-inflammatory agents. Additional compounds in this class are indomethacin, tolmetin, phenylbutazone, and sulindac. These agents have become very popular in their use to treat arthritis and other related diseases.

The side effects of nonsteroidal anti-inflammatory drugs are very similar. Some are allergic reactions (rash, marrow suppression). Others are dose related (central nervous system sensory disturbances, such as tinnitis). Still others are extensions of the pharmacologic action of the drug itself (sodium retention). In general, all nonsteroidal anti-inflammatory agents should be used with added caution by the elderly patient, because side effects are more frequently encountered in this age group. Side effects are individual, however, and because varying effects are seen in each patient, a drug that produces side effects in one may be well tolerated by many others.

Colchicine is primarily indicated for the treatment of acute gout or for the prevention of recurrent gouty attacks (colchicine is extremely effective in shortening the length of the gouty attack). The most predictable and common side effect of the oral drug is gastrointestinal distress, such as diarrhea and cramping.

In addition to the anti-inflammatory agents, a wide variety of analgesics are employed in the treatment of musculoskeletal disorders. Some of the common agents used are acetaminophen, propoxyphene, ethoheptazine, pentazocine, codeine, and zomepirac. Although these agents are very effective in the relief of pain, they are not anti-inflammatory agents, therefore, their use is for only symptomatic relief of pain. The primary concern with some of these agents (propoxyphene, codeine, pentazocine) is the potential for the abuse as well as their overall central nervous system depression. Elderly patients again may be more sensitive to these effects.

Additional compounds used to treat arthritis include chloroquine phosphate and hydroxychloroquine sulfate, gold compounds, penicillamine, corticosteroids, and several cytotoxic agents.[4] Some of the side effects associated with these agents can be severe. The most feared side effect with chloroquine phosphate, for example, is occular damage. Skin rash and bleaching of hair are also common side effects. A concern with gold therapy is thrombocytopenia, a serious blood disorder. Cytotoxic agents (Cytoxan, Immuran) can depress blood counts severely.

ANTIANXIETY AGENTS

The elderly individual may be subject to several unique stresses as a result of social situations and physical disease resulting in symptoms of anxiety. These symptoms may be quite variable. Physical symptoms such as palpitations, fatigue, headache, gastrointestinal distress, and pain may be the only complaints presented. In addition, though, there are psychologic complaints which may or may not be noticed. Such behavioral changes include instability, insomnia, distractibility, and nervousness.

Psychologic support and changing the environment may be all that is necessary to treat some elderly patients. Merely showing interest in patients may generate improvement. Involvement in social activities should be encouraged by the physician and carried out by family, friends, and professional workers. If these efforts are not successful, though, pharmacologic therapy may be necessary.

The anxiolytic agents (tranquilizers) are used most frequently in treating anxiety.[4] In general, these drugs have sedative-hypnotic properties. The most frequently prescribed anxiolytics are the benzodiazepines (for example, Valium, Librium, Tranxene, Ativan). Benzodiazepines are generally considered safer and more effective in treating anxiety than the older antianxiety drugs, such as meprobamate or the barbiturates (Phenobarbital and Butabarbital). These other agents also produce stronger adverse effects on psychomotor functions, such as incoordination, mental confusion, and drowsiness, than do the benzodiazepines.

Beta-blocking agents relieve the somatic symptoms of anxiety, such as tremors or palpitations. However, they do not alter the sense of anxiety.

Antihistamines (Atarax, Vistaril) have a sedative effect and are therefore sometimes used in treating anxiety. Again, depression of the central nervous system is a major adverse reaction of these agents. Barbiturates such as Phenobarbital and Butabarbital have long been used to treat anxiety. These drugs depress the central nervous system, causing drowsiness, impaired mental function, and other undesirable effects. Overdose is a major danger with these agents.

SEDATIVES/HYPNOTICS

Insomnia is the most common sleep disorder; it has many causes and can take various forms: difficulty falling asleep, difficulty staying asleep, and waking up too early and being unable to return to sleep. Although average sleep time decreases only slightly with increased age, complaints of disturbed sleep increase from 8 percent (18 to 19 years) to 26 percent (older than 60 years). Medical problems, including organic brain syndrome, Parkinsonism, stroke, nocturnal angina, hypertension, and depression may all disturb sleep.[1] Many other factors, unfortunately, also can contribute to sleep disturbances in the elderly patient. These include irregular schedules, daytime napping, and nightly reliance on sedatives.

The sleep-inducing drugs are classified as barbiturates and nonbarbiturates.[4] The barbiturates are less desirable because they are addictive and have been used to commit suicide. Furthermore, they (and most other sleep medications) are effective only for limited periods, perhaps only 2 weeks. Despite this, though, recent studies indicate that about 17 percent of prescriptions for insomnia are for the barbiturates (Eskabarb, Amytal, Nembutal, and Seconal).

More than half the prescriptions for sleep-inducing drugs are now flurazepam (Dalmane). It is less addictive than barbiturates and is effective for longer than 2 weeks. Other benzodiazepines also may be prescribed for short-term treatment of insomnia, but only Ativan is specifically indicated for this purpose. Restoril is the most recent drug to compete with flurazepam as a sedative-hypnotic agent. It may have less "hang-over" tendencies associated with it. Chloral hydrate is a milder sedative-hypnotic. None of the medications should be taken with alcohol.

Toxicities caused by benzodiazepines or barbiturates may be particularly troublesome in elderly patients.[17] As with any central nervous system depressant, excess sedation may cause difficulty in coordination, resulting in falls that can result in fractures. Patients may become confused and disoriented. Elderly patients also may develop paradoxical aggressive behavior, especially when taking the benzodiazepines.

Treatment of occasional insomnia that is not primarily caused by depression consists of avoiding daytime napping, no late sleeping, no sleep-disturbing behavior at bedtime (for example, bill paying, arguing, watching active television shows), and no caffeinated beverages. If necessary, occasional bedtime use of hypnotics in low doses can be helpful.

The anticholinergic activity of these drugs is primarily a source of discomfort to the elderly patient. They may be of greater concern because mouth dryness makes for difficulties with dentures or blurred vision may further isolate an individual.

Extrapyramidal effects associated with the use of the neuroleptic agents are most common in the elderly. Such effects include acute dystonias, akathisias, and parkinsonism. These reactions often occur early in the course of neuroleptic therapy and usually respond to either decreased dose of the drug or the addition of an antiparkinsonism agent (anticholinergic agent).

The parkinsonism reaction is a condition similar to Parkinsonism, the disease, with the signs and symptoms being the same. The reactions seen with acute dystonias are of sudden nature and consist of bizarre muscular spasms frequently affecting the muscles of the head and neck. These effects seem to occur more frequently in the young than in the elderly.

Akathisia is a very disquieting effect. It is a subjective state of desiring to be in constant movement. These effects occur early in the course of treatment and are related to drug dose. Unfortunately, it may appear in subtle forms, one of which manifests itself as an anxiety state.

Tardive dyskinesis is a late-appearing neurologic syndrome associated with antipsychotic drug use. It occurs more frequently in older patients, and an incidence as high as 20 percent has been reported in chronically institutionalized patients. It is characterized by stereotyped involuntary movements consisting of sucking and smacking of the lips, lateral jaw movements, and fly-catching dart-ing movements of the tongue. There may be choreiform and purposeless, quick movements of the extremities. All these movements disappear in sleep, as they do in Parkinsonism. The unfortunate aspect of this adverse reaction is that sometimes it is irreversible.

Neuroleptic agents are drugs that have antipsychotic action, affect psychomotor activity, and have little hypnotic activity. These drugs are used to treat major mental disorders characterized by derangements of personality and loss of contact with reality, which are often accompanied by delusions or hallucinations. Schizophrenia and organic brain syndrome with psychosis (dementia) are two of the major psychiatric disorders found in the elderly.[7] The neuroleptic agents are used to treat these two conditions.

The three major classes of neuroleptic drugs used in the United States are phenothiazines, thioxanthenes, and butyrophenones. The pharmacology of these drugs is similar, and the choice of therapy is sometimes based on an attempt to minimize adverse effects.

Many of these drugs are available for use in the United States today. Among the phenothiazines there are chlorpromazine (Thorazine), thioridazine HCl (Mellaril), perphenazine (Trilafon), prochlorpromazine (Compazine), fluphenazine (Prolixin), and trifluoperazine (Stelazine). These agents are the most widely used of the antipsychotic agents.[17] Chlorprothixene (Taractan) and thiothixene (Navane) are of the thioxanthine class of drugs, which are less potent than their homologous phenothiazines. The butyrophenones are the third class of neuroleptic agents, and heloperidol (Haldol) is its prototype. This agent is structurally unlike the phenothiazines but does have many of the same pharmacologic activities.

The pharmacologic properties of this class of drugs are diverse. They will be considered here as a whole. Many of the adverse effects of these drugs are related to their pharmacologic effects. It is important to discuss the activity of this group of drugs in depth because of the wide use of these agents in the elderly. The potential adverse effects or toxicities of these agents are also of special concern to the health care provider and will be discussed later.

The major therapeutic effects of the neuroleptic drug are in the central nervous system. These include psychomotor slowing, emotional calming, and affective indifference. Apparently the behavioral effects of these drugs in normal persons are adverse, resulting in dysphoria and impairment of intellectual performance.

Sedation seems to occur more frequently with chlorpromazine and thioridazine. This effect parallels the hypotensive effect that occurs because of alpha-adrenergic blockage. Both these problems, sedation and hypotension, may be disadvantageous for the elderly patient on long-term therapy with these agents. Tolerance of this sedative effect may occur after several weeks of treatment.

The relatively weak anticholinergic actions of the neuroleptic drugs are primarily a concern because they manifest themselves as adverse drug reactions. Visual blurring frequently occurs at therapeutic doses of these drugs. Other anticholinergic effects include dry mouth, urinary retention, and constipation.

The neuroleptic drugs are potent inhibitors of the chemoreceptor trigger zone. Thus they have the ability to inhibit emesis (vomiting). Compazine is most commonly used for this purpose.

The phenothiazines affect the heart by direct action and indirectly through their anticholinergic and alpha-adrenergic blocking actions. Haloperidol produces minimal hypotension and may be favored for patients with cardiovascular problems. Acetophenazine (Tindal) is mildly sedative and hypotensive. It also appears to have minimal extrapyramidal side effects and is well tolerated in the elderly patient.

The elderly are more sensitive to both the therapeutic effects and the adverse effects of the neuroleptic drugs.[17] Adverse effects include the following: sedation, hypotension, anticholinergic effects, extrapyramidal disorders such as tardive dyskinesia, and cardiac and endocrine abnormalities.

The cardiac effects of the neuroleptic drugs include electrocardiographic abnormalities and cardiac arrhythmias. The endocrine effects include galactorrhea and amenorrhea in women, gynecomastia in men, and decreased growth hormone release. None of these endocrine problems appears to be a major concern for the elderly individual.

Judicious use of neuroleptic drugs by elderly patients who are agitated or paranoid may be beneficial for the patients as well as for those in their immediate environment. In the light of the potential toxicities, it is imperative that the health care provider dealing directly with these patients be aware of these adverse reactions and report signs of them to the proper physician. It is sometimes difficult to specifically discern among these features but, for the health of the elderly patient, it is important to try.

ANTIDEPRESSANT THERAPY

Feelings of sadness and grief are part of normal everyday life. At times, everyone experiences sadness, demoralization, and the grief of personal loss. But when these feelings lead to decreased ability to function and to cope with normal life or when they have no identifiable cause, they may represent so-called pathologic depression. There is a high incidence of depressive illness in the elderly population.[6] Frequently, depression accompanies the physical illnesses of the elderly patient. The depressive states in the elderly are often of greater severity and longer duration and are more resistant to therapy than those in the younger population.

In most cases of depression, attempts to alter lifestyle or attitudes are ineffective. Instead, medical treatment is usually necessary, and in many persons, especially manic-depressives, this need is lifelong. In the elderly population the tricyclic antidepressants are usually used.

For persons suffering from recurrent depression, electroconvulsive (shock) therapy is often more effective than drugs in producing a cure. Controversy surrounds this approach to depression, and unless suicide is an imminent risk, it is generally not the initial treatment of choice. Monoamine oxidase inhibitors, such as Marplan and Nardil, are used much less often in the elderly, too, because of their potential for adverse reactions. This potential is increased for elderly persons whose compliance is suspect and who may be receiving multiple drug therapy.

The most widely used antidepressant agents are the tricyclic antidepressants, which work through the central nervous system. About two thirds of patients taking tricyclic antidepressants (TAD) experienced decreased or total disappearance of the depression in one month. This group of drugs includes amoxapin (Ascendin), doxepin (Adapin, Sinequan), amitriptyline (Elavil, Endep), desipramine (Norpramin), nortriptyline (Pamelor), trimipramine (Surmontil), and imipramine (Torfranil). Some antidepressants, such as Etrafon and Trivail (perphenazine with amitriptyline), and Limbritrol (chlordiazepoxide with amitrityline), offer combinations of antidepressant and antianxiety agents.

The TADs are chemically similar to the phenothiazines discussed in the last section. They share some of their pharmacologic properties, too. For example, the TAD are sedative drugs. Anticholinergic effects, antihistaminic effects, and alpha-adrenergic blockade are all similar effects. Anticholinergic effects include blurred vision, drying of the mouth, urinary retention. Antihistaminic effects, on the other hand, might involve sedation and weight gain. Orthostatic hypotension is the primary side effect of alpha blockade.

Parkinsonism is a slowly progressive disorder of middle or late life. About 200,000 persons in the United States are affected by Parkinsonism. It is especially prevalent in older people, affecting about 1 percent of the population over the age of 60 years.

Parkinsonism consists of decreased movement, tremor, and dementia. Movement gradually degenerates from slowed movements (bradykinesis) to the inability to initiate movement (akinesia) caused by hypertonicity (increased rigidity in the muscles). Parkinsonism generally incapacitates a person in 5 to 10 years, although some persons remain functional for 20 years or more. Two other signs commonly found in Parkinsonism are excessive salivation and a "pill-rolling" tremor of the hands.

As the disease progresses, mental faculties may degenerate. First the cognitive and perceptual abilities are impaired, then occasional memory lapses and confusion occur. The patient may be subject to episodes of depression.

Treatment of Parkinsonism may be with levodopa or carbidopa, anticholinergic or antihistaminic drugs, amantadine, or dopa agonists such as bromocriptine.[11] Physical therapy and treatment of other medical conditions to maintain good health are also useful in reducing disability in some patients.

Levodopa is the most important drug used in the therapy for Parkinsonism disease. The drug is effective only after it has penetrated the central nervous system, where it is converted to dopamine. Unfortuately, 95 percent of the levodopa administration does not go into the brain; instead, it acts on peripheral nerves or is broken down to other biologically active agents such as epinephrine. Therefore, levodopa given by itself produces unwanted side effects such as disturbances of heart rhythm, nausea, vomiting, depression, euphoria, or anxiety. A few of these problems are ameliorated by combining carbidopa with the levodopa (Sinemet). Carbidopa inhibits the enzymes that break down levodopa in the peripheral system, thus minimizing systemic toxicity. The psychiatric side effects may still occur.

Anticholinergic agents seem to have secondary status for the treatment of Parkinsonism. These drugs are much less effective than levodopa. Useful anticholinergic drugs include benzotropine (Cogentin) and trihexyphenidyl (Artane). In patients with mild symptoms, these drugs are usually tried first, with levodopa or Sinemet being added later. Better success can sometimes be obtained by adding antihistamines or the antiviral compound amantadine (Symmetrel) to either anticholinergics or levodopa. Two frequently used antihistamines are diphenhydramine (Benadryl) and chlorphenoxamine (Phenoxene). Finally, bromocriptine is a dopamine receptor antagonist that has been shown to be useful in the treatment of Parkinsonism, alone or in combination forms.

ANTICONVULSANT THERAPY

Epilepsy is a condition characterized by recurring seizures caused by disturbances of the electrical activity of the brain. In the elderly the most common cause of seizures is cerebrovascular disease associated with hemiplegia (paralysis of one side of the body). Dementia is also frequently related. The incidence of epilepsy, unfortunately, seems to increase after age 60. It is difficult to pinpoint the exact reason for this. Investigations to determine the cause of seizures is undertaken as an individual study of each particular patient. This ensures that the patient will receive the proper therapy for his or her clinical situation.

HORMONAL AND ENDOCRINOLOGIC AGENTS

This group of agents includes the estrogens, insulin, the oral hypoglycemic agents, thyroid agents, and the corticosteroids. The incidence of symptoms of disease from endocrine dysfunction increases considerably with advancing age. A few of these changes can be viewed as a normal part of the aging process, but other problems obviously represent disease. For example, estrogen withdrawal during the menopause is a normal aging process, but diabetes, which is more common in the elderly, is a disease. Either problem may or may not necessitate pharmacologic intervention.

Estrogens are among the drugs most widely used by elderly persons. They are prescribed most frequently for the treatment of menopausal symptoms in women but are also used in osteoporosis and metastatic breast cancer in women as well as prostatic carcinoma in men. Many diseases may be adversely affected by estrogen therapy, including diabetes mellitus, seizures disorders, migraine headaches, multiple sclerosis, myocardial infarction, cerebrovascular disease, pulmonary embolism, and some forms of hyperlipidemia.

Insulin is a very important drug used in the treatment of diabetes. Its use by the elderly patient presents several special problems. First, symptoms of overdosage (causing hypoglycemia) may be more subtle, such as headache, decreasing memory or cognitive ability, and personality changes. Another problem is the administration of insulin. Insulin has to be injected subcutaneously. The physical skills and mental ability of self-administered insulin can be an obstacle for some patients. Eventually some elderly patients need the daily help of another person to administer insulin and other medications.

When dietary changes do not work and insulin is not warranted, the oral hypoglycemic agents have sometimes been used by some elderly patients to reduce blood sugar levels. The controversy regarding the efficacy and safety of these agents assumes special importance for older patients. Although the ability to lower blood glucose levels with sulfonylurea (an oral hypoglycemic) is usually reduced in the older patient, severe hypoglycemic reactions to these agents has occurred. Also, there is evidence that sulfonylurea drugs may increase the risk of cardiovascular disease. Other agents that fall into this class include Chlorpropamide (Diabenese), tolbutamide (orinase) and tolazamide (Tolinase).

The preferred drug to treat a deficiency of thyroid hormone is L-thyroxine (Synthroid, Levothroid). Elderly patients are particularly sensitive to the effects of this drug. Dosages given to elderly patients are usually small to avoid sudden and excessive metabolic demands, especially on the heart. Toxic effects of thyroid hormone include palpitations, tremors, diarrhea, nervousness, insomnia, heat intolerance, fever, and angina pectoris.[9]

Corticosteroids are a group of substances made in the outer part of the adrenal gland, a small organ that lies above the kidney. They belong to the larger family of steroid hormones, such as testosterone in the man and progesterone in the woman.

The indications for pharmacologic use of glucocorticoids by the elderly are similar to those for younger patients. However, the prevalence of certain diseases that often require steroid therapy is increased in the elderly. Rheumatoid arthritis is an example. Oral steroids include hydrocortisone, Decadron, Medrol, and prednisone. There are also topical steroids used for skin rashes.

When these drugs are used properly, they are very effective. However, the potential for adverse effects is always present and many times warrants the discontinuation of therapy or sometimes reduced dosages for those on maintenance therapy. Such adverse effects include predisposition to infection, poor wound healing, sodium and water retention, hypertension, diabetes, obesity, osteoporosis, myopathy, cataracts, easy bruising, and psychotic reactions. In view of these problems, other methods of therapy are usually tried before corticosteroid therapy is given. Sometimes there is no alternative and patients need to be on one of these medications. When this is the case, all health professionals should be on the lookout for the potential side effects. If infection occurs or if there is a wound that will not heal, the patient should be referred to a physician.

Drug Interactions/Adverse Reactions

When a patient is given a medication to treat a disease, there are several things that occur. First, the drug exerts its therapeutic effect (drug's activity). This is the effect that is desired and the purpose for which the drug is given. Secondly, the drug also exerts undesirable effects. These are side effects or adverse reactions.

Some side effects are expected and unavoidable, but others may be unexpected. Most of the expected side effects are temporary and need not cause alarm. In other situations, this may not be necessarily true. In all circumstances, health care providers should familiarize themselves with potential side effects of drugs that patients are receiving. Watch for these side effects and symptoms. It may be necessary for the physician to be notified.

Drug interactions are also adverse reactions of medications. Drug interactions occur when the effect of one drug is inhibited or potentiated by the prior or concurrent administration of another drug.[18] Recent literature appears to indicate an increased number of adverse drug reactions caused by interactions. Geriatric patients, in particular, experience a risk of drug interactions because there is an increased likelihood of clinical disorders that will necessitate multiple drug therapy.

It is impossible to remember all possible drug interactions; the list is too long to be memorized. What can be done, though, is to learn a few of the basic interaction mechanisms which will help in anticipating and dealing with problems when they arise. There are several mechanisms of drug interactions. They are briefly mentioned as follows.[19]

1. *Opposing Pharmacologic Effects.* Pilocarpine, prescribed by an ophthalmologist, is an example of a cholinergic drug. Its effects may be altered when an anticholinergic such as propantheline (Pro-Banthine) is given for a gastrointestinal disorder by another physician.

2. *Similar Pharmacologic Effects.* The best-known example is the interaction between alcohol and sedatives or tranquilizers. Although the potential interaction may not be dangerous in one individual, it could be lethal in another. Patients should be alerted to this fact.

   Drugs that differ considerably in their primary pharmacologic activities may exhibit the same adverse effects. Many patients being treated with antipsychotic agents, such as chlorpromazine (Thorazine), are given an antiparkinson agent, such as trihexyphenidyl (Artane). This is to control the extrapyramidal effects of the former. In addition, this same patient may be taking a tricyclic antidepressant such as amitryptyline (Elavil). All these agents possess anticholinergic activity as a side effect. The additive effect could lead to annoying and troublesome problems, especially for the elderly (anticholinergic effects include dry mouth, blurred vision, urinary retention, constipation, and elevated intraocular pressure). Furthermore, the drug interaction could develop into a delirium and be mistaken as an increase in psychiatric symptoms, which might be treated by increasing the dosage of the offending agent. This example points out the difficulty in distinguishing symptoms of the disease from the effects of the drug.

3. *Alterations of Gastrointestinal Absorption.* This type of drug interaction may develop through different mechanisms. For example, the ph of the

stomach affects how a drug is absorbed. If Ecotrin, an enteric-coated aspirin, is given concomitantly with antacids (which increase the pH), the coating may disintegrate sooner than it is supposed to, resulting in the release of the drug in the area it is trying to avoid. Chelating (a process by which positive metal ions tie up the ring structure of the particular drug and form a chelate complex, thereby forming an unabsorbable product) is another mechanism; for example, tetracycline given with antacids containing calcium is poorly absorbed because the calcium binds to the tetracycline. Changes in gastrointestinal motility can affect drug absorption. For example, anticholinergics act to decrease gastrointestinal motility. This can either reduce absorption or increase absorption, depending upon the particular drug involved.

4. *Stimulation of Metabolism.* Many drug interactions result from the ability of one drug to stimulate the metabolism of another. It has been demonstrated, for example, that phenobarbital can increase the rate of metabolism of warfarin (Coumadin), which results in a decreased response to the anticoagulant. Other investigations show that phenytoin (Dilantin) and phenobarbital increase the rate of metabolism of vitamin D. This would explain why some individuals develop osteomalacia while on this therapy. Vitamin D supplements may be necessary to avoid this problem.

5. *Inhibition of Metabolism.* For example, tricyclic antidepressants, such as amitryptyline (Elavil), may decrease the rate of metabolism of the anticoagulant warfarin.

6. *Displacement of Drugs from Protein-Binding Sites.* Because there are only a limited number of protein-binding sites available to a drug in the plasma, a competition will exist between two drugs that tend to bind the same proteins. The drug that has the greater affinity for the binding site will displace the other from plasma or tissue proteins. The drug that is displaced then may exert toxic effects if it was given in normal doses to the patient. Phenylbutazone (butazolidin) does this to warfarin. The anticoagulant effect of warfarin is increased, which could result in hemorrhaging.

7. *Alteration of Urinary Excretion.* Probenecid blocks the tubular excretion of penicillin and maintains higher penicillin levels in the body longer than normal. Urinary ph can alter drug excretion; salicylates, for example, are reabsorbed into the body in the presence of an acidic urine.

8. *Interaction at the Adrenergic Neurons.* A few drugs alter the way chemicals are handled around the adrenergic (sympathetic) nerve endings. For example, monoamine oxidase inhibitors (isocarboxazid and tranylcypromine) cause greater-than-normal amounts of norepinephrine to be stored up. When sympathomimetic agents (amphetamines) are given together with these drugs, the greater quantity of released norepinephrine can cause hypertensive crisis or cardiac arrhythmias.

9. *Alteration of Electrolyte Levels.* Digoxin is a medication given to elderly patients. When it is given together with some diuretics (for example,

Lasix), the potential for digitalis toxicity may be increased because the diuretics tend to deplete the body's potassium, making the heart more sensitive to the effects of digitalis. Potassium supplements usually prevent this potential problem.

Certainly this discussion of drug interaction is not all inclusive. As stated previously, it would be impossible for anyone to memorize the long list of possible interactions. Keying in on some basic causes, though, might provide an individual with some knowledge to ascertain whether a drug interaction is likely to occur. Open communication between all health professionals is of utmost importance. Pharmacists are the most knowledgeable about drug reactions and interactions. If an interaction/reaction is suspected, call in the consultant pharmacist to evaluate the circumstances and allow him or her to make recommendations to the attending physician. Although we are not advocating that physical therapists should be solely responsible for recognizing drug complications, we do feel that it is important to note changes in patient behavior or activity, especially when a new drug is started or an old one is stopped.

CONCLUSION

Drug therapy will continue to be the "treatment of choice" for most diseases and illnesses. If the current trend continues, today's younger and middle-aged people will rely on even greater amounts of drugs than does the current elderly population. This necessitates a greater awareness and understanding about the effects of drugs on the human system by all health care professionals.

Drug therapy of the elderly population places responsibility on all health care professionals. The potential for adverse reactions is increased in elderly persons owing to the combination of the effects of aging and the number of drugs prescribed.[21]

Although final responsibility for drug therapy rests with the attending physician and secondary responsibility usually with the nurse, each person in the health care delivery system can share responsibility for the patient's well-being. Your conversations and interactions with your patients can be a valuable source of information about changes (unwanted or undesirable side effects, symptoms of overdose, behavioral changes) that may escape the attention of other health professionals.

REFERENCES

1. HALLAS, G: *Understanding aging: The physiology of growing older*. Journal of Practical Nursing 21–26, April, 1979.

2. BASEN, MN: *The elderly and drugs—problem overview and program strategy*. Public Health Rep 92(1):43, January–February, 1977.

3. *The Handbook of Nonprescription Drugs*. American Pharmaceutical Association, 2215 Constitution Avenue, Washington, DC, 20037.

4. BRESSLER, R, BODGONOFF, M, GENELL, J: *The Physician's Drug Manual: Prescription and Nonprescription Drugs*. Doubleday & Co, Garden City, NY, 1981.

5. STAPLES, B: *Learning about the elderly: Closing the gaps*. Am Pharm 20(5):19, 1980.

6. PETERSON, D, WITTINGTON, F, PAYNE, B (EDS): *Drugs and the Elderly: Social and Pharmacological Issues*. Charles C Thomas, Springfield, IL, 1978.

7. FINCH, C AND HAYFICK, L (EDS): *Handbook of Biology Aging*. Van Nostrand Reinhold, New York, 1977.

8. WALLACE, D AND WATANABE, A: *Drug Effects in Geriatric Patients*. Drug Intell Clin Pharm 11:597–602, 1977.

9. LYLE, WM AND HAYHOE, DA: *A literature survey of the potentially adverse effects of drugs commonly prescribed for the elderly*. Am J Optom Physiol Opt 768–778, June, 1976.

10. ARMSTONG, WS JR, ET AL: *Analysis of Drug-Drug Interactions in a Geriatric Population*. Am J Hosp Pharm 37(3):385, March, 1980.

11. CONRAD, K AND BRESSLER, R: *Drug Therapy for the Elderly*. CV Mosby St. Louis, 1982.

12. SHIELDS, EM: *Introduction to Drug Therapy for Older Adults*. Journal of Gerontological Nursing 8–13, March–April, 1975.

13. GAETA, M AND GASTANO, R: *The Elderly: Their Health and the Days in Their Lives*. Kendall/Hunt, Dubuque, 1977.

14. LONG, JW: *The Essential Guide to Prescription Drugs*. Harper & Row, New York, 1980.

15. HAMMOND, JJ AND KIRKENDALL, WM: *Anti-hypertensive Drugs for the Aging*. Geriatrics 34(6):27, June, 1979.

16. LAMY, P: *Misuse and Abuse of Drugs by the Elderly*. Am Pharm 20(5):14017, 1980.

17. PRIEN, RF: *Problems and Practices in Geriatric Psychopharmacology*. Psychomatics 21(3):213, March, 1980.

18. ROBINSON, DS: *Pharmokinetic Mechanisms of Drug Interactions*. Postgrad Med 57(2): 55, 1975.

19. HALE, WE ET AL: *Drug use in a geriatric population*. J Am Geriatr Soc 27(8):374, August, 1979.

20. BUTLER, R: *The Gray Revolution and Health*. Am Pharm 20(5):9, May, 1980.

21. CHAPRON, D AND LAWSON, F: *Drug prescribing and care of the elderly*. In REICHEL, W (ED) *Clinical Aspects of Aging*. Williams & Wilkins, Baltimore, 1978.

CHAPTER 14

SEXUALITY AND THE ELDERLY

MOLLY LAFLIN, M.S.

BEHAVIORAL OBJECTIVES

Upon completion of this chapter, the reader will be able to
1. Describe normal age-related changes in the human sexual response cycle.
2. List the barriers to sexual expression among the elderly.
3. Discuss techniques that enhance sexual participation among older persons.
4. Recognize the sexual implications of certain illnesses and treatments.
5. List possible sexual implications attributable to prescription drug use.
6. Recognize the complications associated with sexual expression among nursing home patients.

Contrary to popular humor, sex after 60 is not the province of "dirty old men" nor is it the wishful invention of sexologists. Sexuality exists, in one form or another, throughout life. Age affects the strength of one's sexual response, but there is certainly no uniform chronologic age at which sexual interest, ability, and activity cease.

Many elderly people maintain a lively interest in sex. In fact, a study of men whose average age was 71 found that 75 percent had sexual desires.[1] A longitudinal study of men over age 60, begun in 1954 by the Duke University Center for the Study of Aging and Human Development, found a gradual decline in the reported frequency of sexual intercourse with advancing age. Yet 40 percent to 65 percent of the subjects between the ages of 60 and 71 still reported having sexual intercourse with some frequency. An interesting finding was that about 15 percent of the subjects showed increasing patterns of sexual interest and activity.[2]

ROLE OF REHABILITATION SPECIALISTS

Your job as a rehabilitation specialist is to help people learn to function at their optimal levels despite physical setbacks. Generally patients seek your care or engage your services out of a need to reduce pain and/or to increase mobility. Although the focus of your treatment plan is the presenting symptom, it is the patient as a whole person who must be treated. It is important to be sensitive to the social and emotional, as well as the physical, implications of treatment, disease, and injury.

In treating a woman with an arthritic hip, for example, if you overlook the sexual implications of the patient's condition, either because of personal embarrassment or an assumption that elderly people are not interested in sex, then you are not treating the whole person. You need to be open to discuss the sexual implications of illness and treatment with your elderly patients without pushing them to deal with areas in which they are uncomfortable. You have to walk the fine line between conveying a negative attitude about sex through silence or embarrassment and being too confrontive and shocking. Your primary concern is to treat patients as individuals, with dignity, and with the realization that sexuality, though it is generally not as vigorous among the elderly as among young people, is still part of the total person at any age.

AGE AND SEXUAL RESPONSE

Though there is no age-related end point for sexual functioning, there is an age-related general slowing of the human body, which in turn slows the sexual response cycle. The general effects of aging are listed below.

Men
1. Penile erection takes more time and may not be as hard as before; direct penile stimulation may be required.
2. Testicles elevate later and to a lesser degree.
3. Ejaculatory control increases; ejaculation may take place every third sexual episode, owing to less preoccupation with orgasm. (Lack of orgasm decreases the refractory period.)
4. Sex flush occurs less frequently.

5. Ejaculation is less powerful, and orgasm is often less intense.
6. Rectal sphincter contractions during orgasm occur less frequently.
7. Penile contractions during orgasm may be fewer in number.
8. Loss of erection after ejaculation and testicular descent occur rapidly.
9. Refractory period between ejaculations is longer.

Women
(Most sexual changes in women are associated with a decline in female hormones.)
1. Vaginal lubrication takes longer.
2. Reduction in the expansion of the vaginal barrel in length and width.
3. Lining of the vagina begins to thin and becomes easily irritated.
4. Bladder and urethra may become irritated during intercourse.
5. Vaginal secretions become less acid, increasing the possibility of vaginal infection.
6. Uterus does not elevate as high.
7. Clitoral size decreases and clitoral hood atrophies as does fat pads over the mons.
8. Orgasmic phase is shorter.
9. Capability for multiple orgasm remains.
10. Resolution phase occurs more rapidly.

The old adage "what you don't use, you lose" appears to apply to sex. Older women who have a history of regular sexual intercourse once or twice a week tend to experience fewer symptoms of sexual dysfunction than women with patterns of infrequent sexual activity. Despite steroid insufficiency, the women who maintain active sex lives continue unimpaired vaginal lubrication capacity, and the regular contractions during intercourse and orgasm retain vaginal muscle tone. Contact with the penis helps preserve the shape and size of the vaginal space.[3]

Knowledge of the normal physiologic changes associated with aging can greatly enhance adjustment and enjoyment of sexual expression. For example, women suffering sexual dysfunction or other problems associated with loss of female hormones may wish to discuss the advisability of estrogen replacement therapy with their physicians. An elderly couple that understands it is normal for an older man not to ejaculate every time he has sex can relax and enjoy the advantage of more frequent erections, the side effect of decreased refractory periods resulting from less frequent ejaculations.

LACK OF PARTNER

Not everyone has the opportunity to maintain a sexually active life despite an interest in doing so. There are now four unmarried women over the age of 65 for each unmarried man in the same age range. If all the unmarried men over the age of 65 married women over the age of 65, there would still be almost 6.8 million women without husbands. Sheer numbers indicate a great deal of unmet sexual need among the elderly.[4]

Grown children of widows and widowers often actively discourage their parents from seeking new partners or behaving as sexual beings.[5] Sometimes these "children" are fearful of loss of inheritance, but more often they are fearful of a change that seems uncomfortable and perhaps even morally reprehensible.

In a society that associates sexual attractiveness with youthful bodies and sexual activity with marriage, it is difficult for many older people to overcome their own prejudices without having to deal with such overwhelming societal pressure. The folkloristic view of old age as impotent, uninterested in sexuality, and sexually nonfunctional becomes, for many elderly people, a self-fulfilling prophesy. Homosexuality and masturbation are only a couple of the options open to the elderly who are without partners, but more often than not societal pressure eliminates these choices from active consideration.[6]

SEX AND ILLNESS

Lack of a partner probably accounts for a great many of the elderly who discontinue sexual activity, but illness also steals the sex lives of many.

Sexual activity may be limited by specific disabilities, but fortunately sexuality and the expression of love and caring do not have the same limitations. Rather than focusing on the losses associated with illness, more attention should be paid to what is possible. The psychosocial impact of disability generally has a greater negative impact on sexuality than the physical limitations of the disability itself. An emphasis on confidence building and new forms of sexual expression can be a great help to people suffering from debilitating illnesses.

Arthritis, with its joint deformities, possible contractures, and pain; cancer, with its pain and devastating treatments of surgery, chemotherapy, and radiation; neuromuscular diseases with their muscle atrophy, abnormal muscle tone, and movements can cause a person to feel unattractive and sexually unappealing. These negative feelings impede the development of emotional and physical intimacy. Any illness associated with decreased endurance or pain can be expected to limit sexual desire and activity. Even transient ill health is likely to produce enough anxiety to deter libido and sexual expression. These anxieties and negative self-perceptions must be dealt with so that patients can begin to take pleasure in what is left rather than dwelling on what has been lost.

For many people the key to maintaining personal sexual fulfillment is the ability to adjust old patterns to successfully meet ongoing changes. Intercourse in the traditional man-on-top position may have been very satisfactory for a person in his or her youth, but gradual experimentation over time is likely to uncover a variety of positions and practices that are equally if not more enjoyable. Examples of techniques that have increased sexual participation for many elderly people include

1. Sexual positions (such as side lying or sitting) that do not require support of the body on isometrically contracted arm muscles (Figs. 14-1 to 14-7)
2. Sexual positions that do not put pressure on joints or areas of the body prone to pain or muscle strain (Figs. 14-1 to 14-10)
3. Oral-genital stimulation (Fig. 14-11)
4. Digital stimulation of genital area by partner (Figs. 14-12 to 14-13)
5. Masturbation
6. Use of vibrators
7. Use of penile prostheses in cases of organically based impotence
8. Massage
9. Use of water-soluble lubricant such as K-V jelly during sexual intercourse or masturbation
10. Hugging, kissing, stroking, and talking (Fig. 14-14).

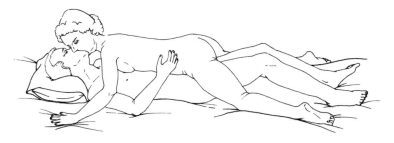

Figure 14-1. In this position the man does not have to expend energy supporting his weight on his arms.

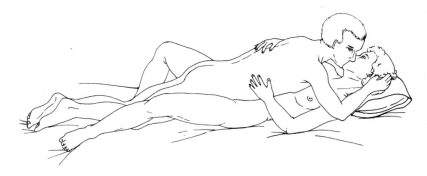

Figure 14-2. In this position the woman does not have to spend a lot of energy supporting her weight on her arms.

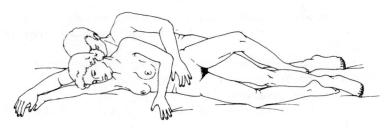

Figure 14-3. In this position, neither partner has to expend excess energy by over-working muscles to support weight.

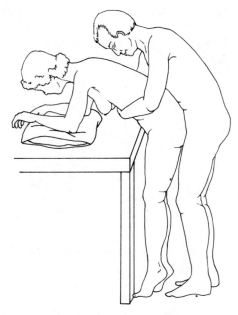

Figure 14-4. This position might be comfortable for someone with limited joint motion. Rear entry by man is supported by the woman.

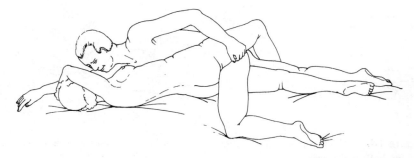

Figure 14-5. In this position, neither partner has prolonged pressure on joints.

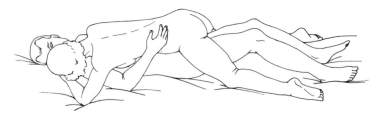

Figure 14-6. In this position the man does not have prolonged pressure on his joints.

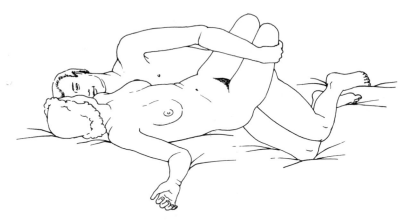

Figure 14-7. Both partners are in good positions with support and no sway-back.

It is not feasible in this chapter to detail the sexual implications of all the major diseases and to give specific suggestions for sexual adjustment. Books have been written on just these areas of sexuality. Several disabilities warrant brief discussion, however, because they are so prevalent among the elderly.

Arthritis

There is evidence indicating that regular sexual activity helps rheumatoid arthritis, probably because of adrenal gland production of cortisone and because sexual activity tends to lessen stress.[7]

Possible functional problems include contractions, joint degeneration, pain, and loss of mobility. A list of suggestions for dealing with these problems follows:

1. Exercise program to increase joint mobility
2. Use of heat (hot shower, hot-water bottle, or heating pad) prior to sexual activity

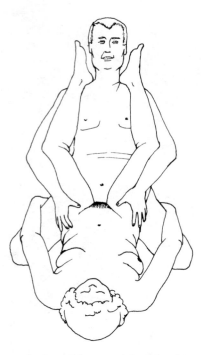

Figure 14-8. A woman who is unable to straighten her hips might use this position.

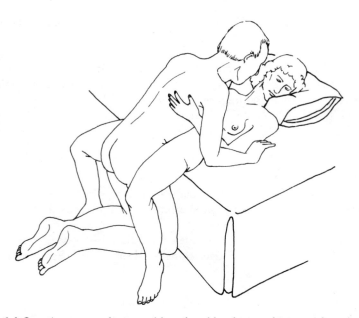

Figure 14-9. A woman who is unable to bend her hips and/or straighten her knees might find this position comfortable.

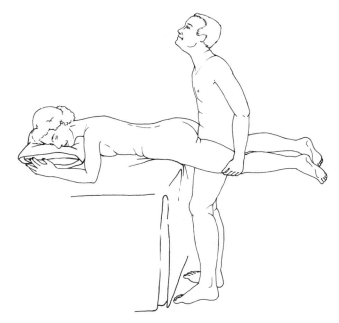

Figure 14-10. This rear-entry position might be useful for a woman who is unable to bend her hips or knees.

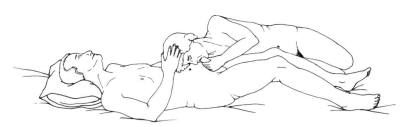

Figure 14-11. With age more direct genital contact is usually required to stimulate and to maintain sexual excitement. Fellatio (oral stimulation of man's genitals) may be used as a prelude to intercourse or as an independent activity. Cunnilinctus (oral stimulation of woman's genitals) is an alternative to intercourse or part of foreplay.

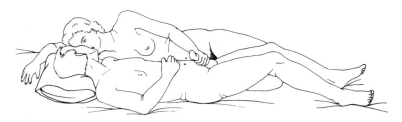

Figure 14-12. Digital stimulation often helps stimulate and maintain erections.

SEXUALITY AND THE ELDERLY

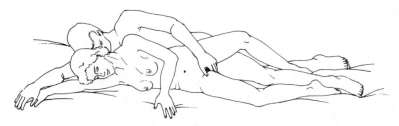

Figure 14-13. Digital stimulation is helpful in stimulating vaginal lubrication. Some women prefer it to intercourse, and others prefer it as a prelude to intercourse or as a means of reaching orgasm after intercourse.

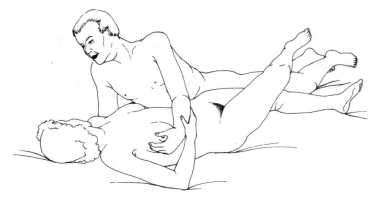

Figure 14-14. Sexual expression is not limited to genital stimulation. Hugging, kissing, stroking, and talking are all part of sexual communication.

3. With permission of attending physician, use of aspirin, taken prophylactally for pain prior to sexual activity
4. Communication with partner about position limitations (alleviates partner's fear of causing pain and patient's fear of being hurt)
5. Avoidance of positions that put prolonged pressure on the involved joints
6. Experimentation with adaptive positions and/or alternatives to intercourse, such as mutual masturbation or oral sex
7. Use of a waterbed
8. Setting aside a rest period before engaging in sexual activity helps prevent fatigue (one of the hallmarks of rheumatoid disease).

Hysterectomy

Numerous studies have shown that hysterectomy and loss of ovarian hormones have virtually no effect on sexual desire, sexual performance, or sexual response.

Disturbances in sexual activity in most instances are due to irrational fears and the psychologic effects of surgery in the genital area.[8]

Cancer

One of the three leading causes of death in the United States, cancer elicits fear and horror in most people. A diagnosis of cancer can cause severe depression and anxiety. The psychologic turmoil associated with coming to terms with the disease must be dealt with before intimate sexual relations can be achieved.

Possible functional problems include deformity caused by surgery, pain, low endurance, nausea, and changes in overall physical appearance owing to weight and hair loss. A list of suggestions for dealing with these problems follows:

1. Use of non-weight-bearing positions to avoid fatigue
2. Mutual masturbation or oral sex
3. Timing sexual activity around a pain-medication schedule so that pain is not a limiting factor
4. Incorporation of massage or deep breathing into foreplay to help relax and to relieve pain
5. Taking a less active role
6. If breathing is difficult when lying down, having sex in a sitting position, propped up on pillows, or in a large comfortable chair.

Heart Disease

Coronary attacks lead many people to give up sex altogether under the assumption that it will endanger their lives. However, the truth is that the oxygen usage (or "energy cost") for sex (average couple taking 10 to 16 minutes for the sex act) approximates climbing one or two flights of stairs, walking rapidly at a rate of 2 to 2½ miles per hour, or completing many common activities, such as driving a car.[9] Therefore, a patient who can comfortably climb one or two flights of stairs or take a brisk walk around the block is ready to resume sexual activity—usually 4 to 5 weeks after the coronary attack, provided there are no complications. Other sexual activities, involving stroking, touching, and embracing, are possible in any event.[10]

Possible functional problems include fear of sudden death during sex, low endurance, and erectile problems caused by medication. A list of suggestions for dealing with these problems follows:

1. Learning that the likelihood of a coital coronary is very small
2. Taking a less active role, decreasing performance anxiety
3. Masturbation (cardiac cost is less than that of intercourse)
4. Use of energy-conserving, non-weight-bearing sexual positions (sitting, side lying, and so forth)

5. Avoidance of sexual activity when anxious or fatigued
6. Avoidance of sexual activity in extremely hot, humid, or cold settings (to eliminate the energy expenditure involved in maintaining body temperature)
7. Increase in time spent in foreplay to allow the heart to warm up gradually
8. Improvement of overall fitness/endurance through a medically supervised conditioning program
9. Consultation with physician if medication affects libido, lubrication, or erectile capacity (medication should not be discontinued without medical consultation).

Stroke

An estimated 500,000 cerebrovascular accidents occur each year in the United States, and more than 200,000 survivors are added to the stroke population annually. Recent research on a population of 35 indicates that although the majority of stroke survivors maintain consistent levels of sexual desire and believe that sexual function is important, most will experience sexual dysfunction following stroke.[11] The dysfunction is occasionally related to fear of causing another stroke, even though it is extremely unlikely that further strokes can be produced through sexual exertion.[12]

Possible functional problems include communication problems, contractures, loss of mobility, perceptual problems, sensation loss, and tremor and visual problems. A list of suggestions for dealing with these problems follows:

1. Use of nonverbal communication
2. Sharing fantasies in writing
3. Exploration through touch and smell rather than depending on vision
4. If vision is impaired on only one side, asking partner to stay on the seeing side
5. Experimentation with comfortable positions
6. Use of a waterbed
7. Use of a vibrator if hands are weak and/or uncoordinated (vibrator may be strapped to hand)
8. Emphasizing stimulation of areas that are still sensitive to touch.

Diabetes

Diabetes mellitus is common in later life. Most diabetic men are not impotent, but it is one of the few illnesses that can cause chronic impotence. Although sexual interest and desire may continue, impotence occurs two to five times as often in diabetes as in the general population. Most cases of diabetic-produced impotence are reversible. If the disease has been poorly controlled, there is a fair chance that proper regulation thereafter will improve potency. Unfortunately, when impotence occurs in well-controlled diabetes, it may be permanent.[13] In women, one study found that 35 percent of the diabetic persons interviewed, versus 6 percent of the nondiabetic persons inteviewed, reported complete absence of orgasmic response during the year preceding the inquiry. Orgasmic dysfunction developed gradually and was directly correlated with the duration of diabetes.[14]

Possible functional problems include impotence, sensation loss, and vision problems. A list of suggestions for dealing with these problems follows:

1. Anxiety reduction
2. Consultation with a physician about possible problems associated with use of medications
3. Seeking pragmatic counseling if impotence is psychogenic
4. Consultation with a physician concerning need for penile prostheses (inflatable implements and flexible and semirigid prostheses are available if the impotence is organically based)
5. A hard doughnut-shaped rubber device slipped over the partially-erect penis can be helpful in maintaining an erection, available in shops dealing with sexual materials (rubber bands are sometimes used for this purpose, though it is not recommended)
6. Asking partner to emphasize stimulation of areas still sensitive to touch
7. Communication through touch and smell and imagination to make up for vision loss.

Prostatitis

Many physicians believe that chronic prostatitis—inflammation of the prostate gland—can be caused by, among other things, too infrequent sex. Treatment includes antibiotics, warm sitz baths, prostatic massage, more frequent sexual intercourse, and, in some severe cases, prostatectomy. Though prostatectomy does not generally interfere with erection and ejaculatory sensation, if often produces sterility by means of "retrograde ejaculation" into the bladder.

SEX AND DRUG USE

Although elderly persons currently make up 14 percent of the population, because of increased incidence of illness they consume 30 percent of all prescription drugs.[15] All too often elderly patients are not informed of the sexual implications associated with the use of certain prescription drugs. A few physicians are uncomfortable discussing sexual issues, and many erroneously assume that there is no need to discuss such things with their elderly patients. The consequences of not discussing sexual implications of drug use can be quite serious. For example, a man who does not know that some medications for hypertension can produce erectile problems or decrease libido may blame himself and become very depressed or attribute the dysfunction to problems in the relationship with his wife.

The generic drugs listed in Table 14-1 are capable of affecting some aspects of sexuality.[16] As would be expected, the principal therapeutic effect of each of these is on the nervous or circulatory system. As with any drug effect, the nature and degree of altered sexual function will vary greatly from one individual to another. Although such effects may occur at any age, they are usually more frequent and more troublesome after the age of 50. Suspicion of the possiblity of such a drug response should result in consultation with the attending physician regarding the advisability of modifying treatment.

SEX IN NURSING HOMES

Although the vast majority of the elderly in this country live in homes or apartments, approximately 5 percent of people over the age of 65 live in nursing

TABLE 14-1.   Generic drugs affect sexuality

DRUG NAME OR FAMILY	POSSIBLE EFFECTS
alcohol	reduced potency in men, delayed orgasm in women
amphetamine	reduced libido and potency
bethanidine	impaired ejaculation
clonidine	reduced libido
debrisoquine	reduced potency, impaired ejaculation
dextroamphetamine	reduced libido and potency
disulfiram	reduced potency
guanethidine	reduced potency, impaired ejaculation
haloperidol	reduced potency
levodopa	increased libido (in some men and women)
lithium	reduced potency
methyldopa	reduced libido and potency
oral contraceptives	reduced libido (in some women)
phenothiazines	reduced libido and potency, impaired ejaculation (occasionally)
phenoxybenzamine	impaired ejaculation
primidone	reduced libido and potency
reserpine	reduced libido and potency
sedative and sleep-inducing drugs (hypnotics) when used on a regular basis	reduced libido and potency
thiazide diuretics	reduced libido (occasionally, in some men)
tranquilizers (mild)	reduced libido and potency
tricyclic antidepressants	reduced libido and potency

From Long,[16] p 879, with permission.

homes or other long-term care institutions. Cole's study of elderly patients in nursing homes found that at least 50 percent wanted sexual activity.[17] The percent who engage in sexual acts is much less, though, because most nursing home patients are treated like children with no option for the privacy necessary for conjugal visits, masturbation, or even kissing or holding hands. Activities of daily living evaluations, which assess everything from patients' bowel movements to dental hygiene, rarely include information about sexual adjustment. The goal of skilled nursing care staff is generally to encourage and to facilitate optimal functioning of residents physically, emotionally, and socially. Avoiding the topic of sexuality tends to perpetuate the myth that sexual expression among the elderly is perverted and sick. In reality, sex can be an expression of pleasure, love, joy, intimacy, and a continuing reaffirmation of life. The healing quality of being touched, held, and caressed does not diminish with age.

A 1974 federal regulation concerning skilled nursing facilities states, "A married patient in a long-term care facility shall be assured privacy for visits by his or her spouse and married inpatients may share a room unless medically contraindicated and so documented by the attending physician in the medical record." The regulation states further that "the patient may associate and communicate privately with persons of his choice." States are required to implement these federal regulations in their health codes if they receive federal funds.[18] Administrators of long-term care institutions are having to come to grips with the increasing emphasis on patients' rights, including rights to privacy with regard to sexual expression. This is not an easy task.

Specific policies regarding sexual expression may pose administrative problems, including the answers to the following questions:

1. How is privacy insured for the roommate of a sexually active person living in a semiprivate room?
2. How is privacy insured without allowing doors to be locked?
3. How are patients who do not want sex protected from those who do?
4. Should the facility provide "sex therapy rooms" or waiting rooms for roommates or a specifically designated unit for patients interested in sexual activity?
5. Should visitors be allowed to spend the night?
6. Should extra-wide beds be available?
7. Who is liable if a patient doesn't use siderails during sex, falls out of bed, and breaks a hip?
8. Should intellectually impaired patients be allowed sexual activity?
9. Should the wishes of the family or the patient come first?

Recommendations for promotion of healthy sexual expression in nursing homes have been suggested, including the following:

1. Recommending books to patients, having them available in the institution, and making provisions for books to be read to those patients un-

able to read; examples of such books are *Joy of Sex* by Comfort, *Sex after Sixty* by Butler and Lewis, and *Sexuality and Aging* by Solnick
2. Including sexual history in the activities of daily living assessments
3. Instituting a patient education program outlining sexual activity related to medical problems of the elderly
4. Listening for verbal and nonverbal cues of sexual concerns
5. Insuring confidentiality
6. Avoiding personal shyness about the subject; although sex is a very personal and private matter, it does not need to be a taboo topic
7. Being aware of the nonverbal message sent by the staff
8. Emphasizing what is left rather than what has been lost
9. Redirecting inappropriate sexual expression to more healthy outlets, not punishing.

CONCLUSION

Sexuality isn't just genital stimulation. It encompasses the entire realm of human contact and communication; it is the way people define and present themselves. Sexual expression can enhance both self-esteem and a positive self-image. Health care providers can enhance quality sexual adjustment to aging and illness by conveying a humanistic, pleasure-oriented view of sexuality rather than a performance-oriented view. Discussion of aspects of health, illness, and treatment that affect sexuality conveys an understanding of sex as an expression of self, not a compartment of self used up in youth.

As a rehabilitation specialist you have the opportunity, without proselytizing, to foster a view of sexual expression as an enriching experience that can open communication and increase intimacy and self-esteem. A little reassurance against their own false expectations and the hostility of society can go a long way in promoting healthy sexual adjustment for elderly patients.

It is worthwhile to keep in mind that despite the decreased speed and agility associated with growing older, the elderly generally have a great deal of free time, as well as life experience to bring to sexual expression. For some, old age is a cold winter with no refuge, but for others it is the harvest of a life's learning and loving.

REFERENCES

1. KAPLAN, HS: *The New Sex Therapy.* Brunner/Mazel New York, 1974, p 104.

2. PFEIFFER, E, VERWOEDT, A, WANG, HS: *Sexual behavior in aged men and women.* Arch Gen Psychiatry 19:753, 1968.

3. BUTLER, RN AND LEWIS, MI: *Sex After Sixty.* Harper & Row, New York, 1976, p 14.

4. LUDEMAN, K: *The sexuality of the older person: Review of the literature.* Gerontologist 21:203, 1981.

5. POC, O AND GODOW, HG: *Can students view parents as sexual beings.* The Family Coordinator 26:31, 1977.

6. LUDEMAN, K: The sexuality of the older postmarital woman: A phenomenological inquiry. (Unpublished dissertation).

7. BUTLER, RN AND LEWIS, MI: *Sex After Sixty.* Harper & Row, New York, 1976, p 32.

8. DRELLICH, MG: *Sex after hysterectomy.* Medical Aspects of Human Sexuality. November, 1967, p 62.

9. BUTLER, RN AND LEWIS, MI: *Sex After Sixty.* Harper & Row, New York, 1976, p 27.

10. STEFFL, BM: *Sexuality and aging: Implications for nurses and other helping professionals.* In SOLNICK, RL (ED): *Sexuality and Aging.* University of Southern California Press, 1978, p 139.

11. BROY, GP ET AL: *Sexual functioning in stroke survivors.* Arch Phys Med Rehabil 62:286, 1981.

12. BUTLER, RN AND LEWIS, MI: *Sex After Sixty.* Harper & Row, New York, 1976, p 30.

13. BUTLER, RN AND LEWIS, MI: *Sex After Sixty.* Harper & Row, New York, 1976, p 30.

14. SCHIAVI, R: *Sexuality and medical illness: Specific references to diabetes mellitus.* In GREENE, R (ED): *Human Sexuality, a Health Practitioner's Test.* Williams & Wilkins, Baltimore, 1979, p 203.

15. BUTLER, RN AND LEWIS, MI: *Sex After Sixty.* Harper & Row, New York, 1976, p 48.

16. LONG, JW: *The Essential Guide to Prescription Drugs: What You Need to Know for Safe Drug Use.* Harper & Row, New York, 1982.

17. LEDEBUR, J AND STRAX, TE: *Geriatric Sexuality Manual for Patients, Spouses, and Family.* Department of Physical Medicine and Rehabilitation, Philadelphia Geriatric Center, Philadelphia.

18. *Federal Register. Skilled Nursing Facilities.* Department of Health, Education and Welfare 39:193, Part 2, October 3, 1974.

CHAPTER 15

RESEARCH AND THE ELDERLY

CAROL R. SCHUNK, R.P.T., M.S.

BEHAVIORAL OBJECTIVES

Upon completion of this chapter, the reader will be able to
1. Identify topic areas pertinent to gerontologic research.
2. Recognize the positive and negative aspects of research designs in aging studies.
3. Explain reliability and validity.
4. Evaluate clinical measurement instruments as a potential source of research data.
5. Develop the concept of functional quality of life as a goal of research on the aged.
6. Describe the importance of the professional's role as a consumer or participant in research related to elderly.

Research on aging is unique in that everyone is a potential subject. Data collected today not only affects the current population over 65 years but also is in the best interest of the older people of tomorrow; research on the elderly is a self-serving activity. Research can provide information to enhance a high quality of life physically and mentally for the older population. A broad-based approach to research is a necessity, owing to the multiple dimensions of aging and the numerous professional disciplines involved. Although the focus of a study might be quite specific, such as basic cellular changes, the overall impact of data collected can be quite general. Whether the gerontologic researcher studies current status or future needs, the end result is geared toward the concept of an optimal quality of life for the elderly population.

There is a current need for services for the elderly, often putting researchers and service providers in the position of competing for funds. The field of aging cannot afford the opposition but needs to develop a symbiotic, not competitive, relationship between the two components of research and service. Research of today provides the services of tomorrow, just as today's services are based on yesterday's research.[1] Owing to the lack of centralized information regarding funding and ongoing programs, planners and administrators must consult a wide range of sources with diverse data when initiating services. Programs developed in accordance with the findings of specific studies, which lack the integration of additional data addressing the total concept of aging and its related problems, will not be in the best interest of the population. For example, if a rural nursing home developed a recreation program based on a single study from an urban elderly population, the chance of success is limited. Consequently, the plea for a national source of information with coordination of the multiple aspects of aging is a valid request in order to enhance the care provided by rehabilitation professionals.

Whether a person who works with the elderly is actively involved in research or a consumer of research, it is necessary to have a basic understanding of the research data available. The ability to analyze studies critically allows appropriate application in the clinical setting. Aging research requires special considerations because of the complicating factors involved with using age as a variable. Health care providers play an integral role in providing services to the elderly; consequently, research oriented around therapeutic activities is essential. An optimal quality of life is often very dependent upon the intervention of professionals involved with the over-65 population. For instance, Kane and Kane[2] found in reviewing the literature that the best predictor of the morale of elderly persons is their physical health. Consequently, therapists who deal with the physical aspect directly contribute to providing optimal quality. How can health care providers help but be involved in research?

TOPIC AREAS

Men and women age biologically, socially, and psychologically; therefore it is necessary to interrelate data from each theory when studying the elderly. According to Kane and Kane,[2] biologic aging refers to the "set of processes such that an individual organism becomes increasingly likely to die the longer he lives even in a favorable environment." If the environment is altered, the biologic age of humans may be changed, but the force of mortality or the increased probability of dying with increased age is a constant. Research focusing on the biologic aspects question whether aging is a result of individual cell physiology or a combination of the body systems' changes.

Psychologic aging is the difference in the persons's adaptive capabilities as he or she moves through time, including dealing with the environment, other people, and one's own emotions. Changes cited in psychologic aging research that affect the developmental process include information processing, sensation, perception, learning, motivation, and thinking.

Social aging refers to the social roles and related habit systems that are acquired over one's lifetime.[3] In other words, how do social support systems affect the older person's aging? Research in social aging is very broad based because the total population must be studied in order to examine the perceived roles and support available to the elderly. In essence, social aging as opposed to psychologic or biologic aging is almost controlled by the nonelderly.

A primary concern in gerontologic research, whether it is in the biologic, psychologic, or social area, is establishing norms for the older population. It is difficult to determine if research data are significant when there are no accepted baselines for the elderly. For example, testing muscle strength on an elderly individual without a concept of what is normal given the person's age and activity requirements doesn't provide the therapist with useful information. Consequently, a primary topic area in research on aging is the development of standards for the older population.

Professionals involved in geriatric rehabilitation are in a unique position of combining the biologic, psychologic, and social aspects of aging. The focus in rehabilitation is on function, which includes information from all three areas and directly relates to the person's quality of life. For example, a research study in a skilled nursing facility might investigate the independence level of arthritic patients who use a cane for ambulation versus those who do not use a cane. Biologically the energy expenditure is a factor, psychologically the individual's ability to adapt to the concept of needing an assistive device plus motivation will influence utilization, and socially the environmental barriers and attitudes of society toward the use of a cane are contributing aspects. On the surface level it might be obvious that the cane provides independence, however, the functional use is influenced biologically, socially, and psychologically.

Even the focus of chart audits for Therapy Quality Assurance has been reoriented to emphasize the functional goals of treatment. Instead of the topic for an audit being cerebrovascular accident, professionals are now looking at the problem from the patient's point of view, seeing immobility or depression as the primary problem.

In an attempt to help the elderly achieve the highest level of independence, rehabilitation research with the emphasis on function is a major contribution to the improvement of the quality of life and a primary focus for continued investigation.

Quality of life is used as an overall concept around which to organize the topic areas of gerontologic research. Looking at optimal aging as the desired outcome, health care professionals can provide data relevant to their specialty area and also contribute to the total knowledge of improving the conditions of life. The dimensions of the quality of life, as described by George and Bearon[4] include subjective evaluations and objective conditions. Life satisfaction (a sense of well-being) and self-esteem (a sense of self-worth) are the two subjective dimensions. The objective conditions described are general health, functional status, and socioeconomic status. These components of the quality of life serve as appropriate topic areas for aged research by health care professionals.

DEMOGRAPHY AND BIRTH COHORTS

Demography is the science of population dynamics. Relevant to the elderly, demography focuses on the large statistical group within the population who are 65 years and older. According to Cutler and Harootyan,[5] the three demographic processes which are basic to the understanding of population are migration, mortality, and fertility. Migration is the changes an individual makes in his or her residence during the life cycle, and mortality is defined as the rates of deaths from various causes. Fertility, or birth rate, is important in its relationship to a primary demographic indicator used in aging research, the birth cohort, which identifies all those people born at a particular time, whether it is a given day, month, year, or any interval of time. Identification of a group of people by birth cohort ensures a similar set of life experiences historically, economically, politically, and socially. The demographic characteristics of a cohort of older people can be traced back and utilized when analyzing present needs and trends. For example, the influence of the Depression on the 1900 to 1910 birth cohort may explain particular educational or economical factors of those who are current members of the aged population. Other demographic indicators are the dependency ratio—the arithmetic representation of the relationship between the portion of the population that is dependent (young and old) to the working population—and the sex ratio. Factors of fertility, mortality, sex ratio, and dependency ratio are constant within a birth cohort, but each succeeding cohort is different in composition. Therefore, comparisons between cohorts are difficult because all the demographic indicators and processes are changed. Cutler[5] views historical and social changes as a succession of birth cohorts traveling through society, each representing a varying set of circumstances.

METHODOLOGY

The complex nature of aging has direct implications when selecting an appropriate research design. Designs often associated with developmental aging research are the cross-sectional and longitudinal studies.[6] Using age as the independent variable, longitudinal studies follow a group of people for a prolonged period of time. Using a pretest, posttest design, each subject is assessed as a younger person and as an older person, thereby taking into account events in early life which may result in specific circumstances in old age.[7] For example, studying the perceptual abilities of a group at ages 20, 40, 60, and 80 years allows analysis of age as a variable in changes in perception. Criticisms of the longitudinal study include the impractical amount of time involved, problems with subject drop out, and sociocultural changes. The National Institute on Aging[1] points out that, besides the time-consuming aspect, the lack of foresight to collect appropriate data at the beginning of a longitudinal study may present problems when the cohort ages, inasmuch as there is no way to go back in time and to ask additional questions. Longitudinal studies are difficult to carry out because it takes a long time to get results and the subsequent rewards.[8] Schaie[7] goes so far as to state that "unless experimental isolation is possible or it can be assured that the dependent variable is not influenced by external events, the single cohort longitudinal design is weak and should be avoided." For example, to conclude that an individual's limitations in range of motion are the result of aging based on a longitudinal study may ignore the effects of decreased activity as a cause for limited range of motion.

Cross-sectional studies examine differences between two populations by observing the groups, one older and one younger, at the same time. The method is short term, easy, and with minimal financial implications; however, the ability to attribute differences between groups to age is difficult. The impact of sociocultural variables or other historical events is impossible to separate, given a one-time observation. Schaie[7] feels that the cross-sectional method is appropriate only if there is strong evidence for the absence of cohort differences and that potentially influential demographic variables are controlled. The latter is a difficult task, given the tremendous complexity of sociocultural variables.

Several alternative designs are presented by Schaie[7] to minimize the acknowledged problems of the two methodologies described. In order to ask questions relative to age without following a group's life course, he proposed an all-purpose design. This design uses cross-sectional and time sequential analysis to differentiate the presence of cohort and age differences. He also suggests minimizing the problems of longitudinal methodology by converting to cohort sequential method, which controls for historical events by following two or more cohorts over equivalent age ranges but different time ranges.

Much of the research in aging follows one of the two designs discussed above. Although some of the data are valid and contribute to our more general, conceptual understanding, therapists must become critical evaluators in order to apply specific findings to the treatment of the aging patient and to be able to develop a sense of what is an appropriate design, given the complexities of using age as a variable.

VALIDITY AND RELIABILITY

When research answers a specific question about the elderly, the matter is not a closed case. It is up to the researcher in planning the design and ultimately to the consumer of the research to decide how good the answer is. Validity reflects the ability of a measurement to identify the characteristics it was intended to assess. Payton[9] attaches terms appropriateness, truthfulness, and supportableness to the concept of validity, emphasizing the fact that a measuring tool is not valid in itself. It is valid only when it is used for the particular measurement for which it was designed.

Reliability, usually used in reference to a measurement tool, reflects the ability to obtain the same results with repeated measurements. In cases in which reported results are confined to specific conditions within one facility, the test instrument may be reliable but will not contribute to overall data on the elderly because it is not repeatable outside the setting.[2] For example, if a measurement instrument were developed to measure social functioning before and after subjects participated in a social skills class but the use of the instrument were dependent upon a highly trained staff to analyze the social skills, the results would not be appropriate to generalize to other settings without similar personnel.

The relationship between variables in adult development and aging also needs to be examined to maximize accuracy. Issues of concern when relating variables are the internal validity and the external validity. According to Payton,[9] a study is internally valid when the differences measured in the dependent variable are accounted for by differences in the independent variable. The goal is to have no other explanation for an outcome than the presumed causal events. If there are alternative interpretations, then the internal validity is jeopardized.[10]

There are specific threats to internal validity of which the researcher and consumer of research should be aware. History, or the passage of time and events happening during that period, may affect results. For example, if an individual becomes ill while participating in a study, decreased performance in mobility cannot be attributed only to the lack of therapy. Testing is another threat to internal validity, because a person may learn something about the test itself by repeated sessions. Consequently, it may be false to assume that someone's mental status has improved because of group support when the person simply remembers how to take the test from previous experience. The death rate, or mortality, is a threat to internal validity that poses problems with aged research, especially with longitudinal studies. If the effects of a support group on adjustment of older individuals following the death of a spouse is the research question, mortality must be considered as a threat to internal validity.

Sampling becomes a critical matter with external validity when a researcher wants to generalize from the sample to the general population.[9] When the observed relationship exists only for a specific group or circumstances, the external validity is affected. Threats to external validity such as treatment, persons, settings, and measures are difficult to completely control but must be minimized whenever possible.

MEASUREMENT AND RESEARCH

If the status of the aged is to be improved, effective assessments of the physical state, adaptive behavior, and emotional state are necessary. The interrelationship of these three areas is reflected by the individual's independence in performing activities of daily living. Thus appropriate measurement should be focused on the individual's level of independence. As many of the techniques for measuring human function are based on the norms for young adults or children, there is an effort to construct alternative test forms for different age levels.[7] To say an 84-year-old individual is independent in wheelchair activities is very different from making the same statement about a 24-year-old person who is confined to a wheelchair. The functional needs of each patient are different and should be reflected in the assessment tool and data analysis method utilized by the researcher.

Health care providers use assessment instruments frequently but often neglect the potential of using the assessment procedure as a source of research data. In their text *Assessing the Elderly*, Kane and Kane[2] discuss the relationship of measurement to research, highlighting factors that allow an assessment to serve a dual purpose of evaluating patient status and providing data for research. Identifying measurable characteristics or anticipating desired outcomes will provide the guidelines for choosing appropriate methodology. Optimal reliability and validity of the assessment tool are the key to collection of sound data which can then be effectively applied to clinical practice. Situational factors that may cause variance should be identified to enhance the researcher to interpret findings realistically. The appropriateness of the selection of the measurement, whether it is a longitudinal or cross-sectional design, will determine the extent of application of the research findings beyond the research setting.

The choice of the measurement technique is influenced by the role of the service provider. Health care professionals can be divided into two general categories. The first group includes physicians and other professionals who encounter elderly patients in the course of clinical practice but who do not confine their practice to the aged. Measurement tools used by this group must be relatively easy to use and readily available; however, the use of one tool for all ages encountered will produce only skewed results. If an orthopedic physical therapy clinic uses range of motion norms standardized on a young adult population, there may be attempts to stretch out a 70-year-old person's extremities beyond ranges of motion considered normal for that person's age group. Therefore, individuals who treat the older population on a part-time basis should be aware of the research available and the normal characteristics of this age group.

The relatively new body of professionals who specialize in geriatrics via experience or education composes a second group. It is hoped that members of this group will provide much of the needed future research. Ongoing assessment of patient progress provides a wealth of potential research data given an appropriately standardized and tested measurement tool.[2] This information is collected throughout the duration of the patient's treatment program and requires only accurate record keeping. Although the primary focus of measurement is usually quality of care, geriatric specialists must keep in mind the all-encompassing spectrum of possible topics to study. Staff morale and effective training of caretakers are two topics in which the effects on patient care are indirect. Staff attitudes and their ability to perform their duties in treating the geriatric patient will influence the overall standard of life for the aged.

Although difficult to distinguish from psychologic and social aspects, physical function is usually the area of emphasis for measurement tools utilized by rehabilitation therapists. The therapist may evaluate mobility, but conclusions on the patient's overall status or potential include psychologic and social factors such as motivation, family support, and environmental barriers. Kane and Kane[2] cite one evaluation form which divides physical functioning into (1) physical health or the degree of fitness, (2) Activities of Daily Living (ADL), and (3) instrumental ADL, which is defined as the more complex activities associated with independent life, such as riding a bus.

Currently there are several measurement instruments that assess physical functioning in relation to ADL. Although preexisting instruments may not meet all the needs of a facility, using a format that is utilized in other places allows comparison of data and contributes to the collection of background information on aging. Kane and Kane[2] describe several of the existing measurement tools, including the Katz Index of ADL, PULSES (profile physical condition, upper limbs, lower limbs, sensory abilities, and social factors), Barthel Index and Barthel Self-Care Ratings, the Kenny Self-Care Evaluation, and the PACE II (patient appraisal and care evaluation). If more facilities adopt similar standardized instruments, the research data available are bound to expand. Even if consistent definitions were used for common terms, therapists would be able to generalize research findings from patient to patient or clinical setting to clinical setting. The functional orientation of rehabilitation therapy is the ideal orientation for bridging the gap between multiple settings: hospital or long-term care and community-based services. Measurement tools designed to enable therapists to collect data easily and to apply results to multiple diagnoses and settings will contribute to improving services for the elderly.

Given the problems associated with the collection of information via longitudinal studies, Glenn and Zody[8] advocate the use of national survey data for gerontologic research. Information collected in national surveys provides a longitudinal view of trends, attitudes, and demographic characteristics which could contribute to the background knowledge about the elderly. Surveys that repeat questions at various intervals over a period of time include the Survey Research Center at the University of Michigan, National Opinion Research Center, and American Institute of Public Opinion (Gallup Poll) among others. Gathering procedures, especially sampling issues, should be carefully examined if conclusions are drawn on data available from only a few polls.[8] Researchers interested in characteristics related to aging can use the characteristics of the adult population as a baseline. If trends associated with the older group move in an opposite direction of those identified with the total population, the consideration of age as a variable is justified. Consequently, there is a wealth of data available from national surveys which can contribute to enhancing the knowledge about the elderly and can provide answers to research questions.

CONCLUSION

The health care professional's responsibility in providing service to the elderly should include participation in research if the care is to be effective. The emphasis in rehabilitation therapy on function is a justifiable response to the current trend away from a disease orientation in treating the elderly patient. The study of function is suitable to a multivariate approach that takes into consideration the complex nature of aging. The therapist must be familiar with methodology appropriate to gerontologic research and concepts such as validity and reliability. This will allow the professionals who work with the elderly to become educated consumers of research even if they do not participate in the research directly. Given the global objective of improving the quality of life for those over 65 years and the importance of physical health in happiness, continued research in rehabilitation is essential.

REFERENCES

1. NATIONAL INSTITUTE ON AGING: *What is Aging Research?* NIH Publication, No. 82-2301, September, 1982.
2. KANE, RA AND KANE, RL: *Assessing the Elderly.* Lexington Books, Lexington, MA, 1981.
3. BIRREN, JE: *Research on aging: A frontier of science and social gain.* In BRANTL, UM AND BROWN, MR (EDS): *Readings in Gerontology.* CV Mosby, St Louis, 1973, p 20.
4. GEORGE, LK AND BEARON, LB: *Quality of Life in Older Persons, Meaning and Measurement.* Human Sciences Press, New York, 1980.
5. CUTLER, NE AND HAROOTYAN, RA: *Demography of the aged.* In WOODRUFF, DS AND BIRREN, JE (EDS): *Aging: Scientific Perspectives and Social Values.* Van Nostrand, New York, 1975, p 31.
6. WILLIS, SL AND BALTES, PB: *Intelligence in adulthood and aging: Contemporary issues.* In POOR, LW (ED): *Aging in the 1980's. Psychological Issues.* American Psychological Association, Washington, DC, 1980.
7. SCHAIE, KW: *Quasi-experimental research designs in the psychology of aging.* In BRITTON, SE AND SCHALE, KW (EDS): *Handbook of the Psychology of Aging.* Van Nostrand Rheinhold, New York, p 39.
8. GLENN, ND AND ZODY, RE: *Cohort Analysis with National Survey Data.* Gerontologist 10:233, 1970.
9. PAYTON, OD: *Research: The Validation of Clinical Practice.* FA Davis, Philadelphia, 1979.
10. HULTSCH, DS AND DEUTSCH, F: *Adult Development and Aging.* McGraw-Hill, New York, 1981, p 30.

CHAPTER **16**

AGING AND THE DYING

ANTONIA LEONARD, O.T.R.

BEHAVIORAL OBJECTIVES

Upon completion of this chapter, the reader will be able to
1. Identify the appropriate therapeutic relationship with an elderly dying patient.
2. Recognize important issues in caring for the elderly dying patient.
3. Describe the historical development of society's view of dying.
4. Develop an understanding of a personal view of dying.
5. Design an appropriate rehabilitation program for the elderly dying patient.
6. Define the hospice concept.

In recent years the topics of aging and dying have been studied from many perspectives. The research has led to the development of a new area of clinical practice within the health care system, the care of the dying patient. Physicians, nurses, social workers, and other health professionals have developed specialized skills in response to the needs of dying patients. Rehabilitation professionals are now becoming more aware of the need to understand the processes of aging and dying and that their roles can contribute in a unique way.

Providing rehabilitation services to aging, dying patients presents a twofold challenge. The first challenge requires an integration of knowledge in areas of both aging and dying. Thus far in this text the aging process has been described in depth with an emphasis on the rehabilitation needs of the elderly. It is equally important to understand that the culmination of the aging process is dying, or as Kübler-Ross[1] refers to it, "the final stage of growth." Rehabilitation professionals must be able to recognize the special needs of the elderly patient approaching the final life experience.

The second challenge offers the opportunity of expanding upon traditional roles within the field of rehabilitation. The training of various rehabilitation disciplines emphasizes the restoration of function and physical well-being. When restoration is not possible, adaptation and compensation become the focus in helping patients to participate in life as fully as possible. In working with the dying person, the same goal, that of full participation in life until death, can be applied. It is the process of intervention that changes.

The focus of this chapter an overview of the process of dying as experienced by the aged person. No attempt will be made to give a formula for treatment; rather, insights on the modification or adaptation of basic rehabilitation principles will be explored. The ultimate purpose of this chapter is to create a climate for future learning which should take place as clinicians encounter the dying person in clinical settings.

DYING IN SOCIETY

The human experience of dying is an inevitable part of life. What changes, however, are the social conditions surrounding the aging and dying processes and the behaviors and attitudes reflected by society and the individual. Vischer[2] writes, "Realization that life must come to an end varies enormously from not only one individual to another and from one social group to another but even from one cultural or historical group to another."

In order to appreciate the social context of aging and dying today, it would be important to understand how the social context has changed over time. Two social phenomena that have been identified by sociologists are (1) the life expectancy and cause of death, and (2) the social structure and circumstances in which dying occurs.

One of the greatest accomplishments of 20th century has been the lengthening of the life expectancy by nearly 30 years. During earlier periods of history the rate of increase was much slower than in modern society. For example, from prehistoric times until the mid-17th century the average life expectancy increased from 18 to only 36 years.

What accounts for the dramatic increase can be attributed to advances in medical science and technology. Lerner[3] reports that the leading cause of death in 1900 was from communicable diseases. Infant mortality was prevalent. It was not uncommon for people to die at an early age from communicable diseases without predictability or prevention. With only limited medical knowledge, society was unable to control death brought about by epidemics, famine, and even war.[4]

During the late 19th century, as technology advanced and medical science discovered ways to control many diseases, the average life expectancy lengthened and greater numbers of people lived into old age. Today the average life expectancy is 70 years. According to Lerner,[3] the leading cause of death is now attributed to the chronic, degenerative diseases associated with the aging process. With the influence of public health education, even greater numbers of people living to old age can be expected in the future. Dying has become a phenomena closely associated with aging more than ever before in history.

The manner in which societies have dealt with their dying members reflects the value of life to the society. In the premodern-era, death of an individual was not only a loss to the individual's family but also a loss to the local community. The impact of death was compounded by the fact that communities were of smaller scale and each person's role was important to the life of the community.

In earlier societies death was a more personalized phenomena. People often died in their own homes surrounded by family and friends. Burial frequently took place on one's own land or in a nearby churchyard. The daily life of the community was often interrupted, and work ceased for the day in order to pay respect to the deceased and family. Dying was experienced at the center of home and community.

The social circumstances of death in modern society contrasts sharply to earlier periods. With increased urbanization and the advent of the nuclear family, individuals are often part of a much broader social group. Within large corporate structures, the work of an individual represents a much smaller contribution to the total system. The aged person is often retired from the work force or public service.

In modern society most people no longer die at home. About three quarters of deaths occur in hospitals and nursing homes.[5] Families are no longer primarily involved in the care of dying members. Instead, the dying are surrounded by a host of medical personnel. Funeral directors see to the details of burial while the general life of the local community remains uninterrupted by the event of death. Dying has now become an experience of old age and is often on the periphery of the social experience.

In modern society death and dying have not always been topics of study and discussion. Death has been not only physically removed from the core of society but also psychologically separated from everyday life. As Fulton[6] states, "Death, like a noxious disease, is a taboo subject, and as such it is both the object of much disguise and denial." General discussions of statistics, fatal diseases, and philosophic argument are permissable, but death on a personal level is often shunned as a topic. These inhibitions still prevail among many health care professionals who care for the dying in hospitals and institutions.

It was in such a climate as this that Dr. Elizabeth Kübler-Ross began the work of revolutionizing the field of death and dying. Colleagues, at first, seldom referred their terminally ill patients to her service because she attempted to discuss this sheltered topic.[7] Largely through her work, and that of others who followed, the social conscience has been awakened to the needs of the dying.

THE PERSONAL EXPERIENCE OF DYING

Most of what is known about death comes from those who have entered the final stage of life. Many terms have been used to describe dying, such as a journey, an event, and a human experience. For those learning about dying or caring for the dying, it is worthwhile to describe it as a process. Although various commonalities exist among the dying, the phenomenon of dying is a uniquely individual experience.

Glaser and Strauss[8] described the span of time from the point one learns that death is imminent to the moment of death as the "dying trajectory." The dying person, the family, and the health care team each perceive the course of dying based upon what may be expected to occur. When the dying trajectory is of long duration, the patient may fear a long, lingering death. Families may experience the mourning process. Rehabilitation professionals may anticipate the decline in a patient's ability to participate in various physical activities. In many cases the actual process may be different from anticipated.

Kübler-Ross[7] was the first to describe the stages of dying. In her theory, the stages of isolation and denial, anger, bargaining, and depression must be worked through in order to reach the final stage of acceptance. These stages may be reached in a different order, or various stages may not be reached at all. In addition, the powerful forces of life experience, personality, outlook on life, pain, and physical deterioration also influence the individual's ability to deal with dying.[9] A variety of emotions may interplay at any time. It is not enough to be able to identify the emotional responses. The rehabilitation professional must be able to help the patient cope with feelings and bring them to expression in a supportive, accepting atmosphere.

Among the elderly are those who have begun the process of dying without the presence of a terminal diagnosis. Aging itself is a process that closely parallels that of the terminally ill patient. The elderly are usually retired from the work force. During this time, one often reflects upon life's accomplishments and regrets what is undone. It is a time to put personal affairs in order and to make peace with oneself and others. Participation in life continues but with less emphasis on physical performance and more on experiencing the "essence of life."

In contrast to the younger terminally ill patient, the older patient has frequently experienced many of the losses even before entering the process. Many have experienced the loss of family and friends. Many may have already experienced physical deterioration and loss of control of bodily functions. One of the most difficult aspects is the feeling of aloneness often realized in the institutional setting. It is even possible that the feelings of isolation and abandonment can hasten the onset of withdrawal from life before physical deterioration demands. How often do rehabilitation professionals encounter elderly patients who do not appear "motivated" for therapy? It is important to understand the patient's present life situation in many cases. Perhaps the patient is experiencing anger or depression. It may be a point at which reflection is more important that participation.

The needs of the dying are important to understand from the perspective of the individual. Often the rehabilitation professional can assist the dying person in meeting these needs. The dying have the need for personal expression and choice. There is the need to live out one's life as one chooses as much as this is possible. There is a need for comfort, both physical and emotional. Finally, there are the needs to live with integrity and the feeling of fulfillment and to die with dignity.

CARING FOR THE DYING

One of the current issues generated within the health care system is the proper method of caring for the dying. It has long been recognized that hospitals are places of cure with emphasis on the preservation of life. Nursing homes provide medical, nursing, and supportive services but are usually not structured to provide for the special needs of the dying. The home is often the preferred setting, yet many individuals have no one to care for them. Others are in need of specialized nursing service which families cannot provide at home. More vital than the question of setting is how the care should be administered.

One answer to this dilemma comes to us from Europe, where specialized treatment for the dying has long been established. The hospice concept of care is new to this country but is being recognized widely and is being applied to the care of the terminally ill. One reason for its effectiveness is that the purpose of the hospice is solely to care for the dying in a manner that promotes the quality of life. Hospice care can be provided in many settings, including hospitals, in the home, as a free-standing inpatient facility, or as part of long-term-care facilities.

Hospice is an organized program of services containing basic elements.[10] One of the primary elements is to control pain—physical, emotional, or spiritual—so that the patient can continue to participate in life as fully as possible. It is a physician-directed program which emphasizes the interdisciplinary team approach, including the rehabilitation disciplines. The person is encouraged to maintain as much control of everyday life as possible. Both the patient and the family are the center of concern. Even after the patient's death, staff remain in contact with the family as part of a bereavement program.

Hospice programs were developed for those whose prognoses are terminal within a relatively defined time. The chronically ill do not often qualify for admission into these programs, because they are not designed for providing long-term care. Although hospice programs may not be appropriate for persons with a long-term illness, the hospice concept has potential for application in special programs which might be designed for the chronically ill population.

Two important issues faced by the dying and the health care community concern the rights to live and to die. Advanced medical technology has now made it possible to extend life through artificial support systems. By extending life it is hoped that cure may be found or that the individual may have more time spent living and sharing with loved ones. A number of individuals maintain the right to refuse extraordinary measure to prolong life. The concern is that although the body continues to function, the quality of life may be lost.

It is far beyond the scope of this chapter to discuss the moral, legal, and ethical considerations raised in these issues. Rehabilitation professionals perhaps will face these issues personally or clinically. Patients may discuss the fear of dying or the fear of living by artificial systems. It would be important to disclose this information to physicians and families or to encourage the patient to do so. Regardless of the individual's decision, services must always be rendered with respect for the patient's right to choose and with respect for the dignity of the individual's life.

APPLICATION OF THE REHABILITATION PROCESS

The Treatment Setting

Rehabilitation professionals provide service to dying patients in a number of clinical settings, including hospitals, long-term-care facilities, hospices, and home-care agencies. Patients may be referred at any time during the course of illness, although more often in the early and middle phases of dying. The particular setting often defines the length of involvement; it should never determine the quality of intervention.

In long-term care and hospice there is a greater opportunity for extended involvement in the care of the dying. Here the therapist can directly affect the process of physical decline. With knowledge and understanding of the frustrations associated with restricted mobility and dependency, the therapist contributes to supporting the patient at each declining level. It is a challenge to professional creativity to help the patient utilize remaining abilities. When this is not possible, the therapist offers emotional support by allowing the patient to express feelings and concerns.

In home care and hospital settings, the length of service may be limited by the need for service based upon regulatory statutes. The patient may remain in the hospital for the duration of a specific medical treatment. In home care the involvement is usually based on the patient's potential for improvement at a specific level. The therapist must make the most of this time by selecting specific goals with the patient that can be met during this period. One can also act as a resource to patients and families by sharing knowledge of available resources and providing guidelines for dealing with specific physical and functional problems.

The Therapeutic Relationship

During the course of training, rehabilitation professionals learn about the "therapeutic relationship" between patient and therapist, which sets certain boundaries of interaction and obligations on each side. The therapist offers understanding, privacy of information, and professional skills; the patient reciprocates with a certain amount of trust, effort, and the provision of necessary background information. These occur to varying degrees, depending upon the personality, responsibility, and openness of both parties.

In working with the dying patient, the therapeutic relationship takes on new meaning. More than clinical service, the patient needs human compassion. Therapists have the privilege of sharing in the patient's dying. This requires that one reciprocate with caring and acceptance.[12] It is especially important to realize that professional does not mean impersonal. In paraphrasing a story from Fischer, LeShan[13] writes,

> He tells the story of the schizophrenic girl being seen at a hospital staff conference. When asked "How do you like the people here?" she replied, "There are no people here. There's just doctors, nurses and patients."

Components of Intervention

Typically, patients referred for rehabilitation services are given an evaluation to determine problems upon which the goals of therapy are based. To varying degrees patients may not be physically able to undergo lengthy testing sessions which drain energy especially during the later phases of disease. One should set realistic limits on the scope of the evaluation without sacrificing that which is necessary. Pertinent information may be obtained through observation, medical records, and staff and families.

The dying patient should always be given some choice in goal setting. Terminally ill patients may possess limited amounts of strength and endurance. The patient may desire to spend this energy on activities of personal importance. Although ambulation is possible, the patient may choose to use a wheelchair, reserving strength for visits with friends or for attending an outside event. The substitution of one activity for another should be looked upon carefully during earlier phases of the dying process. It may well be that the patient is disguising any number of feelings in relinquishing a realistic goal.

The treatment session can be one of the most important components of intervention. It is the setting for meaningful exchange, in which the dying patient may choose to share inner experiences more than to participate in a therapeutic regimen. In the course of performing physical and occupational tasks, the patient may ask questions concerning the possibilities of future disability.

The length and content of each session should remain relatively flexible because patients might not be capable of performance at the scheduled time. There are often fluctuations in strength and endurance, depending on a number of factors, including pain, emotions, and preoccupation. The patient may have a particular request for help in a specific area not on the therapist's agenda. Over time, it becomes clear that the therapist is asked by the patient for help in living until death, rather than in preserving abilities.

Patients in the final stages of dying need the therapist's support more than ever. Although the technical portion of intervention may not be needed, patients may feel abandoned when left alone by those who interacted so closely during their more functional states. Unless the setting prohibits it, effort should be made to continue the supportive aspect of therapy, even if only through brief visits.[14]

The Interdisciplinary Team

The rehabilitation professional often functions as a member of an interdisciplinary team. Each member contributes knowledge of a particular aspect of life according to experience and training. Usually disciplines are clearly defined, but in working with the dying patient roles may overlap, with any one team member emerging as "primary" caregiver. One team member may have established a rapport with the patient, who chooses to disclose some deeply personal feelings. The patient may be more comfortable discussing emotional difficulties with the nurse rather than with the psychologist. To complement this situation, the psychologist might assume a consultative role to the nurse and patient.

Each team member is responsible for providing one particular aspect of care, but all must approach the patient holistically. The team can act as a mutual support group, sharing personal feelings as well as professional views. In this way the role of the rehabilitation professional is expanded, and the therapist receives the opportunity to gain insights not only in the knowledge of the dying process but also into areas of human nature and behavior exceeding the boundaries of the profession.

MEETING THE CHALLENGE

The question is often asked, "What education and experience do I need for working with the dying?" I began work with the dying in a long-term-care facility and hospice program immediately after completing undergraduate training in occupational therapy, so my answer is somewhat biased. As stated at the beginning of this chapter, knowledge of the processes of aging and dying is essential, along with basic rehabilitation skills founded in adequate practical experience. It is beneficial to have some experience in the art of active listening. Many courses are offered in counseling, death and dying, and aging on university campuses and in adult education centers. Hospice programs frequently have training programs for their staffs. On-site visits to clinical settings where the rehabilitation staff are active members of the oncology team might be useful. The education sought should be based on a personal assessment of need and upon the particular setting for potential practice. Experience can be gained in many settings even at the entry level by taking time and effort in understanding dying clients. One can always learn from the dying. One also can learn from the living.

Openness to the experiences of all patients and to all people will be a source from which to reflect and to grow.

Some qualifications are essential to working with the dying. One cannot work effectively in any setting with personal strong inhibitions concerning death. To varying degrees, many people may be inhibited in talking about death as a personal experience. If these inhibitions are overpowering, it becomes difficult to share in patients' experiences and to help them cope with fear and frustration. As soon as one begins to face personal mortality, the door begins to open. Comfort with the dying is gained with experience and openness.

One must choose to work with the dying to be effective. Many rehabilitation professionals work with dying patients assigned to the caseload. Only those who choose to do so really work with their patients' dying.

When I first started out in hospice care, I asked myself, "What can you do for this patient? She is not going to be able to take care of herself anymore." This question may be asked of the rehabilitation professional by those both within and outside the disciplines who try to stereotype the roles. As a professional, one does not carry around a table from which to select a treatment for the corresponding problem. Instead, one learns how to assess patients on many levels and to explore creatively any number of solutions to the problem. In working with the dying, creativity in both problem solving and role definition is essential. Although the purpose of intervention may not be to restore function or physical well-being, it is well within reason to enhance the quality of life if only for a short period.

The role of the rehabilitation professional in working with the dying person has much potential. Perhaps the greatest challenge is to become involved and to explore that potential. There is nothing to lose and much to learn about dying and living.

REFERENCES

1. KÜBLER-ROSS, E: *Death: The Final Stage of Growth*. Prentice-Hall, Englewood Cliffs, NJ, 1975.

2. VISCHER, AL: *Growing Old*. Houghton-Mifflin, Boston, 1967, p 187.

3. LERNER, M: *When, why and where people die*. In SHNEIDMAN, E (ED): *Death: Current Perspectives*. Mayfield Publishing, Palo Alto, CA, 1976, p 146.

4. GOLDSCHIDER, C: *The mortality revolution*. In SHNEIDMAN, E (ED): *Death: Current Perspectives*. Mayfield Publishing, Palo Alto, CA, p 167.

5. ELDER, RG: *Dying and Society*. In CAGHILL, RE: *The Dying Patient: A Supportive Approach*. Little, Brown, & Co, Boston, 1976, p 5.

6. FULTON, R: *Death and Identity*, rev ed, Charles Press, Bowie, MD, 1976, p 3.

7. KÜBLER-ROSS, E: *On Death and Dying*. Macmillan, New York, 1969.

8. GLASER, B AND STRAUSS, AL: In SHNEIDMAN, E: *Death: Current Perspectives*. Mayfield Publishing, Palo Alto, CA, p 210.

9. SHNEIDMAN, E: *Death: Current Perspectives.* Mayfield Publishing, Palo Alto, CA, p 446.

10. MARKEL, W AND SINON, V: *Hospice Concept* 28:4, August, 1978.

11. RUSSELL, E: *Freedom to Die: Moral and Legal Aspects of Euthanasia.* Human Science Press, New York, 1975, p 59.

12. LESHAN, L: *Mobilizing the life force: An approach to the problem of arousing the sick patient's will to live.* In LESHAN, D AND LESHAN, L (EDS): *Psychosomatic Aspects of Neoplastic Disease.* JB Lippincott, New York, 1964, p 6.

13. FISHER, GM: In LESHAN, D AND LESHAN, L (EDS): *Psychosomatic Aspects of Neoplastic Disease.* JB Lippincott, New York, 1964, p 7.

14. LEBAN, M: IN KRUSEN, F (ED): *Krusen's Handbook of Physical Medicine and Rehabilitation.* WB Saunders, Philadelphia, 1982, p 961.

CHAPTER 17

PRACTICAL ASPECTS OF FINANCING REHABILITATION FOR THE ELDERLY

KATHRYN SCHAEFER, M.P.A., R.P.T.

BEHAVIORAL OBJECTIVES

Upon completion of this chapter, the reader will be able to
1. Identify and analyze financial incentives and deterrents as they have impact on consumer demand for therapy.
2. Discuss guidelines and regulations of the Medicare insurance program as it affects funding for therapy programs.
3. List professional lobbying strategies.
4. Identify the need for lobbying on behalf of rehabilitation for the elderly.
5. Outline an approach to a lobbying strategy to improve and to maintain government funding of therapy services for the elderly.
6. Analyze the basic principles involved in financing a therapy service as a business venture, including budgeting and planning as management tools in a nursing home.

The following section of this chapter explains how health care in the United States is financed for the elderly and for the general population. This section also explains the impact of health insurance on the types of health care services that are offered to and demanded by the elderly.

Health care in the United States is financed by health insurance, self-payment, or a combination of the two. Health insurance is guaranteed payment to an individual for certain predetermined health care services for a predetermined fee. Health insurance companies offer a variety of health insurance plans from which an individual may choose. As a general rule, the higher the fee, the greater the number of health care services that are guaranteed payment. The most common private health insurance companies are Blue Cross/Blue Shield, Aetna, Prudential, and New York Life insurances. Medicare is the federally funded public health insurance for persons over the age of 65 and the permanently disabled. Medicaid is the public health insurance funded by the federal and state governments that provides health insurance for the poor. Most persons in the United States are covered by one form of health insurance or another. Children, as long as they are dependents of their parents, are covered by their families' insurance policy. Adults who work are usually covered by a group insurance plan which is purchased by their employer and is considered a benefit of employment. Adults who are permanently disabled or over the age of 65 are covered by Medicare. Persons who do not fit into one of the above categories may purchase health insurance independently, or they may pay for health care services as they use them.

Health insurance reimbursement directly and indirectly affects the relationship that exists between the elderly patient and his or her therapist. In order to understand how health insurance reimbursement affects the patient/therapist relationship, understanding the economic principle of demand theory is useful. Demand theory explains why consumers choose to spend their money on one good or service instead of another good or service.[1] The service we provide is therapy, and the amount of therapy that a consumer will demand is influenced by the price of the service, the amount of satisfaction that he or she perceives he or she will receive from the service, and other goods or services that he or she could buy with the same money. If we assume that people purchase only things that they believe will provide them with satisfaction, then when a person suffers from an illness or injury, it is possible that his or her satisfaction can be increased by purchasing some therapy. However, the need for therapy does not necessarily generate demand for therapy services.[2] The consumer must weigh a number of important trade-offs. The value of improved health through therapy must be weighed against a loss of satisfaction from other goods and services that can no longer be purchased (Fig. 17-1). The less wealthy the consumer, the more essential are the goods he or she must trade in exchange for better health and the less likely he or she will be to choose to purchase therapy. Although the poverty of the elderly has steadily decreased over the last 20 years, approximately one fourth have an inadequate income. When treating the elderly, remember to

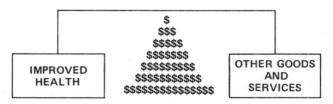

Figure 17-1. Illustrated here are the economic choices of the elderly.

keep in mind that they may have to choose between receiving therapy and other essential goods and services, such as food and clothing. This necessity of choice will have impact on the expectations they have toward the therapy they receive.[2]

The more services that are covered by the consumer's health insurance policy, the lower the out-of-pocket price to the consumer, the fewer trade-offs for other goods he or she will have to make, and the more likely he or she will be to purchase therapy services. Medicare reimburses for certain therapy services for persons over the age of 65. Those persons will be more likely to purchase the services that Medicare covers and less likely to purchase those services that it does not cover.[1]

The average retired person who lives on a fixed income is more likely to demand health care that is paid for by his or her health insurance than he or she is to demand health insurance care services that he or she must pay for out of pocket. For example, Medicare will pay for outpatient physical therapy but not for outpatient occupational therapy. The elderly person who has a stroke, is discharged from the hospital, requires outpatient therapy, and lives on a fixed income is more likely to demand physical therapy than he or she is to demand occupational therapy, simply because Medicare pays for it and it is therefore affordable. Because outpatient physical therapy is more affordable than outpatient occupational therapy to the elderly individual who is insured by Medicare, there is more demand for the outpatient physical therapy services than there is for the outpatient occupational therapy services.[1]

When there is a greater demand for a service, that service grows and is allocated more funding and staffing by the institution in which it is located. Therefore, it is clear that the large insurance companies have a significant impact on the health care industry. The health care services that the insurance companies choose to reimburse are those services that are more likely to grow.

These incentives and constraints which are placed on the elderly consumer to purchase therapy often influence his or her response to the therapy he or she is receiving and his or her interpersonal relationship with the therapist. The elderly consumer who is living on a low fixed income finds that nonreimbursed therapy is more costly to him or her in relationship to the other goods he or she could purchase than it is for the consumer with more discretionary funds. The more costly that therapy is to the elderly consumer, the more likely he or she is to demand quick results, inasmuch as therapy has a greater value to that person in relationship to other goods. In a case such as this, the therapist should recognize that the patient's incentive is toward self-care and a need for independence from the therapist. Patient education, mutual goal setting, involvement of family, and reliance on a home program become particularly important to the elderly patient with few funds for therapy. In order for the elderly patient to participate in self-care, he or she must understand, through education, the nature of the illness or disability.

People learn through repetition and reinforcement. Elderly patients who may have reduced functioning of one or more of the five senses especially appreciate instructions given verbally and in writing, which are reviewed and discussed during each treatment session.

In mutual goal setting, the therapist asks the patient what it is that he or she expects to accomplish as a result of therapy. The therapist then incorporates the patient's expectations into the treatment plan, and together the patient and therapist determine a set of treatment goals that are realistic and acceptable to the patient.

If the elderly patient is unable to afford continuous treatment, family or friends can often be called upon to assist in a home treatment program between periods of reevaluation by the therapist. Although this type of arrangement may be less than ideal, it may be the most practical solution to the complex problem of inadequate financial resources. Regardless of the complexity or simplicity of the financial situation, the patient's activities outside the therapy sessions are a critical factor in the improvement of the patient's health.

All activities, from speaking and eating to dressing and walking, are exercises that reinforce certain movement patterns. Because the purpose of therapy is almost always to improve the elderly individual's movement patterns and to help that person achieve an independent level of functioning, all activities he or she engages in will reinforce either appropriate or inappropriate movement patterns. Therefore, outpatients should have a home program and it should be reviewed at least briefly at each treatment session. An institutionalized patient should have his or her time away from the clinic analyzed by the therapist so that personal activities enhance the therapy program. The elderly patient's family or friends can be instructed in how best to help the patient achieve appropriate movement patterns during times when the patient is not supervised by the therapist. In this way, the patient is able to achieve therapeutic results more rapidly and at a lower cost.

Most insurance plans require the consumer to pay part of the cost of purchasing the health services. This partial payment is called cost sharing and can take the form of a deductible, coinsurance, copayment, or indemnity payment. A deductible is one of the most common forms of cost sharing in which the consumer pays all expenses up to a certain point at which insurance coverage begins. The deductible is usually around $100. Coinsurance is also commonly found in insurance policies. Coinsurance requires the individual to pay a predetermined percentage of the insured expenses. Coinsurance usually requires the patient to pay 20 percent. Copayment is less common and requires the consumer to pay a fixed charge per unit of insured service. Indemnity payments provide the consumer with a fixed payment per unit of service used, regardless of actual charges. Cost sharing is used by insurance companies because they believe that increasing out-of-pocket cost to the consumer at the time that the service is rendered will deter use of the service, thus reducing demand and overall expense to the insurance company.

Medicare uses two forms of cost sharing: the deductible and the coinsurance. Persons who are insured by Medicare pay the first $100 of their reimbursable health care bills each year, and then they pay 20 percent of the remainder of the bills. The purpose of cost sharing is to reduce the individual's incentive to use "free" services. If the patient must pay part of the bill, the patient will use only the services that are necessary, thus reducing overutilization of services and health care expenses.

It is important that the therapist understand the financial constraints placed upon the patient, because these constraints do have impact on the way the patient views the service being rendered, what he or she expects from the service, and whether or not he or she will demand the service at all.[3]

MEDICARE

The major health insurer of the elderly is Medicare. Medicare is a federally funded and administered health insurance program for eligible persons over the age of 65 and for the permanently disabled. It was passed into law in 1965 as Title XVIII of the Social Security Act. Medicare consists of two parts, A and B.

Part A is hospital insurance, which covers inpatient hospital care and subsequent care in a patient's home or a skilled nursing facility. Part A is primarily paid for by Social Security tax funds.[3]

Part B covers physician services, outpatient hospital care, home health care, other health-related services such as therapy, and durable medical equipment. Part B requires an annual deductible fee of $100 and then covers 80 percent of the cost of allowable services or supplies. Part B is a supplemental health care policy and is paid for by a monthly premium of money from those who are enrolled in the program.[4]

Although the Medicare legislation was passed in 1965, efforts to establish a national health insurance program in the United States have been promoted since 1912. Debate over the merits and demerits of such a federally funded program still rages today. The arguments for and against the program remain essentially the same as in 1912. As a general rule, the politically liberal favor the Medicare program. They tend to believe that it is a society's responsibility to care for the health of its people. The politically conservative, however, favor private insurance coverage for the elderly. They tend to believe in the individual's right and responsibility to care for himself.[4]

Providing a nationally funded health insurance for the elderly was a compromise between the conservative and liberal views. Persons over 65 who had contributed to Social Security were presumed to be in greater need for nationally funded health insurance than was the general population because the older people were retired, earned less, and needed more medical care. In the early 1960s, just prior to the passage of the Medicare program, the elderly had less coverage under private health insurance owing to their high-risk status and lack of job-related insurance. Conservative factions could no longer unilaterally defeat the arguments of the growing voice of the elderly, and thus the Medicare legislation was passed.[4]

Medicare is now an established right of elderly citizens. The debate is no longer over whether or not the nation should provide health care for the elderly but how much it can afford to provide. In other words, which health care benefits are included or excluded from coverage. Liberals still tend to argue for greater coverage based on society's responsibility to its elderly sick. Conservatives argue for less coverage based on the individual's responsibility to care for himself. What results is a compromise of the two views and complicated, often difficult to understand, benefit packages and regulations designed to distribute the benefits and to prevent abuse.

Physical therapy, occupational therapy, and speech-language pathology are covered, reimbursable benefits for the elderly who are insured by Medicare. The regulations that govern the reimbursement packages for each of the therapies are similar in some respects and different in others.

Some of the regulations that are shared by the three therapies follow. The elderly patient who is receiving therapy must be under the primary care of a physician, who is responsible for the overall care of the patient and the supervision of the therapy. This physician must sign a plan of treatment for the elderly patient who is receiving outpatient care. The plan of treatment must be reviewed and signed by the physician every 30 days. The physician must also see the outpatient at least every 30 days. Another similarity among the Medicare regulations for physical, occupational, and speech therapy is the requirement that therapy be rendered through an organization that has been approved by Medicare. All therapy services must be reasonable and necessary in order to qualify as a Medicare benefit.

Any therapy procedure that is routine and provided solely for an individual's general welfare, rather than for the therapeutic improvement of a specific condition, is not a reimbursable benefit. Another similarity among the reimbursable benefits provided to the elderly by Medicare is universal coverage for hospitalized beneficiaries and outpatients receiving therapy following inpatient hospitalization. All three therapy services provided in a nursing home are also reimbursable.

A few of the differences in reimbursable benefits for the three therapies follow. Services provided by the independently practicing occupational therapist are not reimbursable. However, physical therapy provided by an independent practitioner is reimbursable up to $500 per year. Home care provided by physical and speech therapists is reimbursable, but occupational therapy provided in the home is covered only if physical or speech therapy are also required.

Health care professionals should be aware of the benefits due their elderly patients in order to serve them best.[2] For example, an independently practicing physical therapist who receives a referral for treatment for an elderly person who is insured through Medicare and who has been discharged recently from a hospital may advise the patient to receive treatment from the hospital if he or she is going to require prolonged rehabilitation past the $500 annual reimbursement limit for services provided by independently practicing physical therapists. Because there is no such limit placed on reimbursement for outpatient care provided in a hospital following hospitalization, the patient will have less out-of-pocket expenses for the therapy.

Because there is a direct correlation between available funding and availability of services, therapists should be aware of Medicare regulations and pending changes in the regulations that affect funding. Ultimately, the elderly patient suffers from lack of funding for the care he or she needs. Ultimately, it is the responsibility of the health care professional to help protect the therapy needs of the elderly consumer through professional lobbying efforts.

LOBBYING IN THE GOVERNMENT FOR CHANGES IN MEDICARE

Lobbying is the act of influencing legislators to support a particular point of view. The American Physical Therapy Association, the American Occupational Therapy Association, and the American Speech-Language-Hearing Association all keep an eye on legislation that affects the elderly in the event that it may have impact on elderly persons who need physical, occupational, or speech therapy. The job of the association lobbyist is to identify such legislation, to determine whether the potential impact of the legislation is positive or negative, and to influence legislators either to support or to help defeat the legislation.

The importance for the individual therapist to understand the role of the association lobbyist cannot be underestimated.

Although the therapist must be aware of Medicare regulations and guidelines in order to help the elderly patient receive maximum benefit from insurance, the therapist should not let the regulations dictate the kind of care he or she provides. Medicare guidelines, and even the laws, are often changed. Those of us who are in contact with patients every day know the needs that Medicare does and does not meet. We can influence changes in Medicare by educating our patients and the public in general to voice their needs to their representatives in Congress and to the media constructively. Our patients can help us help them influence Medicare guidelines through the lobbying efforts of our professional organizations. Because Medicare is federally mandated and regulated, the way to influence reimbursement for therapy services is through a strong lobbying effort.

Each therapist who recognizes need for a change in the Medicare regulations or guidelines should notify the professional association lobbyist of changes that he or she perceives are needed in order that the lobbyist is well armed with information for a strong lobbying effort. Through the efforts of consumers, professionals, and interested taxpayers, Medicare does change. For example, in the 1960s and 1970s, the Medicare incentive was toward institutionalization in hospitals and skilled-nursing facilities because that is where the elderly would be receiving covered treatment. The combined voice of the elderly, who prefer their home environment to that of an institution, and that of taxpayers, who realize that home health care can be more cost effective (economical) than institutional care, helped change Medicare's reimbursement emphasis. The 1980s are bringing increased benefits to the homebound Medicare recipient whose health care needs can be met equally in the home and in an institution.

A lobbying effort must have several thrusts aimed at the several decision-making levels in government. The first level, which is the most difficult and expensive to influence, is the legislative level. The legislators—that is, the senators and congressmen who sit on health and finance committees and subcommittees—first must be convinced that there is a need for the law to be changed. There are various ways to convince legislators of the importance of a particular issue. One way is through direct verbal contact with the senator or congressman. To be effective, during that contact the lobbyist must know the legislator's voting record and use that knowledge to form arguments toward the sympathies of the legislator. The lobbyist must also know the needs of the legislator's voting constituency. If the legislator is convinced that a large segment of voters are interested in an issue, that issue gains greater importance in his or her eyes.

For example, Florida has a much larger geriatric population than does Maine. Inasmuch as the legislator is a representative of the people who elected him or her to office, it stands to reason that a legislator from Florida would be more interested in issues affecting the elderly than would a legislator from Maine. But arranging for an appointment with a legislator can be next to impossible for a lobbyist unless members of the group the lobbyist represents have demonstrated that they are a strong and interested constituency. This can be done through constituent letters, phone calls, and visits. Not to be overlooked is the importance of convincing the legislator of the strength of the support of the group through campaign contributions.

Even if an appointment with a legislator can be arranged, it is just as important to meet with the assistant who handles health legislation. The assistant is the person who researches the issues and advises the legislator concerning the impact that the legislator's actions will have on the law, on the constituency, and on the chances for reelection. Once the legislator is convinced that an issue should become a law, he or she introduces a bill to the Senate or House of Representatives. The bill is then sent to the appropriate House or Senate committee to study the bill.

Once the bill to effect a change in the law moves out of committee, it is debated and voted on by the legislature. At this point all legislators should be involved in the lobbying process.

When the bill is approved by the House and Senate and is signed by the President, it becomes law and cannot be changed except by another change in the law.

Because this process is so complex and time consuming, laws are usually written in general terms in order that they can withstand the passage of time. The specific details of the law's regulations are developed and passed by the agency that is charged to enforce it. In the case of Medicare, the Health Care Financing Administration (HCFA), which is a division of the Department of Health and Human Services, is charged with enforcement. Therefore the second level of the lobbying effort should be aimed toward the policy makers of the regulating agency. The lobbyist should make himself or herself useful to the bureaucrat by providing the bureaucrat information that will help him or her make policy decisions. The Health Care Financing Administration negotiates with local health insurance companies across the country to process claims and to enforce regulations locally. These insurance companies are called Third Party Intermediaries. These Third Party Intermediaries exhibit a certain amount of discretion in interpreting HCFA's regulations on a case-by-case basis. If a claim for reimbursement is denied, a Medicare subscriber may appeal the decision on an individual basis.

An understanding of the various levels of the making of a law and its enforcement is useful to the health care practitioner who wants to try to change the law or the way the law is interpreted through lobbying at the various levels. A therapist can better serve patients if he or she understands the legislative process that creates the laws under which the patients are reimbursed. The therapist who understands this legislative process can better influence legislation at its various levels of implementation. And the therapist can better understand the need to support the lobbying efforts of the professional organization at the federal and local levels (Fig. 17-2).

FINANCING THERAPY AS A BUSINESS VENTURE

The financing of physical, occupational, and speech therapies for the elderly includes not only the income generated by the service but also the management of the expenses and the growth of the therapy service.

A therapy service providing care for the elderly, whether it is physical, occupational, or speech, is a business venture. For example, the purpose of the business of running a nursing home is to provide a community service that generates an income sufficient to meet expenses and to provide for the growth of the institution. The financial health of a therapy service in a nursing home requires that the therapy department head have an intimate understanding of the services' income and expenses. Although an advanced degree in accounting and bookkeeping is not necessary, knowledge of a few basic principles from those fields is critical for the department director. The therapy department head in a nursing home has access to professional accountants and bookkeepers who guide and assist him or her, but the ultimate responsibility for the fiscal integrity of the business lies within the therapist's running of the department.

The nursing home must rely on its revenue-producing departments for sufficient income to perpetuate itself and to grow, or the institution, unless heavily endowed, will eventually die. Nursing homes are highly labor intensive, which means that salaries comprise a large portion of total expenses. Most of the labor in nursing homes is not directly income producing, such as housekeeping, nursing, maintenance, and administration. Therefore, the income-producing departments—such as physical therapy, speech pathology, and occupation therapy—must generate income to help defray the expenses incurred by the nursing home as a whole.

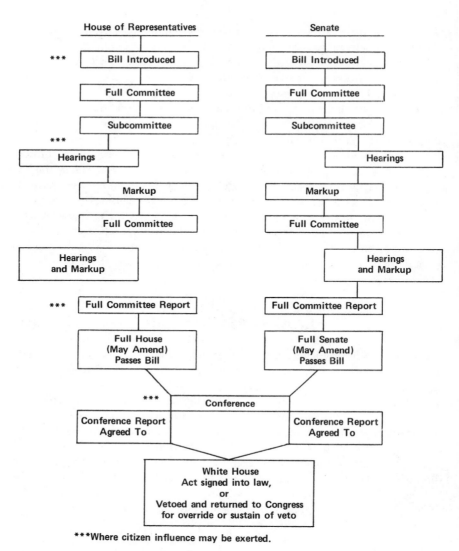

House of Representatives   Senate

***   Bill Introduced   Bill Introduced

Full Committee   Full Committee

Subcommittee   Subcommittee

***   Hearings   Hearings

Markup   Markup

Full Committee   Full Committee

Hearings and Markup   Hearings and Markup

***   Full Committee Report   Full Committee Report

Full House (May Amend) Passes Bill   Full Senate (May Amend) Passes Bill

***   Conference

Conference Report Agreed To   Conference Report Agreed To

White House
Act signed into law,
or
Vetoed and returned to Congress
for override or sustain of veto

***Where citizen influence may be exerted.

Figure 17-2. Diagrammed here is a typical journey for legislation in Congress. (From American Association of Museums, with permission.)

BUDGETING

Because therapy departments are income producing, it is important for the therapy department head to understand the relationship between income and expenses. The study of this relationship is a departmental budget. The budget is a listing of income less expenses for a particular period, usually a month. Items included in the budget are revenue, direct expenses, and indirect expenses. Revenue is the income generated by the department, which includes income from treatments rendered and from other sources, such as the sale of equipment.

Direct expenses are easily identified as regular monthly expenses, such as wages. Indirect expenses are costs that are allocated to the department's share of operating the facility. For example, a nursing home allocates to the therapy department its share of the heat, light, and housekeeping costs, which are usually allocated on the basis of percentage of square feet used by the department to the total square feet of the building.[2]

The budget compares income and expenses by subtracting the total expenses from the total revenue, which produces the net revenue. The net revenue is the department's profit. The net revenue must be a positive number in the long run in order for the department to remain financially viable.[2]

All the items listed in the budget are totaled and are compared with other months. The department director evaluates any significant changes and determines the reason for the change. For example, if the net revenue for the Comma Nursing Home were usually around $2000 and it increased to $4000 one month, the department director would look for changes in the individual revenue and expense items. If the cause of the increase in net revenue were due to a $1500 increase in treatment income and there were no comparable increase in labor expense, it would be clear that the physical therapy department had been twice as productive during that month. The nursing home administrator would want to know if the department had been twice as productive because the department usually had been overstaffed and only now had worked up to capacity or if the regular staff had been overworked during that month. Careful monthly evaluation of all budgeted items is crucial to the administration of a well-run, fiscally sound therapy department.

PLANNING

In addition to managing the ongoing activities of the therapy department, it is also important for the therapy department head to plan for future growth of the department. When planning a new service in a nursing home or evaluating an existing service, ask yourself why the service exists. Answering the following questions is a first step in planning your service. What is the community or potential elderly community it may serve? Is there a need in the elderly community that is not filled or that can be filled better by a therapy service? What type of service will best fit the need? How will the service be funded?[2]

By answering these questions, you may find that the need is greater than or different from what you anticipated. If that is the case, your entire approach to planning the development of the service will change.[2]

The third step in planning a therapy service in a nursing home is publicizing its availability. To do this effectively you must identify who is most likely to send patients to you. Generally, the primary publicity target for the therapist is the referring physician. The secondary target is the elderly consumer, the potential patient. Once you have identified the major publicity targets, decide what kind of advertising to which they respond best. Ask yourself, "If I were a physician (or a consumer of therapy services), what would make me want to buy the service?" Answer that question with several advertising approaches, decide which will be the best approaches, and try them.

The last step in planning your therapy service is evaluating the results of your efforts. You can do this by comparing volume and/or income data over time and looking for peaks that correspond with your promotional efforts.

Another practical example of this planning process follows. Imagine that you are a physical therapist who runs a weekly exercise class in a retirement residence. You learn from members of the class that several residents needs physical therapy and can't find a therapist. You have a general idea that there may be a need for a physical therapy service in or near the residence. The first step in this marketing process is to establish need. You take a survey of all residents to determine how many needed physical therapy in the last 5 years, whether they received it, where they received it, and whether they were satisfied. Then you evaluate other potential competition. Your competition may be the physical therapy department of area hospitals, local physical therapists in private practice, home health agencies, or physicians who have physical therapists in their offices. Find out the type of service that is offered by each competitor, the fees they charge, and, if possible, the level of satisfaction of the patients. Use your imagination and think of all the possible functions of a physical therapy service in the community, including direct patient care provided in an office, prevention programs, and home health care. Determine the demand for each of these functions, then analyze your ability to fill the demand. The optimum even is designing a physical therapy service that fits the established demand.

As soon as you decide to start developing the physical therapy service, start informing other professional practitioners of the services you are planning. Solicit continual input from all sources concerning their perception of the need for your service.

When you are ready to open for business, send formal announcements to area physicians, other area health care professionals, the residents of the retirement home, and any other potential group of consumers. You may want to have an open house. Visit and chat with physicians and area health care professionals. Make yourself visible in the community. Advertise in the yellow pages within the limits of your professional guidelines. Then provide the best quality service possible.

As time goes by, evaluate your volume and revenue statements at least monthly to determine the effectiveness of your ongoing planning efforts. The growth and long-term health of your therapy service for the elderly depends on an effective planning process.

CONCLUSION

Health care reimbursement mechanisms, Medicare regulations, lobbying legislators, budgeting therapy services, and planning therapy services all contribute to the financing of therapy services for the elderly. The therapist whose education includes an understanding of these financing aspects of therapy is better prepared to serve the elderly patient. The income generated through Medicare reimbursement provides an opportunity for the elderly to have access to services that they might otherwise be unable to afford, yet the restrictions of the current system might also be the reason older persons do not receive many of the desperately needed services.

Because many therapists desire better control and utilization of their services, financial incentives, lobbying strategies, and marketing are essential to therapists' education. This chapter has presented an overview of the most important issues a therapist should be aware of in order to manage the financing of a physical, occupational, or speech therapy service effectively.

ADDENDUM

Since this chapter was written, Medicare has changed its method of reimbursement for Part A hospital coverage from the system described in the text (reimbursement of services rendered) to a system of payment to the hospital of a fixed amount for each diagnosis. This fixed dollar amount is divided among the hospital services as the hospital sees fit. This change has implications on patient care incentives and interdepartmental coordination of care.

Nursing homes and outpatient Medicare reimbursement mechanisms remain as described in the text. Other, nonfederal, insurances still reimburse for services rendered in hospitals.

REFERENCES

1. LUKE, RD (EDS): *Issues in Health Economics.* Aspen, Rockville, MD, 1982.
2. RAPOPORT, J, ROBERTSON, RL, STUART, B: *Understanding Health Economics.* Aspen, Rockville, MD, 1982.
3. DAVIS, CK, ET AL: *Medicare: Special Pullout Section (Part I).* Rx Home Care 4:7, 1982, p 31.
4. DAVIS, CK, ET AL: *Medicare and You.* Chenning L. Bete, Greenfield, MA, 1976.

BIBLIOGRAPHY

ADMINISTRATION ON AGING, OFFICE OF HUMAN DEVELOPMENT SERVICES: *Statistical Notes from the National Clearinghouse on Aging.* US Department of Health, Education and Welfare, Washington, DC, 1978.

BALL, PM.: *The fortieth year of social security in America.* In SEBASTIAN, CL (ED): *Papers from the Economics of Aging: Toward 2001.* Institute of Gerontology, Ann Arbor, 1976.

CELEBREZZE, AJ: *The Older American.* US Government Printing Office, Washington, DC, 1963, p. 14.

CHULIS, GS: *Medicare: Use of Skilled Nursing Facility Services.* US Department of Health, Education and Welfare, Washington, DC, 1976.

DENKOVICH, LE: *Government's Nursing Home Rules—Better Care or More Bureaucracy?* Medical Economics 12:11, 1980.

DONABEDIAN, A: *Benefits in Medical Care Programs.* Harvard University Press, Cambridge, MA, 1976.

EBERSOLE, P AND HESS, P: *Toward Healthy Aging, Human Needs and Nursing Response.* CV Mosby, St Louis, 1981.

FELDSTEIN, P: *Regulating Health Care: The Struggle for Control.* Academy of Political Science, New York, 1980.

HYMAN, J: *Empirical Research on the Demand for Medical Care.* Inquiry 8(1):71, 1971.

IGLEHART, JK: *The Cost of Keeping the Elderly Well.* National Journal 10:10, 1978.

KLARMAN, HE: *The Economics of Health.* Columbia University Press, New York, 1965.

MANCINI, M: *Medicare: Health Rights of the Elderly.* American Journal of Nursing, No. 10, 1979.

Medicare Provider Manual. US Department of Health Education and Welfare, Washington, DC, 1978.

MUSHKIN, S. (ED): *Consumer Incentives for Health Care.* Prodist, New York, 1974.

NEWHOUSE, J AND PHELPS, CE: *Price and Income Statistics for Medical Care Services. The Economics of Health and Medical Care.* Macmillan, London, 1974.

SILVERS, JB AND PRAHALAD, CK: *Financial Management of Health Institutions.* Spectrum, New York, 1974.

SILVERSTONE, B AND HYMAN, H: *You and Your Aging Parent.* Pantheon Books, New York, 1976.

SMITH, DB: *Long-Term Care in Transition: The Regulation of Nursing Homes.* AUPHA Press, Washington, DC, 1981.

TOPICAL LAW REPORTS: *Medicare and Medicaid Guide*, Vol 1–4. Commerce Clearing House, Chicago, 1982.

TRAGER, B: *Home Health Care and National Health Policy.* Haworth Press, New York, 1980.

US GOVERNMENT PRINTING OFFICE: *The Federal-State Effort in Long-Term Care for Older Americans. Nursing Homes and "Alternatives."* Washington, DC, 1979.

WALTHER, R: *Economics in the Older Population.* In WOODRUFF, D AND BIRREN, J (EDS): *Aging.* D. Van Nostrand Company, New York, 1975.

CHAPTER 18

IMPLICATIONS FOR THE INDIVIDUAL AND THE COMMUNITY

CAROLYN E. CRUMP, M.A.
CAROLE BERNSTEIN LEWIS,
R.P.T., M.S.G., M.P.A., Ph.D.

BEHAVIORAL OBJECTIVES

Upon completion of this chapter, the reader will be able to
1. Outline the impact the medical care system can have on an elderly individual's health status.
2. List the major federal and state programs that provide funding for long-term health care services to the elderly.
3. Describe the demographic trends that will affect the health care delivery system.
4. Highlight the current problems and issues that must be addressed in order to improve the current medical health care system.
5. Define and describe the array of services that are considered long-term health care.
6. Present several examples of programs working to coordinate long-term health care services for the elderly.

HEALTH PLANNING: THE FUTURE FOR THE ELDERLY

The World Health Organization (WHO) defines health as "a state of complete physical, mental and social well-being, not merely the absence of disease or infirmity."[1] To provide health care for the elderly patient that is consistent with the

WHO's definition, geriatric practitioners working in the area of rehabilitation must investigate the concept of preventative medicine, which may lead to optimal health.

An illustration of the concept of preventative medicine is Rogers' Health Status Scale[2] (Fig. 18-1). Optimal Health, the first category, is the state of health described in the WHO definition. This category of health status does not contain degrees of illness or disability. Instead, it is viewed as a state of complete physical and social well-being. This category of health status is seldom maintained for a prolonged period of time by an elderly individual.

The second category, Suboptimal Health, describes the health status of the general public. A person in the Suboptimal Health category may appear healthy, but this person may have a nutritional, psychologic, or physiologic problem that is unrealized. An example of someone in this area would be a middle-aged woman who has developed the early stages of diabetes mellitus but has not yet experienced any symptoms.

Overt Illness or Disability, Approaching Death, and Death are the third, fourth, and fifth categories of health status. These last three health status categories are the main tenents of the traditional medical model. The majority of today's physicians practice under this medical model which has as its goal the cure of disease and the treatment of disabilities.

The Health Status Scale is a useful tool for identifying the elderly individual's need for rehabilitation. Figure 18-1 illustrates how sharply health deteriorates as one passes through the health status categories. When the health of the elderly individual begins to deteriorate, it may decrease at an alarming rate. It is the rehabilitation professional's job to assist the older person in maintaining or

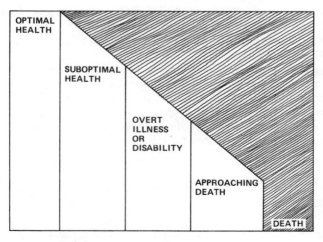

Figure 18-1. Illustrated here is the Health Status Scale. (Adapted from Rogers, ES: *Human Ecology and Health.* Macmillan, New York, 1960.)

achieving optimum health through preventative medicine or rehabilitation. But the way the current medical system is designed, little preventative information is available to the elderly.

At present most of the elderly perceive themselves as belonging to the Optimal Health category, when in reality they may be suffering from poor vision, osteoporosis, an inadequate social support system, an unsafe home enrivonment, muscle tightness and weakness, arteriosclerosis, or poor nutrition. Unfortunately these conditions that place an individual in the Suboptimum Health category are not recognized or diagnosed until the person has sustained a serious injury. For example, an elderly woman who was perceived to be healthy was diagnosed as having osteoporosis, glaucoma, and high blood pressure only after a severe fall in which she sustained a hip fracture. According to the health scale in Figure 18-1, she would be in the Overt Illness category only after her hip fracture. Unless her total health status is assessed before she returns home with a walker, she will have a limited recovery. If the elderly woman is not rehabilitated, her health will begin to deteriorate.

It is the goal of preventative rehabilitation to understand and to integrate the Roger's Health Scale to provide optimum health care to the elderly population. The two processes of prevention are understanding and anticipating complications that will arise and taking the appropriate steps to deter their occurrence.[3] Geriatric rehabilitation professionals need to develop assessment tools that will identify the elderly who are at risk in the community before they reach the illness category. Assessment tools must also be used as an individual prepares to return home after a hospital stay. For example, the elderly woman described above could have received a screening questionnaire before she was sent home from the hospital. Her support systems and safety factors would have been assessed by this questionnaire. Developing individual assessment tools for community, home, hospital, and long-term care needs is a challenging task, but it will provide the information rehabilitation professionals need concerning their elderly patients. A few tools for this area have already been developed, such as the Pulses Profile, the Lawton Activities of Daily Living Profile, and the Barthel Index.[4-6] However, the individualized assessment devices need to be more specific and meaningful.

The rehabilitation professional must possess the following in order to prevent an elderly individual's health from deteriorating: (1) the ability to assess the situation accurately; (2) the knowledge to choose the appropriate intervention; (3) the skills to execute treatment and to evaluate its use, and (4) the time, space, and appropriate environment to accomplish the assessment and to provide the proper guidance and care.

The knowledge and skill to choose and to execute appropriate interventions can be acquired only through study and experience. Reading texts, taking courses, and sharing and practicing techniques of geriatric rehabilitation will improve a professional's knowledge base and skills. Finally, the critical issue of time, space, and environment can be influenced only by examining and redesigning our health care system.

THE HEALTH CARE SYSTEM

It is important for professional health care individuals to have some understanding of the legislative issues and financial implications surrounding the health care delivery system. To some extent Congress, through health care legislation, influences whether the medical profession is able to reach its goal of maintaining a large population of healthy, functioning people. The following sections of this chapter review the background of financial implications of health care costs, the needs of older adults, problems of the current system, the cost and importance of long-term health care, and examples of working programs.

The older adult group needs the services of the health care systems more often than any other age group. But is the older adult in better condition both physically and emotionally after receiving outside assistance? How effective is our health care system? Does the system facilitate the goals of the professionals in health-related fields, such as rehabilitation specialists, physicians, and nurses? What programs are available to the older individual in terms of medical care, advice, and psychologic and social support?

Background

During the early 1900s the professionals concerned with public health and medical care emphasized environmental sanitation and the control of infectious and communicable diseases.[7] The need for more comprehensive public welfare programs came about as a result of the Great Depression. The public's demand for assistance was reflected in the policy outcomes during the next half century (that is, from to 1930 to 1980).

The passage of the Social Security Act of 1935 mandated the federal government to assume the responsibility for providing social services to the needy, the aged, the blind, single women with children, and the disabled. However, the initial Social Security Act did not provide medical services. During the 1930s and 1940s the patient's ability to pay for needed health care was enhanced by private health insurance plans sponsored by hospital and physician groups, such as Blue Cross (that is, hospital) and Blue Shield (that is, physician).[8] These health insurance programs provided security and protection from high health care costs to all individuals. Since World War II, employers have been encouraged, through favorable tax laws, to provide their workers with private health insurance. Up until this time health benefits were not part of a worker's taxable income.

Today, many different federal and state programs provide long-term health care services. The principal federal programs that provide these services are Medicaid, Medicare, Title III of the Older Americans Act, and the Social Services Block Grant (that is, Title XX of the Social Security Act).[9] The Medicare and Medicaid programs were enacted in 1965 owing to the great concern for the large number of elderly and needy who did not receive public assistance specifically for medical costs.[10] Medicare was established to provide health insurance to the aged and disabled, and Medicaid provides medical services to low-income individuals of all ages.

The Older Americans Act (OAA), also enacted in 1965, carries a broad mandate (ten specific objectives) to improve the quality of the lives of older persons in terms of income and psychologic, physical, and social well-being. Title III of this act outlines the need for a coordinated aging service system that provides funding enabling older adults to live in their own homes as independently as possible. However, the development of this system is the responsibility of the state government. Although this act was passed in 1965, the development and effectiveness of social services for the elderly has been limited because of the lack of federal funding and variations in initiation from state to state.

Title XX of the Social Security Act, passed in 1975, provides funding to the states to establish a number of home-based and community services to low-income individuals and families. This program can assist families and individuals in maintaining a self-sufficient lifestyle. However, the benefits are not provided nationwide because allocation of Title XX funds for services vary by state and community. The services that could be made available to communities by the state include the following: homemaker services (general household activities), chore services (home maintenance activities), home management (formal or informal instruction, consumer education), and home health aide services (medical care activities provided by nursing aides).

There are many other federal programs that assist persons with long-term health care problems by providing housing, income, nutrition, and transportation needs (for example, HUD Housing Construction and Assistance Programs, Supplemental Security Income, and Veterans Administration programs). Although each of these programs provides some community-based long-term health care services, there is little coordination between these programs.

The Needs of Older Adults

Today the elderly make up 11 percent of the population. However, as a group they are responsible for 29 percent of the nation's total health care costs, and their numbers are continuing to increase.[10] The actual number and percentage of those over 65 increased greatly between 1950 and 1980. In 1950, 8.1 percent of the population was over 65, and in 1980, 10.8 percent, or 24 million persons, was 65 or over.[10] This trend will continue well into the next century, owing to individuals' longer life expectancy. In 1950, 2.6 percent was over 75, and by 1980, 4.2 percent of the population was 75 and older.[11] By the year 2000, it is estimated that 5.3 percent of the population will be 75 years of age or older.[11] These demographic trends have implications for the health care delivery system.[12] The increased number of older adults will cause an increase in the number of those less capable or incapable of caring for themselves.[13]

There will be a higher percentage of individuals who need care, but the numbers of those who provide health care and other services will be decreasing. For example, the reduction in the size of the nuclear family (that is, brothers and sisters) and the increase in two-income families limit the number of older adults who can be cared for at home. Those over 65 demand a higher percentage of the health care resources and, thus, account for a greater percentage of the national health care bill. Therefore the health care system must plan for the increased demand from the older adult, realizing that the most frequent health problems among the aged are multiple, chronic, and often degenerative. These problems have a direct effect on the ability of the older individual to remain independent, and this lack of independence may cause them to be institutionalized. The older adults' subsequent loss of autonomy from institutionalization usually has a negative effect on their self-esteem and in turn the quality of their lives. Thus the elderly have a need for community-based long-term health care services that will enhance the quality of their lives.

Long-term care (LTC) "refers to services needed by persons who have functional limitations."[8] The Department of Health and Human Services defines LTC as a wide array of services provided to individuals over a prolonged period of time because of acute illness, exacerbation of chronic illness, or disability.[14] Historically, LTC was defined in institutional terms. However, over the last 10 years the emphasis has shifted from the services provided in an institution to those provided in the community and home as well.[15] Brody and Masciocchi suggest a model for long-term support systems that defines LTC services on a scale from most restrictive to least restrictive[15] (Fig. 18-2). These services for an LTC support system may include health care, housing assistance, transportation services, social services, legal services, income security, and employment counseling or training.

The elderly are particularly concerned about the financing of long-term care. Most of the funds for LTC are spent on income support and acute health care needs (hospitals and physicians) rather than on community-based health services programs[8] (Table 18-1). It is important that federal and state programs provide different options for health intervention, because the elderly are a heterogeneous group. What the elderly individual requires may not always be a *cure* but rather *care* for a long-term chronic condition. Assessing the type of care required must involve the individual's total environment (that is, social, psychologic, economic, and physical factors). This requires a combination of services because of the complexity and diversity of an individual's environmental needs.

Problems of the Current System

One of the major problems in the current system providing LTC is that it categorizes people into separate eligibility groups by age (for example, the lower limit may be 60, 62, or 65), disability, or income classification. There is little coordination between these entitlement categories. No single program funds a compre-

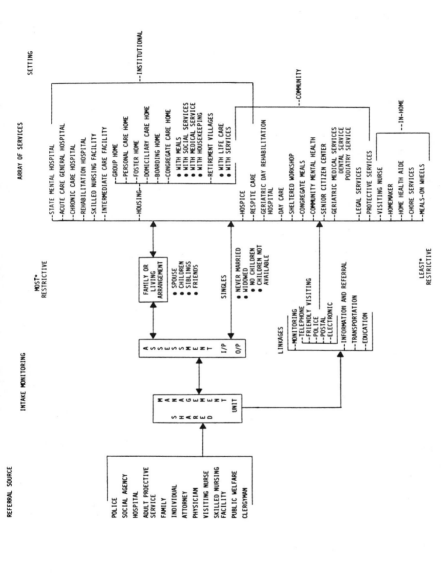

Figure 18-2. Diagrammed here is an inventory of recommended available services appropriate to a long-term care/support system. (From Brody and Masciocchi,[15] with permission.)

TABLE 18-1. Expenditures for selected federal programs fiscal year 1978 (in millions of dollars)

	MEDICARE*	MEDICAID*	OLD AGE SURVIVORS†	DISABILITY INSURANCE†	SUPPLE-MENTAL SECURITY INCOME†	SOCIAL SERVICES BLOCK GRANT‡	OLDER AMERICANS ACT§	VETERANS ADMINIS-TRATION*
Income maintenance			$53,255	$10,315	$6,552			
Basic living services								
Transportation						$ 71	$ 19	
Housing						$ 28	$ 3	
Meals						$ 22	$247	
Chore services (Homemaker/health aide)						$481	$ 17	
Dependency services								
Day care						$ 34	$ 2	
Home health	$ 548	$ 160				$ 98		
Illness/disability services								
Nursing home care	$ 396	$ 7,246						
Physician services	$ 5,548	$ 2,054						
Hospital services	$18,275	$ 6,854						
Total	$24,767	$16,314	$53,255	$10,315	$6,552	$734	$288	

*Gibson, R: National Health Expenditures, 1978, Health Care Financing Review, Summer, 1979, (1–36).

†Social Security Administration, the Social Security Bulletin, Annual Statistical Supplement, 1977–79. Figures shown are for calendar year 1978. Dollar payments for the Old Age Survivors and Disability Insurance programs shown are for retired and disabled workers only. Figures for dependents and survivors have not been included.

‡Planned expenditures rather than actual spending, obtained from State Title XX plans. Technical Notes, Summaries and Characteristics of States' Title XX Social Services Plans for Fiscal Year 1979, Gloria Kilgore and Gabriel Solman, Washington: DHEW/ASPE, June 15, 1979.

§AOA program statistics.

From the 1981 White House Conference on Aging, 1981, p 85, with permission.

hensive array of both institutional (that is, skilled nursing facility, nursing home) and noninstitutional (that is, home care) long-term care services. State plans under OAA and those under Title XX need some administrative coordination. Certain programs provide health care but offer no assistance in social services; others provide acute health care for the elderly but offer little assistance for a chronic condition.

The following example illustrates the fragmentation of the present noninstitutionalized LTC programs. The elderly woman who entered the medical health care system with a broken hip, mentioned earlier, needed to receive LTC and social services addressing all her problems. However, she received only medical treatment for her hip. If she had tried to contact the appropriate social services, she would have had to make numerous telephone calls and followups. Her chronic conditions required a team of health professionals to treat more than just her fractured hip. Ideally she would have received assistance from a nutritionist, physical therapist, occupational therapist, social worker, internist, ophthamologist, and homemaker. However, in the current system these services are difficult to locate, to identify, and to coordinate. Owing to the fragmentation of these programs, it is difficult for older adults to piece together a comprehensive plan that will help them remain independent.

Another problem with the current system centers around the rules of the Medicare and Medicaid programs. These programs create financial incentives to use nursing homes rather than noninstitutional, prevention-oriented, community-bases services (part-time skilled nursing care, social services, adult day care, counseling, financial advice, transportation assistance, nutritional information, and general health education[10]). Medicare is actually a program that assists those in need of short-term acute care, and it does not cover many preventive health expenses. Therefore, less than 1 percent of Medicare funds are used for home health care.[10]

Despite the wide array of home care services, there is a bias toward the institutionalization of the individual. First, the amount of funding the federal government provides to a community-based alternative is limited by the high costs incurred by the government's bill for institutional care[9] (see Table 18-1). In other words, the federal government spends so much on hospitalization, nursing home care, and physicians' services that little is left for preventive community-based health services.

Second, the lack of adequate funding for the noninstitutional community-based long-term care services limits the number of individuals who can be cared for outside an institution. The traditional medical system is designed to provide acute health care for the sick in institutions rather than on an outpatient or home-care basis and therefore cannot be used to handle the increasing demand for LTC. The short-term medical model simply cannot be used or slightly modified to function as a viable long-term care system.[15] Third, there is a lack of support provided to families or other primary caregivers that would allow a greater number of elderly individuals to remain in their homes. Much of the care to an estimated 5 percent to 10 percent of older individuals living in the community is provided by relatives.[16] There is a need to provide additional support services such as respite care, adult day care to the individual who is the primary caregiver. Providing assistance to the private sector for the care of dependent individuals will aid in meeting the diverse needs of the elderly more equitably.[14]

Because the present health care system is not adequately meeting the needs of the senior adult population, revisions in the current health care services should be addressed. Policy makers such as Senator Packwood (R-OR) outlined the following changes needed in the health care system: (1) limiting the placement in nursing homes of elderly and disabled who could be cared for in their homes; (2) recognition of both the special needs of the family and the service needs of the individual; (3) more comprehensive coordination among the service programs; (4) mandate that people assume a certain amount of personal responsibility for the cost of health and social services, reducing the fiscal responsibility of the federal and state governments; and (5) financing options that would aid and encourage families or individuals to care for older people in their homes.[17] These suggestions should be researched so that administrative details of an optimal long-term health care system can be implemented.

The Cost and Importance of Long-Term Health Care

Cost and financing are the two principal factors that have stagnated the growth and development of a community-based noninstitutional long-term care system.[17] There are several options for organizing and financing health care, but it is unknown how each system might affect both the demand and the total cost of care.[16] For example, there is uncertainty about the potential decrease in the public cost of expanded community-based care. It is possible that increased community-based services will not result in lower health care costs because the homebound elderly will be added to those receiving care. Current statistics indicate that health care costs may increase because 14 percent of the noninstitutionalized elderly have a functional disability. With an increase in community-based services, there will be a large number of these elderly persons seeking these services.[14]

Several studies attempt to compare the costs of community-based or in-home services with the costs of institutional care in order to show that significant cost savings will occur from lowered admissions and earlier discharges.[18] Yet, definite conclusions are difficult because any study of cost effectiveness of home or community-based versus institutional care must consider both public (federal and state programs) and private costs (family and friends' support). It is hard to determine total public costs because of the many federal programs that provide services considered long term. It is even more difficult to gauge costs or values of home services provided privately by family or friends.[19] However, the older individuals gain an improved quality in their lives from community-based services.

What is needed to improve the health and quality of life of the elderly? What is the best way to contain health care costs?[20] It is difficult to answer these two questions because many factors influence the health care delivery system for the elderly. For example, the aged require more acute health care and LTC; the aged are less capable economically, physically, and socially to obtain health care without assistance; and the health care professionals are generally less motivated (financially and professionally) to care for the elderly and also have less training in geriatrics.

What is needed, according to Brehm, is a coordinated and comprehensive system that includes maintaining the optimum health of older adults as well as caring for disease and injuries.[21] In order to accomplish this goal, the medical health care delivery system must be reorganized to develop a system that works to prevent as well as to care for illness. Adequate funding and more programs providing community-based long-term health services are thus required in addition to the Medicare and Medicaid programs. Resources need to be directed toward keeping people healthy.

Garfield stresses the importance of providing an economic incentive for keeping people healthy.[22] The present medical system model, fee for services (paying for services rendered), does not provide an economic incentive for physicians to prevent illness in clients. The fee-for-service model merely serves to regulate the use of the health care system by limiting the number who seek care. An alternative to the fee-for-service model is a prepaid medical care system (that is, paying a predetermined yearly amount) in which the providers (for example, physicians) share in the cost for health care and are therefore motivated to help control costs.[21] An example of this is the Kaiser Permanente System, which uses a combination of prepayment and "whole system management" to minimize health care costs.[22] This type of system facilitates early treatment of symptoms and thus prevents serious illness. This system ultimately reduces health care costs.

Providing noninstitutionalized LTC to the elderly living in the community may increase the nation's total health care bill. Yet community-based LTC appears to have a positive effect on the social, emotional, and mental well-being of the elderly. Examples of several programs providing LTC services will be described in the next section.

Working Programs

The goals of health-care related social services are to help the elderly who are capable of self-care to maintain their independence in a home environment and to provide health care for the elderly who are frail. The Department of Health and Human Services funds various projects related to health care for the elderly. These projects include studies of costs related to health care and of the needs of the elderly in the social services area. These studies are conducted by establishing demonstration projects in which actual programs for the elderly are implemented and evaluated. Part of the funding for the demonstration projects (training, research, social services programs) is provided by the Older Americans Act under Title III.

The demonstration projects either modify an existing program by providing additional services or create a new organization that coordinates and directs the health care resources already available in a community. For example, grants are awarded for programs concerning (1) transportation needs; (2) information and referral for LTC services (that is, channeling); (3) in-home services such as home-maker, home/health aid, and chore maintennance; (4) educational programs; (5) counseling services; and (6) day care centers for the elderly. Services must be provided without regard to income, although the programs may concentrate on those with the greatest social or economic need. The commonalities that exist among the many different demonstration projects providing health-related social services include a multidisciplinary assessment of need, case management, and followup of the client's placement. Including these steps in many of the service programs helps prevent unnecessary institutionalization, thereby helping preserve an individual's personal identity and autonomy.

Examples of programs that might be followed to integrate health and social services at the community level include the Monroe County Long-Term Care Program called ACCESS (Assessment for Community Care Services) in New York State, the Central Connecticut Planning Region (Triage Project), and the Guale Homemaker-Home Health Aide Project in Chatham County, Georgia.[10,18]

The ACCESS program is an information and referral project that helps control nursing home admissions. A team of health care professionals (that is, internist, nurse, medical social worker) evaluates the needs of the individual, outlines alternatives, recommends services, and provides appropriate placement through case management procedures.[10,23] For example, through ACCESS an individual is evaluated during a hospital stay to determine if he or she should be sent home, to a nursing home, or to a skilled-nursing facility. The recommendations by the team of health professionals helps limit the inappropriate placement of individuals into long-term care institutions. The evaluation and placement unit also provides information and referral for services to the older adult which allows the individual to return home with optimum knowledge of the services available in the community.

The Triage Project is a research and demonstration project to determine the effectiveness and cost of using a single-entry model to coordinate the complete LTC needs of individuals. The services provided by the community based on an individual's specific needs were integrated with the person's support system.[24] This program, started in 1974, has helped make providers more accountable for the services they deliver because the assessment and coordination effort is separate from the service delivery. For example, a professional team (that is, nurse, clinician, social service coordinator) assesses the needs of an individual who contacts the Triage Program. The team will then coordinate and oversee the individual's use of agency and community resources to meet the individual's LTC needs.

The Guale Homemaker-Home Health Aide Project was established to eliminate duplication of two agencies providing in-home services to adults in Chatham County, Georgia.[25] The project uses nurses, social workers, homemaker supervisors, and family members to assist the patient in evaluating and coordinating a full range of services available in the community.

The programs mentioned above are examples of how health care services for older people can be improved. Their focus is on community support, home-based care, and service integration. More projects such as these need to be developed to fill the gap in the current health care system.[23]

Challenge to Rehabilitation Professionals

Optimal health is not easy to achieve for any age group. Knowledge, skill, and the appropriate environment are critical ingredients in achieving the highest categories of health (see Figure 18-1). To serve the elderly in the community, the rehabilitation professionals will have to upgrade their clinical knowledge and skill in the area of geriatrics. Additionally they must become aware of the needs of the elderly and the community programs that provide appropriate LTC services to the elderly. Because of their expertise in providing geriatric care, these rehabilitation specialists should be involved in health legislation and the development of health care systems. Rehabilitation professionals should begin to work together to influence health care legislation. They must contribute expertise to all levels of health planning (that is, community, state, and federal), which will ultimately influence the medical care environment.

The aging of America is truly a challenge to rehabilitation professionals because of the increasing need to provide more services to the older adult. Working with the elderly person should provide a challenge to rehabilitation professionals, encouraging them to explore and to expand their knowledge base. This knowledge must then be used to provide assistance and input to federal, state, and community LTC programs that serve the elderly.

REFERENCES

1. WORLD HEALTH ORGANIZATION: *Constitution of the World Health Organization.* Geneva World Health Organization, 1964.

2. ROGERS, ES: *Human Ecology and Health Introduction for Administrators.* Macmillan, New York, 1960.

3. LAWTON, EB: *Activities of Daily Living: Testing, Training and Equipment.* New York Institute of Physical Medicine and Rehabilitation, New York University Bellevue Medical Center, Monograph No 10, 1956.

4. BROWN, ME: *Daily activity inventory and progress record for those with atypical movement.* Am J Occup Ther 4:195, 1950.

5. DENMERSTEIN, AS, LOWENTHAL, M, DEXTER, M: *Evaluation of a rating scale of ability in activities of daily living.* Arch Phys Med Rehabil 46:579, 1965.

6. HOFF, WI AND MEAD, S: *Evaluation of rehabilitation outcome. An objective assessment of the physically disabled.* Am J Phys Med 44:579, 1965.

7. BEATTIE, WM: *Aging and the social services.* In BINSTOCK, RH AND SHANAS, E (EDS): *Handbook of Aging and the Social Services.* Reinhold Publishing, New York, 1976.

8. *Final Report: The 1981 White House Conference on Aging.* US Department of Health and Human Services, Washington, DC, 1981.

9. O'SHAUGHNESSY, C AND REISS, K: *Long Term Care: Community-Based Alternatives to Institutionalization.* Congressional Research Service, Washington, DC, 1981.

10. PEGELS, CC: *Health Care and the Elderly.* Aspen, Rockville, MD, 1980.

11. RUSSELL, LB: *An aging population and the use of medical care.* Med Care 19:633, 1981.

12. SIEGEL, J: *Recent and prospective demographic trends for the elderly population and some implications for health care.* In *Epidemiology of Aging.* US Department of Health and Human Services, Washington, DC, 1980.

13. MEYER, L: *Aging well: A secret scientists are now trying to crack.* The Washington Post, November 4, 1982.

14. *Working Paper on Long-Term Care.* US Department of Health and Human Services, Washington, DC, 1981.

15. BRODY, SJ AND MASCIOCCHI, C: *Data for long-term care planning by health systems agencies.* Am J Public Health 70:1194, 1980.

16. SHANAS, E AND MADDOX, G: *Aging, health, and the organization of health resources.* In BINSTOCK, RH AND SHANAS, E (EDS): *Handbook of Aging and the Social Services.* Reinhold Publishing, New York, 1976.

17. PACKWOOD, R: *Long-term care: Public and private sector policy options.* Journal of the Institute for Socioeconomic Studies 3:13, 1981.

18. *Home Care Services.* US Department of Health and Human Services, Washington, DC, 1981.

19. OUR FUTURE SELVES: A RESEARCH PLAN TOWARD UNDERSTANDING AGING. US Department of Health and Human Services, publication no 78:1443, Washington, DC, 1978.

20. *The 1981 Federal and State Legislative Policy.* National Retired Teachers Association/American Association of Retired Persons. Washington, DC, 1981.

21. BREHM, HP: *Organization and financing of health care for the aged: Future implications.* In *Epidemiology of Aging.* US Department of Health and Human Services, Washington, DC, 1980.

22. GARFIELD, SR: *The delivery of medical care.* Sci Am 222:15, 1970.

23. KERR, JO AND WHITNEY, SE: *Community Intervention for the Elderly.* Institute on Aging, Portland State University, 1981.

24. HODGSON, JH AND QUINN, JL: *Impact of the triage health care delivery system upon client morale, independent living and the cost of care.* Gerontologist, 20:364, 1980.

25. LEE, JT AND STEIN, MA: *Eliminating duplication in home health care for the elderly: The Guale project.* Health and Social Work 5:29, 1980.

BIBLIOGRAPHY

FURUKAWA, C AND SHOMAKER, D: *Community Health Services for the Aged.* Aspen, Rockville, MD, 1982.

HUNT, TE: *Practical considerations in the rehabilitation of the aged.* J Am Geriatr Soc.

MEYER, L: *HMO alive and thriving after scrape with death.* The Washington Post, December 27, 1982.

PACKWOOD, B: *Long-term care: Costs, financing, and alternative services, public and private sector policy options.* National Journal, June 6, 1981.

US Congressional Record, 97th Congress, 1st Session, 127654, April 2, 1981.

WELLS, T: *Aging and Health Promotion.* Aspen, Rockville, MD, 1982.

INDEX

An *italic* page number indicates a figure.
A "t" indicates a table.

Acute brain syndrome—*continued*
recognition of, 28
treatment of, 28–29
Adapin, 285
Adrenalin, in stress response, *247*, 248
Adrenergic blocking agents
alpha, 276
beta, 275, 281
Adrenocorticotropic hormone, in stress
response, *247*, 248
Aerosol drugs, 270
bronchodilator, 278
Affect, inpaired, in organic brain
syndrome, 28
Age pigments, 15
Aging
activity theory of, 21
adaptation to, coping mechanisms for,
252–256
cellular, autoimmune theory of, 15–16
Carrel and Ebeling experiment in, 9
cross-linkage theory of, 13–15, *14*
error theory of, 12
free radical theory of, 15
genetic theories of, 9–13
historical perspective on, 9–10
Hayflick and Moorehead experiment
in, 9–10, *10*
Hayflick limit theory of, 9–11, *10*, *11*
hormonal theories of, 16–17
in vivo vs. in vitro theories of, 16–17
nongenetic theories of, 13–17
programming of, 13
redundant DNA theory of, 12
transcription theory of, 12–13
continuity theory of, recreational
activity planning and, 90
defined, 312
deprivations in, 23
as developmental process, 8
disengagement theory of, 21
as ego development stage, 20–21
ego integration in, 20–21
loss of status in, 23
losses in, 23
most common disorders of, 273–274
negative view of, 22–23
normal vs. pathological effects of, 8
physiologic aspects of, research on, 313
psychologic aspects of, research on, 313
psychosocial aspects of, 19–31
research, 311–319
on biologic aspects of, 312
birth cohorts for, 314
cohort sequential method for, 315

cross-sectional studies in, 315
demographics in, 314
establishing norms in, 313
importance of, 312
longitudinal studies in, 314–315
measurement in, 316–318
of independence, 317
of physical functioning, 318
methodology of, 314–315
national survey data for, 318
on psychologic aspects, 313
on quality of life, 313–314
reliability of, 315–316
sampling in, 316
on social aspects, 313
time sequential analysis in, 315
topic areas of, 312–311
validity of, 315–316
social, research on, 313
stress and, 246–266. *See also* Stress
stress management in, 23–24
subculture theory of, 21–22
task theory of, 22
technological advances and, 8
theories of, 7–18
diversity of, 8
genetic, 8
nongenetic, 8
Agranulocytosis, procainamide and, 274
Akathisia, neuroleptics and, 282
Alcohol
sedatives and, 288
sexual effects of, 306t
tranquilizers and, 288
Aldactazide, 275
Aldactone, 275–276
Aldomet, 276
Allergy, drugs for, 278–279
Alveolar ventilation, in exercise, 186
Alzheimer's disease, 28
Mini-Mental State Exam for, 29, *30*
recognition of, 28
treatment of, 28–29
Amantidine, 285
The American Occupational Therapy
Association, lobbying by, 337–
339
The American Physical Therapy
Association, lobbying by, 337
The American Speech-Language-
Hearing Association, lobbying
by, 337–339
Amitriptyline, 285
warfarin and, 289
Amoxapin, 285

Articulation, 62
  disturbed, in dysarthria, 71
Ascendin, 285
Aspirin
  for arthritis, 279–280
  for colds and flu, 279
  side-effects of, 279
Asthma, drugs for, 278
Astigmatism, 104
Atarax, 218
Atherosclerosis, 168
Ativan, 281, 282
Atrial pressure, systolic, 170
Atrioventricular node, age-related
      changes in, 167
Aural rehabilitation, 66–67
Auscultation, 193–196, *195*
  in lung cancer, 219
Autogenic training, 259–260, 263
Autoimmune theory of cellular aging,
      15–16
Avocational Activities Inventory, 89

BALANCE, hypokinesis and, 145
Balke stress test, 201t
Ball squeezing, after radical mastectomy,
      228
Bandages, for ostoearthritis, 136
Barbiturates
  for anxiety, 281
  for insomnia, 281–282
  side effects of, 282
Barrel chest, 191, *194*
Barthel Index, 318
Barthel Self-Care Rating, 318
Basal cell carcinoma, 237
Bath seat, *53*
Bathing, 160
Bathroom safety, 52–54, *53*, 160
Beclome thasone, for asthma, 278
Beclovent Inhaler, 278
Bed bathing, 160
Benadryl, 279, 286
Benzodiazepines
  for anxiety, 281
  for insomnia, 282
  side effects of, 282
Benzotropine, 286
Bethanidine, sexual effects of, 306t
Bicycle stress test, 201t
BIH protocol stress test, 201t
Biofeedback, 260–261, 263–264
Birth cohorts, 314
Birth rate, 314

Blindness
  diabetic retinopathy and, 107
  glaucoma and, 105
  legal, 107
  night, 106–107
Blocadren, 276
Blom-Singer artificial larynx, 77
Blood pressure
  in exercise, 172, 174
Blood vessels
  fibrotic changes in, 167–168
  morphologic changes in, 167–168
Blue Cross, 332, 348
Blue Shield, 332, 348
Blurred vision, drug–induced, 279, 282,
      283, 285, 288
Bone density, 118
Bone lesions, in multiple myeloma, 236
Bone metastasis
  in breast cancer, 229–230, 229t
  in prostate cancer, 235
Bowling, activity analysis for, 93–94
Bradykinesis, in Parkinsonism, 285
Brain. *See also* Nervous system
  decreased blood flow in, 144
  decreased nitrogen in, 143
  decreased sulfur in, 143
  oxygen consumption by, 144, *145*
Breast cancer
  early signs of, 226
  epidemiology of, 226
  lumpectomy for, 227
  mastectomy for, 227–228
    radical, 227
      complications of, 228–229
    simple, 227
  metastasis in, 229–230, 229t
  survival in, 226–227
  treatment of, 226–227
Breath control, as relaxation technique,
      261, 264
Breath sounds
  adventitious, 193, 196
  auscultation of, 193–196, *195*
  bronchial, *195*
  bronchovesicular, *195*
  in lung cancer, 219
  tracheal, *195*
  vesicular, 193, *195*
Breathing exercises, 196–197
  for relaxation, 261, 264
Broca's aphasia, 69
Bromocriptine, 285, 286
Brompheniramine, 279

Feet, swelling of, in pulmonary disease, 188, *191*
Fellatio, *301*
Fenoprofen, 280
Fertility, aging research and, 314
Firbrosarcoma, 233
Fight-or-flight response, 246
Finger clubbing, 188, *191*
Fitness, defined, 146
Flexibility, loss of, 199–122
    arthritis and, 121–122
    collagen deterioration and, 119–120
    hypokinesis and, 120–121
    prevention of, 14
    range of motion test for, 120
Flexor muscles, tightness of, with hypokinesis, 120
Flu, drugs for, 279
Fluphenazine, 283–284
Flurazepam, for insomnia, 282
Food(s)
    for dysphagia, 153–154
    mucus-producing, 153
Forced expiratory flow, 199t
Forced expiratory volume, 199t
Fork, large-handle, *52*
Fracture(s)
    complications of, 135
    of hip, 135–136
    pathologic, in breast cancer metastatic to bone, 230
        in multiple myeloma, 236
    stress, 136
Free radical theory of cellular aging, 15
Frozen pops, for tongue-palate stimulation, 152
Frozen shoulder, rehabilitation of, 119–120
Functional residual capacity, 184, *185*, 199t

Gag reflex, evaluation of, 150, *150*
Gait
    changes in
        age-related, 129–134
        in amputee, 132–134
        biologic, 130–132
        functional, 132
        neurologic, 145–146
        pathologic, 132–134
    defined, 129
    normal, *131*

in Parkinsonism, 147
    improvement of, 147–148
Gas(es), pulmonary, 184
    in exercise, 186
Gastric ulcers, 277
Gastrointestinal disorders, drugs for, 277
General adaptation syndrome, 246
Generic drugs, 271
Giving-up syndrome, 250
Glaucoma, 105
Global aphasia, 70
Glucocorticoids, 287
Glutathione peroxidase, as age retardant, 15
Glycolysis, neuronal, 144
Glycoproteins, 122
Gold compounds, 280
Gout, colchicine for, 280
Grab bar, for bathtub, 53
Growth hormone, in stress response, *247*, 248
Guale Homemaker-Home Health Aide Project, 356–357
Guanethidine, sexual effects of, 306t
Guided imagery, 259–260, 263

Haldol, 283–284
    sexual effects of, 306t
Haloperidol, 283–284
    sexual effects of, 306t
Hayflick limit theory, 9–11, *10*, *11*
Hayflick-Moorehead experiment in cellular aging, 9–10, *10*
Head, forward, neck flats exercise for, 126–127, *127*
Head and neck cancer
    age and, 222
    of larynx and hypopharynx, 223t, 224
    of nasopharynx, 223t, 224
    neck dissection in, 225
    of oropharynx, 223t, 224
    of paranasal sinuses, 223–224, 223t
    postoperative complications of, 222–223
    postoperative therapy in, 222–223
    postural exercises in, 225
    psychologic counseling in, 226
    types of, 222, 223t
Health
    definition of, 345
    independence in activities of daily living and, 34–35
    optimal, 346
    self-perception of, 347
    suboptimal, 346

AGING: THE HEALTH CARE CHALLENGE

Lipofuscin, 15
  accumulation of, in heart, 167
    in neurons, 143
Liposarcoma, 233
Lipreading, 66
Liquids, thickening of, in dysphasia, 154
Listening, techniques, for expressive lan-
    guage deficiencies, 64
Lithium, sexual effects of, 306t
Lobbying, 337–339
Loneliness, as social stressor, 250
Long-term care
  defined, 350
  financing of, 350
  institutional, 350
  need for, 353
  noninstitutional
    ACCESS program for, 356
    cost of, 354–335
    demonstration projects for, 355–357
    eligibility for, 350–353
    fragmentation of, 353
    funding for, 352t, 353–354
    Guale Homemaker-Home Health
        Aide Project for 356–357
    importance of, 354–355
    improvement of, 354–355
    Medicaid and, 353
    Medicare and, 353
    need for, 353
    programs for 353
    recommended services for, 351
    Triage Project form 356
    working programs for, 355–357
  recommended services for, 350, 351
Longitudinal studies, 314–315
Loniten, 276
Lopressor, 276
Lordosis, exercises for, 127, 128, 129
Lumpectomy, for breast cancer, 227
Lung(s). See also Pulmonary entries
  age-related changes in, 182–184
    functional, 183–184
    pathologic, 184–186
    vs. chronic obstructive pulmonary dis-
        ease, 185, 198
  cancer of, 218–222
    age of onset of, 218
    auscultation in, 219
    breath sounds in, 219
    metastasis in, 218, 229–230
    palpation in, 219
    paraneoplastic syndromes in, 221–222
    percussion in, 219
    physical therapy in, 219–220

postoperative complications in, 219
postoperative sputum retention in, 219
postoperative therapy in 219
post-thoracotomy pneumonitis in, 220
postural drainage in, 219–220
smoking and, 218
symptoms of, 218
response of, to exercise, 186–187
tissue of, age-related changes in, 182–183
ventilation of, mechanism of, 183
Lung capacity, 184, 185
Lung compliance, 183
Lupus erythematosus, systemic, pro-
    cainamide and, 274
Lying-to-sitting maneuver, 159–160
Lymphedema, of arm, after radical mastec-
    tomy, 228–229
Lymphoma, non-Hodgkin's, 233–234
Lyopia, cataracts and, 105

Macular degeneration, 106
Maguire's Trilevel Activities of Daily Liv-
    ing Assessment, 38–50
  problems in, 49–50
  sample of, 39–46
  scoring of, 38–49, 47
Marplan, 284–285
Mastectomy, 227
  radical, 227
    arm edema after, 228–229
    shoulder dysfunction after, 227–228
  simple, 227
Master's stress test, 201t
Maxillofacial prosthesis, 223–224
  after skin cancer surgery, 237
Measurement of oxygen consumption, 204
Medicaid, 348–349
  defined, 332
  expenditures on, 352t
Medicare
  changes in, lobbying for, 337–339
  coinsurance in, 334–335
  cost sharing in, 334–335
  deductible in, 334–335
  defined, 332
  expenditures on, 352t
history of, 335
  for inpatient services, 335, 343
  long-term noninstitutional care and, 353
  for outpatient services, 335
  Part A, 335, 343
  Part B, 335
  reimbursement by, 336–337
    for home care, 337–338, 353
    for occupational therapy, 336

Neuroleptics—*continued*
  chemoreceptor trigger zone inhibition by, 284
  endocrine effects of, 284
  extrapyramidal effects of, 282
  indications for, 283
  Parkinsonism reaction and, 282
  sedative effects of, 283
  side effects of, 282–284
  tardive dyskinesis and, 282–283
  therapeutic effects of, 283
Neurologic disabilities, functional approaches to, 150–160
Neuromuscular disorders. *See also* Musculoskeletal disorders
  bathing in, 160
  dressing in, 159–160
  positioning in, 155–156, *156–159*
  toileting in, 157–159
Neurons(s)
  branching of, 143
  glycolysis in, 144
  lipofuscin accumulation in, 143
  loss of, 142–143
  microenvironment of, 144
Neuropathies, peripheral, cancer and, 221–222
Neurotransmitters, 143–144
Nipride, 276
Night blindness, 107
Nitrogen, decreased cerebral, 143
Nitroglycerin, 275
Nitroprusside, 276
Non-Hodgkin's lymphoma, 233–234
Norepinephrine, accumulation of, monoamine oxidase inhibitors and, 289
Norpramin, 285
Nortriptyline, 285
Nursing home(s). *See also* Rehabilitation
  depersonalization in, 84
  financing of, 339
  importance of resident decision-making in, 84–85, *85*
  routine in, 84
  therapy department in. *See* Therapy service

Occupational therapy. *See* Rehabilitation; Therapy service
Ointments, 271
Old age survivors benefits, expenditures on, 352t

Older Americans Act, 348, 249
  demonstration project funding by, 355–357
Oral contraceptives, sexual effects of, 306t
Oral mucosa, evaluation of, 153
Orbicularis orbis muscle, stimulation of, 151, *152*
Oraganic brain syndrome, 27. *See also* Dementia
  acute, 27
  affect impairment in, 28
  chronic, 27–28
    Alzheimer's 27–28
    arteriosclerotic, 27–28
  cognitive in, 28
  judgment impairment in, 28
  memory impairment in, 28
  Mini-Mental State Exam for, 29, *30*
  neuroleptics for, 282–284
  orientation impairment in, 28
  recognition of, 28
  treatment of, 28–29
Orgasmic dysfunction, in female diabetics, 305
Orientation, impaired, in organic brain syndrome, 28
Orinase, 287
Oromotor assessment, 151–153
  of oral mucosa, 153
  of pharyngeal swallow, 153, *154*
  of soft palate, 152–153, *153*
  of sucking, 151
  of tongue mobility, 151
  of tongue—palate, 151–152, *153*
  of uvula, 152–153, *153*
Orthostatic hypotension, beta-adrenergic blocking agents and, 276
Osteoarthritis, 121–122
  bandages for, 136
  of cervical spine, 137–138, *138*
  cold for, 136
  exercise for, 136–137
  heat for, 136
  of hip, 137
  of knee, 137
  pain in, 136
  of shoulder, 137
  treatment of, 136–137
Osteoarthropathy, pulmonary hypertrophic, cancer and, 221–222
Osteoporosis, 118
Otitis media, 110
Otosclerosis, 110
Overcrowding, as stressor, 249

Pigments, age, 15
Pilocarbine, anticholinergics and, 288
Pleomorphic rhabdomyosarcoma, 231–232
Polymyalgia rheumatica, 123
Polymyopathies, in lung cancer, 221–222
Positioning, in neuromuscular disorders, 155–156, *156–158*
Postural drainage, 196
Posture
  age-related changes in, *126*, 124–125
  evaluation of, 126
  good, 124, *125*
  poor, 124–129
    exercises for, 126–127, *127–129*
    functional causes of, 127
    improvement of, 126–127, *127–129*
    pathologic causes of, 127–129
Potassuim
  decreased muscular content of, 123
  deficiency of
    fatigue and, 125
    thiazide diuretics and, 275
Pheumonitis, post-thoracotomy, in lung cancer, 220
Prednisone, 287
Pre-ejection period, ventricular, 170
Prebycusis, 65, 110–111
  managment of, 66–67
Presbyopia, 104–105
Primidone, sexual effects of, 306t
Proazosin, 276
Procainamide
  for arrhytmias, 274
  side effects of, 274
Prochlorpromazine, 283–284
Proctoform HC, 277
Progeria, Hayflick limit in, 11
Programmed theory of aging, 13
Progrssive relaxation, 259, 263
Prolactin, in stress response, *247*, 248
Prolixin, 283–284
Propranolol, 276
  bronchospasm and, 277
Propoxyphene, 280
Prostate, cancer of, 234–235
Prostatitis, sexuality and, 305
Prosthesis
  extremity, after amputation for pleomorphic rhabdomyosarcoma, 232
  fitting of, 133
  selection of, 133
  upper extremity stress test for, 133
  use of
    energy expenditure in, 133

knee instability in, 133
  success of, 134
  for wheelchair users, 134
maxillofacial, 223–224
  after skin cancer surgery, 237
Protein molecules, crosslinkage of, 13–15, *14*
Protein synthesis, mistakes in, and cellular aging, 12
Pully exercises, after radical mastectomy, 228
Pulmonary capacity, reduced, speech dysfunction and, 61
Pulmonary disease(s). *See also* Lung(s)
  age-related factors in, 277
  auscultation in, 193–196, *195*
  breathing exercises for, 196–197
  bronchodilators for, 198
  bronchopulmonary hygiene in, 196–198
  drugs for, 277–279
  exercise program for, 205–k210
    modality for, 206
    prescription for, 206–209
  exercise stress testing in, 198–204
    beginning of, 202–204
    modality of, 200, 201t
    monitoring parameters in, 200–202, 203t
    patient preparation for, 202
    protocol for, 200, 202t
    setting goals in, 204
    stopping of, 204
  finger clubbing in, 188, *191*
  history taking in, 187, *188*
  humidity therapy for, 198
  musculoskeletal adaptations to, 188, *190*
  palpation in, 189, 191–193, *192–195*
  patient evaluation in, 187–196
    draping for, 188, *189*
  patient observation in, 188–189, *189–191*
  respiratory response in, 182
  secretion clearance in, 198
Pulmonary gases
  delivery and exchange of, 184
  of in exercise, 186
  monitoring of, in stress test, 202, *203t*
Pulmonary hypertrophic osteoarthropaty, 221–222
Pulmonary pH
  age-related changes in, 199t
  monitoring of, in stress test, 200–202
Pulmonary rehabilitation, 181–211
Pumonary secretions
  clearance of, 196–197, 198

bronchodilators for, 198
humidification for, 198
Pulmonary system. *See also* Lung(s)
age-related changes in, 182–184
pathologic, 184–186
vs. chronic obstructive pulmonary disease, 185, 198
response of to exercise, 186–187
Pulse(s), 318
oxygen, in exercise training, 174
taking of, in exercise program, 172
Puritan work ethic, 86

QUALITY of life, dimension of, 313–314
Questran, 275
Quibron Plus, 278
Quinidine, 274

RADICAL mastectomy, 227
arm edema after, 228–229
shoulder dysfunction after, 227–228
Rales, 196
Range of motion test, 120
Reaction time
in assessment of speed, 145
decline in, neurologic factors in, 145
Recreation. *See* Leisure
Rehabilitation
after amputation, 132–134
team approach to, 133–134
anticipating complications in, 347
assessment tools for, 347
aural, 66–67
budgeting in, 340–341
in cancer, 217–218
in dying, 326–328. *See also under* Dying
exercise program in. See Exercise program; Exercise training
family involvement in, 334
financing of, 331–343
as business venture, 339
demand theory and, 332–333
by Medicare, 335–337
by private health insurance, 331–335
functional goals of, 313
home program in 334
impact of health insurance on, 333
medicare reimbursement for, 336–337
mutual goal-setting in, 334
patient instruction in, 333–334
patient-therapist relationship in, effect of health insurance on, 333
prevention, goals of, 347

providing appropriate environment for, 26–27
providing choices in, 26
providing motivation in, 25–27
pulmonary. *See* Pulmonary rehabilitation
reproducible measurement certification in, 26
in sexual dysfunction, 294–295
after stroke, 148
Rehabilitation, professional, qualifications of, 347
Relaxation techniques, 258–266
autogenic training for, 259–260, 263
benefits of, to therapist, 265
biofeedback as, 260–261, 263–264
breath control as, 261, 264
choice of, 264
guided imagery as, 259–260, 263
hypnosis as, 259–260, 263
instruction in, 265
meditation as, 258–259, 263
physical condition and, 264
progressive relaxation as, 259, 263
selected awareness as, 259–260, 263
systematic desensitization as, 261, 262, 264
Reliability, in research, 315–316
Remotivation therapy, for depression, 24–25
Renal function, drug metabolism and excretion and, 272, 273
Reproducible measurement certification, 26
Reserpine, 276
sexual effects of, 306t
Residual volume, 184, 185, 199t
Resonance, 62
disturbed, in dysarthria, 71
Respiration, speech and, 61
Respiratory disease. *See* Pulmonary disease
Respiratory rate, monitoring of, in stress test, 200
Restoil, 282
Retinal detachment, 107
Retinitis pigmentosa, 106–107
Retirement
coping mechanisms for, 256
losses in, 23
as social stressor, 250
Rhabdomyosarcoma, pleomorphic, 231–232
Rheumatoid arthritis, 121–122. *See also* Arthritis
Ribcage, in exercise, 187

Ribonucleic acid, messenger, 12–13
Right hemisphere communication syndrome, 72–75
  management of, 80
Right-left descrimination, 160
Rinne test, for hearing loss, ill
Rocking chair, for sitting balance, 160
Rogers' Health Status Scale, 346–347, *346*
Ronchi, 196
Rosenbek's light step continuum, 73

SAFETY precautions, in activities of daily living, 52–54,
Sampling, 316
Sarcomas, 231–233
Schizophrenia, neuroleptics for, 282–284
Seconal, 282
Secretions, pulmonary, clearance of, 196–197
Sedatives, 281–284
  alcohol and, 288
  sexual effects of, 306t
Seizures, causes of, 286
Selected awareness, 259–260, 263
Selenium, 15
Self-esteem, quality of life and, 314
Self Leisure Interest Profile, 89
Selye's stress response theory, 246–247, *246*
Senility. See Dementia; Organic brain syndrome
Sensory input, decreased, and falls, 149
Serpasil, 276
Sexual activity, in nursing homes, 306–308
Sexual dysfunction
  age-related factors in 294–295
  in arthritis, 299–302
Sexual intercourse. See also Sexuality
  frequency of, 293–294
  positions for, *297–302*
Sexual positions, *297–302*
Sexual potency, reduced, drugs and, 306t
Sexuality, 293–308
  age-related physiologic changes in, 293, 294–295
  arthritis, and 299–302
  cancer and, 303
  diabetes and, 304–305
  drugs and, 305–306, 306t
  frequency of intercourse and, 293–294
  heart disease and, 303–304
  after hysterectomy, 302–303
  illness and, 296–305
  lack of partner and, 295–296

prostatitis and, 305
role of rehabilitation specialist in, 294–295
stroke and, 304
Shock therapy, 284
Shoulder
  dysfunction of, after neck dissection, 225–226
    after radical mastectomy, 227
  exercises for, after neck dissection, 225–226
    after thoracotomy, 229
  frozen, rehabilitation of, 119–120
  osteoarthritis of, 137
Shower, safety aids for, *53*
Showerhead, hand-held, *53*
Sinemet, 285
Sinequan, 285
Sinoatrial node
  age-related changes in, 167
  decreased rhythmicity of, 169
Sinuses, paranasal, cancer of, 222–226, 223t. See also Head and neck cancer
Sitting balance, exercises for, 160
Sitting-from-lying maneuver, 159–160
Skin
  aging of, and protein molecule crosslinkage, 14
  cancer of, 237
Sleep disorders, 281
  drugs for, 281–284
Slophyllin, 278
Smell, age-related changes in, 113
Smoking, lung cancer and, 218
Snellen eye chart, 108
Soap on a rope, 160
Social Security Act of 1935, 348
  Title XX of, 348–349
    expenditures on, 352t
Social services block grant, 348–349
  expenditures on, 352t
Social stressors, 250
Soft palate, evaluation of, 152–153, *153*
Solutions, drug, 271. See also Drug(s)
Somatic cells, 8–9
  continuously proliferating, 9
  fixed postmitotic, 9
  reverting postmitotic, 9
Speech. See also Communication; Voice
  adaptation of, for receptive language difficulties, 63–64
  aphasia and, 67–71
  apraxia and, 73–74

articulation in, 62
central disorders of, 61
chronic obstructive pulmonary disease and, 78–80
dysarthria and, 71–73, 79
esophageal, 77
laryngectomy and, 77–78, 80
peripheral disorders of, 61
phonation in, 61–62
physiology of, 61
process of, 60–61
reception of, 62–64
resonance in, 62
respiration and, 61
self-monitoring of, 64
shaky voice in, 61
slowed, 62
slurred, 62
unintelligible, 62
vocal dynamic changes in, 62
vocal pitch changes in, 61
Speech-language-hearing therapy. *See also* Therapy service
Medicare reimbursement for, 336
Speech preservation, 68
Speech reading, 66
Speed of movement, age-related changes in, 145
Spine
age-related changes in, 125–126
cervical
hyperostosis of, 137–138, *138*
osteoarthritis of, 137–138, *138*
inflexibility of, 119
structure of, 125–126
Spinothalamic pathways, 134
Spironolactone, 275, 276
Spoon(s)
built-up, 155
swivel, 55
Sputum, clearance of, 196–197, 198
Squamous carcinoma, 237
Stance, instability of, 149
Stelazine, 283–284
Steroids
for arthritis, 280
for asthma, 278
indications for, 287
side effects of, 287
Stoma care, 237
Stomach ulcers, of 277
Strength
age-related changes in, and hyopkinesis, 144–145

improvement of, measurement of, 122
loss of, 122–124
energy conservation and work simplification techniques for, 50–51
evaluation of, 124
exercise program for, 124
functional causes of, 123–124
pathologic causes of, 123
practical aids for, 54–55
Stress
alarm reaction in, 246, *246*
change in environment and, 249
coping mechanisms for. *See* Stress management
depression and, 24–25
disease and, 248
exhaustion stage in, 246, *247*
flight-or-fight response and, 246–247
general adaptation syndrome and, 246
hypochondriasis and, 24–25
lack of motivation and, 25–27
management of in clinical setting, 256–268
neuroendocrine response pathways in, 247–248, *247*
physiologic response to, 246, 247–248, *247*
aging and, 248
positive stressors, 248
resistance stage in, 246, *247*
of retirement, minimization of, 256
Selye's theory of, 23
stressors and , 248–252
type A personality and, 249–250
Stress fractures, 136
Stress management, 23–24, 252–256
autogenic training for, 259–260, 263
biofeedback for, 260–261, 263–264
breath control for, 261, 264
coping mechanism identification in, 257
guided imagery for, 259–260, 263
guidelines for, 266
hypnosis for, 259–260, 263
meditation for, 258–259, 263
patient instruction in, 257–258
professional referral in, 257
progressive relaxation for, 259, 263
relaxation techniques for, 258–266
benefits of, to therapist, 265
choice of, 264
instruction for, 265
physical condition and, 264
types of, 258–264
selected awareness for, 259–260, 263

Vitamin D, Dilantin and, 289
Vitamin E, 14–15
Voice
  in chronic obstructive pulmonary disease, 78
  in dysarthria, 71
  hoarseness of, 61
  increased loudness of, 62
  pitch of, changes in, 61
  resonance of, 62
  shaky, 61
Voice sounds, thoracic, palpation of, 191–193
Volunteers, for leisure activities, 95–96
  handbook for, 96
  screening of, 95
  training program for, 96

WARFARIN
Waterbed, 156
Weakness, causes of, 122–124
Wernicke's aphasia, 69–70
Wheelchair, toilet transfer from, 157–159
Word finding, 61
Work importance of, 23, 85–86
Work ethic, 86
World Health Orangization, definition of health by, 345
Wrist, fractures of, 135

XANTHINES, 278

ZOMEPIRAC, 280